Surface and Interface Modification of Graphite and Graphene-Based Materials for Energy and Sensor Applications

Surface and Interface Modification of Graphite and Graphene-Based Materials for Energy and Sensor Applications

Guest Editors

Luca Tortora
Gianlorenzo Bussetti

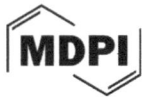

Basel • Beijing • Wuhan • Barcelona • Belgrade • Novi Sad • Cluj • Manchester

Guest Editors

Luca Tortora
Department of Sciences
Roma Tre University
Rome
Italy

Gianlorenzo Bussetti
Department of Physics
Politecnico di Milano
Milano
Italy

Editorial Office
MDPI AG
Grosspeteranlage 5
4052 Basel, Switzerland

This is a reprint of the Special Issue, published open access by the journal *Molecules* (ISSN 1420-3049), freely accessible at: https://www.mdpi.com/journal/molecules/special_issues/chemistry_Tortora.

For citation purposes, cite each article independently as indicated on the article page online and as indicated below:

Lastname, A.A.; Lastname, B.B. Article Title. *Journal Name* **Year**, *Volume Number*, Page Range.

ISBN 978-3-7258-3309-2 (Hbk)
ISBN 978-3-7258-3310-8 (PDF)
https://doi.org/10.3390/books978-3-7258-3310-8

© 2025 by the authors. Articles in this book are Open Access and distributed under the Creative Commons Attribution (CC BY) license. The book as a whole is distributed by MDPI under the terms and conditions of the Creative Commons Attribution-NonCommercial-NoDerivs (CC BY-NC-ND) license (https://creativecommons.org/licenses/by-nc-nd/4.0/).

Contents

About the Editors vii

Preface ix

Heriberto Cruz-Martínez, Brenda García-Hilerio, Fernando Montejo-Alvaro, Amado Gazga-Villalobos, Hugo Rojas-Chávez and Elvia P. Sánchez-Rodríguez
Density Functional Theory-Based Approaches to Improving Hydrogen Storage in Graphene-Based Materials
Reprinted from: *Molecules* 2024, 29, 436, https://doi.org/10.3390/molecules29020436 1

Jung Jae Lee, Su-Hyeong Chae, Jae Jun Lee, Min Sang Lee, Wonhyung Yoon, Lee Ku Kwac, et al.
Waste-Wood-Isolated Cellulose-Based Activated Carbon Paper Electrodes with Graphene Nanoplatelets for Flexible Supercapacitors
Reprinted from: *Molecules* 2023, 28, 7822, https://doi.org/10.3390/molecules28237822 18

Laura Fazi, Carla Andreani, Cadia D'Ottavi, Leonardo Duranti, Pietro Morales, Enrico Preziosi, et al.
Characterization of Conductive Carbon Nanotubes/Polymer Composites for Stretchable Sensors and Transducers
Reprinted from: *Molecules* 2023, 28, 1764, https://doi.org/10.3390/molecules28041764 29

Norazreen Abd Aziz, Mohd Faizol Abdullah, Siti Aishah Mohamad Badaruddin, Mohd Rofei Mat Hussin and Abdul Manaf Hashim
Highly Sensitive Sub-ppm CH_3COOH Detection by Improved Assembly of Sn_3O_4-RGO Nanocomposite
Reprinted from: *Molecules* 2022, 27, 8707, https://doi.org/10.3390/molecules27248707 42

Rossella Yivlialin, Claudia Filoni, Francesco Goto, Alberto Calloni, Lamberto Duò, Franco Ciccacci and Gianlorenzo Bussetti
Optical Anisotropy of Porphyrin Nanocrystals Modified by the Electrochemical Dissolution
Reprinted from: *Molecules* 2022, 27, 8010, https://doi.org/10.3390/molecules27228010 58

Qizhang Jia, B. Jill Venton and Kateri H. DuBay
Structure and Dynamics of Adsorbed Dopamine on Solvated Carbon Nanotubes and in a CNT Groove
Reprinted from: *Molecules* 2022, 27, 3768, https://doi.org/10.3390/molecules27123768 70

Kai Wang, Luoxing Yang, Huili Huang, Ning Lv, Jiyang Liu and Youshi Liu
Nanochannel Array on Electrochemically Polarized Screen Printed Carbon Electrode for Rapid and Sensitive Electrochemical Determination of Clozapine in Human Whole Blood
Reprinted from: *Molecules* 2022, 27, 2739, https://doi.org/10.3390/molecules27092739 93

Min Li, Xiaoying Yin, Hongli Shan, Chenting Meng, Shengxue Chen and Yinan Yan
The Facile Preparation of PBA-GO-CuO-Modified Electrochemical Biosensor Used for the Measurement of α-Amylase Inhibitors' Activit
Reprinted from: *Molecules* 2022, 27, 2395, https://doi.org/10.3390/molecules27082395 107

Ewelina Skowron, Kaja Spilarewicz-Stanek, Dariusz Guziejewski, Kamila Koszelska, Radovan Metelka and Sylwia Smarzewska
Analytical Performance of Clay Paste Electrode and Graphene Paste Electrode-Comparative Study
Reprinted from: *Molecules* 2022, 27, 2037, https://doi.org/10.3390/molecules27072037 121

Claudia Filoni, Bahram Shirzadi, Marco Menegazzo, Eugenio Martinelli, Corrado Di Natale, Andrea Li Bassi, et al.
Compared EC-AFM Analysis of Laser-Induced Graphene and Graphite Electrodes in Sulfuric Acid Electrolyte
Reprinted from: *Molecules* **2021**, *26*, 7333, https://doi.org/10.3390/molecules26237333 . . . . . . **131**

Tajana Kostadinova, Nikolaos Politakos, Ana Trajcheva, Jadranka Blazevska-Gilev and Radmila Tomovska
Effect of Graphene Characteristics on Morphology and Performance of Composite Noble Metal-Reduced Graphene Oxide SERS Substrate
Reprinted from: *Molecules* **2021**, *26*, 4775, https://doi.org/10.3390/molecules26164775 . . . . . . **142**

About the Editors

Luca Tortora

Luca Tortora (LT) is an Associate Professor at the Department of Science of Roma Tre University, a Researcher Coordinator at National Institute for Nuclear Physics (INFN), and an Associated Researcher at the National Research Council of Italy (CNR-IMM). He is Director of the inter-institutional laboratory LASR3 (Surface Laboratory Roma Tre) and group leader of the SMAC "Surface modification and characterization" group at Roma Tre University. He received his PhD in Chemistry at the University of Roma "Tor Vergata" in 2011 working on the synthesis and characterization of metal complexes of pyrrolic macrocycles and their application for chemical sensing technologies. Then, he moved to Roma Tre University and INFN, where he is actively involved in investigating surface/interface reactions through experimental (ToF-SIMS, XPS, FT-IR, AFM, SEM-EDS, XRD, XRF, PL) and theoretical approaches (DFT). More recently, in his group, different approaches for the synthesis of metal oxides and semiconductor nanocrystals have been developed for application in technological, environmental, and cultural heritage fields. LT is a member of the Italian Chemical Society (SCI) and American Chemical Society (ACS). He is also a co-author of more than 100 peer-reviewed papers (+1500 citations; h-index = 23) and has given over 50 talks as an invited speaker in national and international conferences. LT is a reviewer for several journals in the field of material chemistry and a member of the editorial committee of indexed journals. In addition to his research, LT is actively involved in teaching at both undergraduate and doctoral levels, offering courses in general and inorganic chemistry, advanced materials, and surface analysis techniques. He has also supervised multiple PhD and MSc students, fostering the next generation of researchers in the field.

Gianlorenzo Bussetti

Gianlorenzo Bussetti (GB) received his PhD in physics at the University of Roma "Tor Vergata" in 2005, he spent a postdoctoral period at the INSP in Paris and at the Johannes Kepler University of Linz in 2007 and 2008, and qualified as a professor by his Habilitation at the Politecnico di Milano, in 2017. In Rome, GB worked under the supervision of Em. Prof. Gianfranco Chiarotti on the optical properties of semiconductor surfaces prepared under ultrahigh vacuum conditions. The results obtained by the application of surface-sensitive optical probes to organic/inorganic interfaces were awarded the Giulotto's prize in Physics. In the period 2008–2009, GB worked in the Institute of Physical and Theoretical Chemistry (University of Bonn) where, in collaboration with Prof. Klaus Wandelt, a reflectance anisotropy spectroscopy (RAS) system was coupled with an electrochemical STM (EC-STM) to compare both spectroscopic and morphological changes occurring on the electrode surface during electrochemical processes. At the Politecnico di Milano, GB won two projects for setting up a new Institutional facility (SoLINano-S lab) for the microscopic and spectroscopic investigation of liquid/solid interfaces. A specific Ph. D. course has also been introduced at the Politecnico di Milano. Currently, GB's research focuses on fundamental aspects of the physical properties of inorganic (metallic, semiconductor) and organic surfaces under ultrahigh vacuum conditions and in aqueous electrolytes, on the processes acting during the intercalation of stratified materials, and, most recently, on the dissolution reaction of organic crystals. GB has supervised nearly 50 master's/diploma and PhD theses, published about 150 papers, and has co-authored more than 200 presentations at conferences, workshops, and colloquia. He is a member of both the Italian Physics Society (SIF) and the European Physics Society (EPS).

Preface

This Reprint, *Surface and Interface Modification of Graphite and Graphene-Based Materials for Energy and Sensor Applications*, explores the latest developments in carbon-based materials, particularly focusing on their modification for use in energy storage systems and sensor devices. The studies in this collection investigate the synthesis, characterization, and functionalization of graphite, graphene, and their composites, enhancing their performance in applications such as supercapacitors, fuel cells, hydrogen storage, and biosensors.

The Reprint covers a wide range of subjects, from intercalation processes and nanoparticle decoration to cutting-edge surface modification techniques. These modifications have proven essential in optimizing the materials' electrochemical properties, enabling their use in advanced energy systems and sensitive detection technologies. With a blend of theoretical models and experimental data, the work provides new insights into the functionality of graphite and graphene in these crucial applications.

The main objective of this volume is to highlight how surface and interface modifications affect the performance of graphite- and graphene-based materials. By showcasing innovative methods and practical applications, this collection aims to serve as a comprehensive resource for researchers, engineers, and professionals in the fields of materials science, nanotechnology, and renewable energy. It is particularly relevant to those working on the development of more efficient energy storage solutions and next-generation sensors.

The motivation behind this work stems from the urgent need for more efficient and sustainable technologies across multiple sectors, especially in energy and healthcare. Graphite and graphene, with their remarkable properties and versatility, hold great promise for addressing these challenges. The contributions in this Reprint reflect the dedication of leading researchers working to bridge the gap between theoretical predictions and practical applications.

The intended audience includes researchers, professionals, and students in the fields of chemistry, physics, and materials science, as well as industry practitioners exploring new innovations in battery technology, sensing devices, and energy systems.

We extend our sincere thanks to all the authors and contributors for their invaluable work, as well as to the reviewers and institutions whose support has been critical to the success of this Special Issue. Their contributions have ensured the highest standards of quality and relevance, making this collection a valuable addition to the ongoing research in carbon-based materials.

Luca Tortora and Gianlorenzo Bussetti
Guest Editors

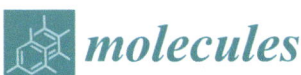

Review

Density Functional Theory-Based Approaches to Improving Hydrogen Storage in Graphene-Based Materials

Heriberto Cruz-Martínez [1], Brenda García-Hilerio [1], Fernando Montejo-Alvaro [1], Amado Gazga-Villalobos [1], Hugo Rojas-Chávez [2] and Elvia P. Sánchez-Rodríguez [3,*]

[1] Tecnológico Nacional de México, Instituto Tecnológico del Valle de Etla, Abasolo S/N, Barrio del Agua Buena, Santiago Suchilquitongo, Oaxaca 68230, Mexico; heri1234@hotmail.com (H.C.-M.); brenda.hilerio@itvalletla.edu.mx (B.G.-H.); moaf1217@gmail.com (F.M.-A.); gazgavillalobos@gmail.com (A.G.-V.)
[2] Tecnológico Nacional de México, Instituto Tecnológico de Tláhuac II, Camino Real 625, Tláhuac, Ciudad de México 13550, Mexico; hugo.rc@tlahuac2.tecnm.mx
[3] School of Engineering and Sciences, Tecnologico de Monterrey, Atizapan de Zaragoza 52926, Mexico
* Correspondence: elvia.sanchez@tec.mx

Abstract: Various technologies have been developed for the safe and efficient storage of hydrogen. Hydrogen storage in its solid form is an attractive option to overcome challenges such as storage and cost. Specifically, hydrogen storage in carbon-based structures is a good solution. To date, numerous theoretical studies have explored hydrogen storage in different carbon structures. Consequently, in this review, density functional theory (DFT) studies on hydrogen storage in graphene-based structures are examined in detail. Different modifications of graphene structures to improve their hydrogen storage properties are comprehensively reviewed. To date, various modified graphene structures, such as decorated graphene, doped graphene, graphene with vacancies, graphene with vacancies-doping, as well as decorated-doped graphene, have been explored to modify the reactivity of pristine graphene. Most of these modified graphene structures are good candidates for hydrogen storage. The DFT-based theoretical studies analyzed in this review should motivate experimental groups to experimentally validate the theoretical predictions as many modified graphene systems are shown to be good candidates for hydrogen storage.

Keywords: decorated graphene; defective graphene; doped graphene; decorated-doped graphene; DFT calculations

1. Introduction

Hydrogen is gaining importance as a clean energy carrier with higher energy density than conventional fuels [1,2]. Although it is the most abundant element in the universe [3], it is not a primary energy source available on our planet. Therefore, various technologies have been proposed that allow for the efficient and safe production, storage, and utilization of hydrogen [4–6]. Currently, hydrogen is obtained from a wide range of resources, such as renewable resources and fossil fuels [7,8]. Unfortunately, the element has a low density under ambient conditions. Consequently, many storage technologies have been developed for storing it with a high density [9,10]. Diverse electrochemical systems with extremely high efficiencies have been proposed to obtain clean electrical energy from hydrogen [11–13].

The existing hydrogen storage technologies are based on liquefaction or compression or a combination of the two. However, the liquefaction and pressurization of hydrogen are not economically viable alternatives for hydrogen storage [14,15]. Hence, hydrogen storage in materials is considered a good storage option [14] because some of the explored materials provide H_2 storage capacities like or better than the requirements prescribed by the U.S. Department of Energy (DOE) [16,17]. Therefore, in recent years, numerous materials have been explored to store hydrogen [18–23]. Among them, carbon-based materials are of high importance because of their suitable properties, such as high specific surface area, low density, and high thermal as well as chemical stability, making them promising materials for hydrogen storage [24,25].

Currently, at the molecular level, owing to advances in density functional theory (DFT)-based methods and computer equipment, novel materials with good performances have been proposed for hydrogen technologies [26–30]. The DFT-based approach has gained greater importance as it maintains a good balance between computational time and accuracy in terms of agreement with the experimental results [31–33].

To date, numerous carbon structures (e.g., graphene, graphite, graphene, nanotube, nanocone, fullerene, nanotorus) have been explored for hydrogen storage at the DFT level, and promising results have been achieved [34–41]. These structures are shown in Figure 1. Although carbon structures are good candidates for hydrogen storage, pristine carbon structures have limited reactivity for hydrogen storage [42,43]. Therefore, to improve the hydrogen storage properties of these structures, diverse approaches such as defect engineering and surface functionalization have been implemented. These strategies allow us to improve hydrogen storage in carbon structures such as graphene, carbon nanotubes, and fullerenes [44,45]. Consequently, the modification of carbon structures through defect engineering and surface functionalization for hydrogen storage is a relevant topic for designing novel carbon-based hydrogen storage materials. Among the structures investigated for hydrogen storage at the DFT level, graphene is the most studied structure. In this sense, there are some review articles that analyze the applicability of graphene for hydrogen storage. For instance, in 2017, some theoretical studies on the hydrogen storage properties of modified graphene were revised [45]. Recently, Singla and Jaggi reviewed the theoretical studies on graphene and its derivatives for hydrogen detection and storage applications [44]. They analyzed the effect of different dopants (i.e., alkali and alkaline earth atoms, transition metal atoms) on the properties of graphene-based structures to improve their hydrogen detection and storage capabilities [44]. These review articles show the importance of modified graphene to be used for hydrogen storage [44,45]. However, to date, there has been no detailed review article that explains in detail the modifications made to graphene structures for improving their hydrogen storage properties. Therefore, in this review, we analyze the DFT-based theoretical advances in the design of novel graphene-based hydrogen storage materials, highlighting the most popular modifications made to the graphene structure to improve the hydrogen storage properties.

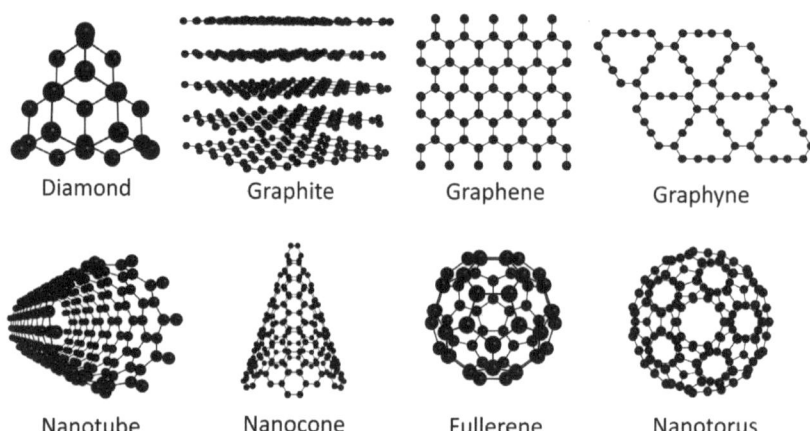

Figure 1. Carbon structures used for hydrogen storage.

2. Hydrogen Storage on Pristine Graphene

One of the first theoretical investigations on the use of pristine graphene to store hydrogen was reported by Ganji et al. [35]. They investigated hydrogen storage on graphene nanoflakes using the B3LYP-D3 method and demonstrated that hydrogen was adsorbed on a coronene surface with a physisorption energy of approximately -0.05 eV. In another study, H_2 interaction on pristine graphene was investigated by using different DFT-based methods that incorporated dispersion corrections. The computed hydrogen adsorption energies on pristine graphene were less than -0.08 eV [46]. The investigated adsorption energies computed were less than the optimal hydrogen adsorption energy (-0.2 to -0.6 eV/H_2) [47–49]. Therefore, to improve the hydrogen storage properties of graphene, graphene modification using methods such as defect engineering and surface functionalization is necessary. These studies also demonstrated that dispersion corrections must be included to explain the interactions of hydrogen on graphene accurately [35,46].

3. Hydrogen Storage on Decorated Graphene

3.1. Hydrogen Storage on Single-Atom Decorated Graphene

The use of decorated graphene is one of the strategies used to improve the hydrogen storage properties of pristine graphene. This approach involves the deposition of single-atoms (Figure 2a) or clusters (Figure 2b) on pristine graphene. Ample reports of DFT studies on hydrogen storage on decorated graphene are available in the literature [50–93]. Single-atom decoration is the commonly used strategy to decorate graphene [50–59,61–93]. Figure 3 shows different single-atoms that have been used to decorate graphene. The commonly used elements for decoration are Li, Ca, Ti, and Pd. Interestingly, several studies have considered dispersion corrections that substantially improve the description of the interaction between H_2 and decorated graphene [50,52,53,56,60,62,68,72–75,81,83,85,86,90,91,93]. When the hydrogen molecule is adsorbed on graphene decorated with single-atoms, hydrogen is adsorbed on the decorating atoms as they function as active centers. Many studies showed that the adsorption energies of hydrogen on decorated graphene were higher than those of hydrogen on pristine graphene, highlighting that most single-atom-decorated graphene systems comply with the DOE requirement for hydrogen storage through physisorption. Other important parameters to consider when exploring new materials for hydrogen storage are gravimetric capacity and volumetric capacity. The 2025 targets set by the DOE are a gravimetric capacity of 5.5 wt.% and a volumetric capacity of 40 g L^{-1} for hydrogen storage systems onboard light-duty vehicles [94]. Interestingly, several of the investigated materials—decorated graphene materials such as Al [50], Ca [53,55–57], Li [64–67,72,88], and Ti [65,83]—possess gravimetric capacities higher than the targets set by the DOE. Thus, these studies show that single-atom-decorated graphene systems are a good strategy to store hydrogen via physisorption.

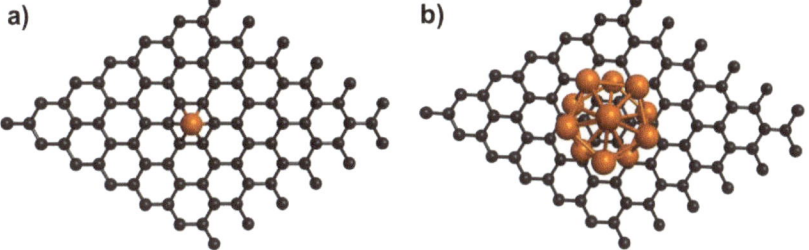

Figure 2. Models of decorated graphene. (**a**) Single-atom-decorated graphene, (**b**) cluster-decorated graphene.

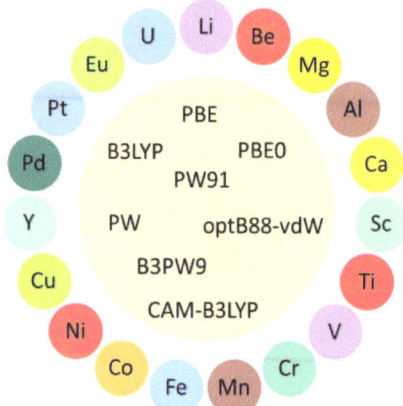

Figure 3. Decorative elements and computational methodologies for decorated graphene.

3.2. Hydrogen Storage in Cluster-Decorated Graphene

Another approach to decorate graphene is by using clusters (Figure 2b). Theoretical studies on cluster-decorated graphene have been reported [60,74,77]. For instance, a theoretical study examined the H_2 interaction on Pd_n (n = 1–6) clusters supported on graphene using the PW91 functional [77] and reported that the H_2 adsorption energy is close to the optimal values for hydrogen storage. In another study, hydrogen storage on Co_4 clusters deposited on graphene was investigated using the Perdew–Burke–Ernzerhof (PBE) functional [60]; the H_2 adsorption energy was close to the values required by the DOE. Recently, H_2 adsorption on Li_n (n = 1–6) clusters supported on graphene was investigated using the PBE functional and dispersion corrections [74]. For four H_2 molecules adsorbed on Li_6 clusters supported on graphene, the computed adsorption energy was -0.31 eV/H_2. Similar to single-atom-decorated graphene, clusters act as active centers in cluster-decorated graphene for hydrogen storage [60,74,77]. Thus, these studies show that the use of graphene systems decorated with clusters or atoms is a good strategy to store hydrogen via physisorption.

4. Hydrogen Storage on Doped Graphene

4.1. Hydrogen Storage on Single-Atom-Doped Graphene

Another route used to modify the properties of pristine graphene is through substitutional point defects such as doping. This approach substantially modifies the reactivity of pristine graphene [95–100]. At the DFT level, different types of doping have been investigated to modify the reactivity of graphene [61,62,79,101–125]. The commonly used route is to replace a carbon atom in the graphene structure with a dopant atom. To date, many studies have explored the development of single-atom–doped graphene for hydrogen storage [61,62,79,101,102,104–112,114–116,118,121,122,124,125]. Figure 4 shows the different single atoms used to dope graphene. The commonly used dopant atoms are N, Ti, Cu, Pd, and Pt. The PBE functional is a popular tool used to study single-atom-doped graphene for hydrogen storage. Similar to research on decorated graphene, several studies on single-atom-doped graphene for hydrogen storage adopted dispersion corrections [61,101,104,112,116,118,121,122,124,125]. Interestingly, many studies showed that the hydrogen adsorption energies on the single-atom-doped graphene fulfill the DOE requirement for hydrogen storage via physisorption. Meanwhile, the gravimetric capacities of several single-atom-doped graphene materials were close to the DOE requirement. These investigations show that the use of single-atom-doped graphene systems is a good alternative for hydrogen storage.

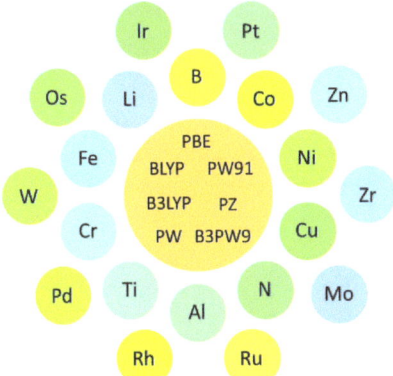

Figure 4. Doping elements and computational methodologies for single-atom-doped graphene.

4.2. Hydrogen Storage for Different Doping Concentrations

Some studies explored the influence of the concentration of doping elements on the hydrogen-storage properties in doped graphene [103,104,109,112,122]. For instance, DFT calculations and molecular dynamics were used to study H_2 adsorption on Li-doped graphene ($C_{17}Li$ and C_7Li). At atmospheric pressure and 300 K, the C_7Li composite could store up to 6.2 wt.% hydrogen, with an adsorption energy of -0.19 eV/H_2 [109]. Interestingly, this material satisfies the DOE requirements. Therefore, it can be a promising material for hydrogen storage. In another study, hydrogen storage on Ti- and Ti_2-doped graphene was investigated using the PBE functional, as shown in Figure 5 [122]. Ti_2-doped graphene was found to be a better material for hydrogen storage than Ti-doped graphene (Figure 5d). Thus, these studies show that the concentration of doping elements plays an important role in determining the hydrogen storage capacity of doped graphene [103,104,109,112,122].

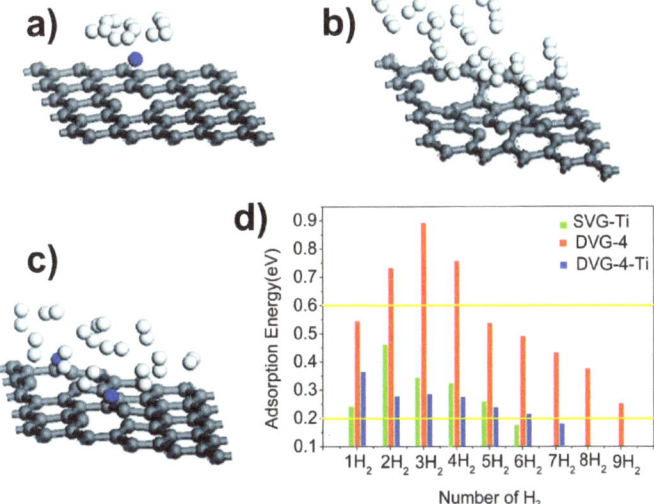

Figure 5. H_2 adsorption on graphene structures. (**a**) H_2 adsorption on Ti-doped graphene (SVG-Ti), (**b**) H_2 adsorption on double-vacancy graphene (DVG-4), (**c**) H_2 adsorption on Ti_2-doped graphene (DVG-4-Ti), (**d**) hydrogen molecule adsorption energies on graphene structures. The values reported between the horizontal yellow lines indicate the optimal adsorption energies for hydrogen storage by physisorption. Reproduced from reference [122].

4.3. Hydrogen Storage on Cluster-Doped Graphene

Hydrogen storage on cluster-doped graphene has been explored [113,115–117,120]. For example, Ti_4- and Ni_4-doped graphene structures were studied for hydrogen storage using PBE functional [113]. It was observed that the Ti_4-doped graphene has a better gravimetric capacity (3.4 wt.%) than Ni_4-doped graphene (0.30 wt.%). In another study, H_2 storage on Pd_6-doped graphene was examined by using the PW91 functional. It was demonstrated that Pd_6-doped graphene is a good material for hydrogen storage [117]. In another study, hydrogen storage was computed on Pd_n-doped graphene (n = 1–4) by using the PBE functional [115]. The variation of the H_2 adsorption energies on the Pd_n (n = 1–4) clusters-doped graphene supported as a function of cluster size is illustrated in Figure 6. The single H_2 adsorption energy increases as the Pd cluster size increases. Also, Pd_4-doped graphene can adsorb four molecules of H_2 while satisfying the requirements of the DOE, making it a good candidate for hydrogen storage.

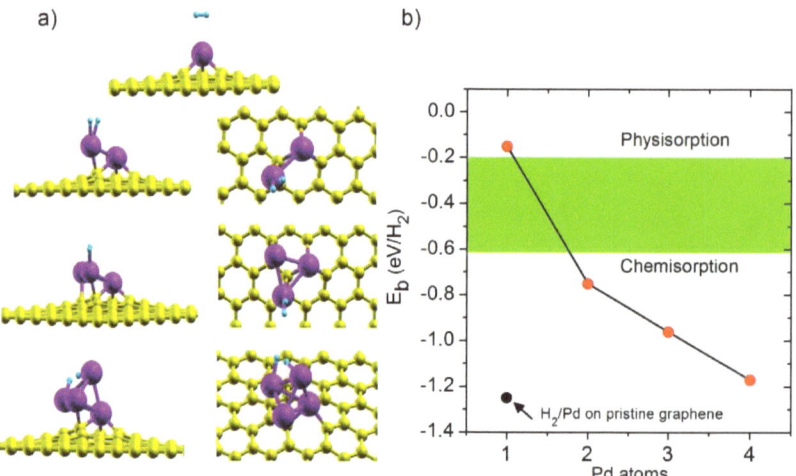

Figure 6. (a) Relaxed structures and (b) variation of the adsorption energies for a single H_2 on the graphene-supported Pd_n (n = 1–4) clusters as a function of cluster size. The adsorption energy for a single H_2 on a Pd atom deposited on a pristine graphene is also given. The energy ranges for chemical and physical H_2 adsorption are marked. Yellow, purple, and cyan circles represent carbon, palladium, and hydrogen atoms, respectively. The optimum energy range for reversible H_2 absorption/desorption is marked in a green rectangle. Reproduced with permission from reference [115].

4.4. Hydrogen Storage on Co-Doped Graphene

Hydrogen storage on co-doped graphene has been investigated by various studies [119,125–131]. In this case, two types of atoms are embedded in the graphene structure. Figure 7 shows the different configurations that have been explored. Numerous co-doped graphene systems, such as B–Pd [119], B–Li [125], 3N–Li [126,128], 3N–Ti [127], 3N–Pd, 3N–Pd$_2$, 3N–Pd$_3$, 3N–Pd$_4$ [129], N–Sc, 2N–Sc, 3N–Sc [130], N–Cu, 2N–Cu, and 3N–Cu [131], have been explored for hydrogen storage. Interestingly, most of these systems meet the DOE requirement for hydrogen storage via physisorption [119,125–131]. For instance, hydrogen adsorption on B-Li co-doped graphene structure was studied using the PBE functional [125]. It was computed that B-Li co-doped graphene can adsorb up to three H_2 molecules with an adsorption energy of -0.19 eV/H_2. Also, the hydrogen storage properties for Ti-3N co-doped graphene structure were computed using the PBE functional considering the van der Waals interactions [127]. The study demonstrated the ability of Ti-3N co-doped graphene to adsorb up to three H_2 molecules with the adsorption energy required by the DOE [127]. In another investigation, hydrogen storage properties for Sc-N,

Sc-2N, and Sc-3N co-doped graphene were studied using the PBE functional considering the van der Waals interactions [130]. The average adsorption energies of H_2 molecules on Sc-N, Sc-2N, and Sc-3N co-doped graphene structures are reported in Table 1. The results show that the H_2 adsorption energy on co-doped graphene increases gradually as the N concentration increases. In terms of gravimetric capacity, N–Sc, 2N–Sc, and 3N–Sc co-doped graphene can adsorb up to six H_2 molecules with adsorption energies of -0.15, -0.17, and -0.19 eV, respectively; see Table 1 [130]. Also, DFT-based theoretical computations were conducted for studying the H_2 adsorption on Cu-N, Cu-2N, and Cu-3N co-doped graphene structures employing the B3LYP functional [31]. It is observed that the Cu-3N co-doped graphene structure is the best candidate for hydrogen storage. These results show that co-doped graphene structures are promising candidates for hydrogen storage.

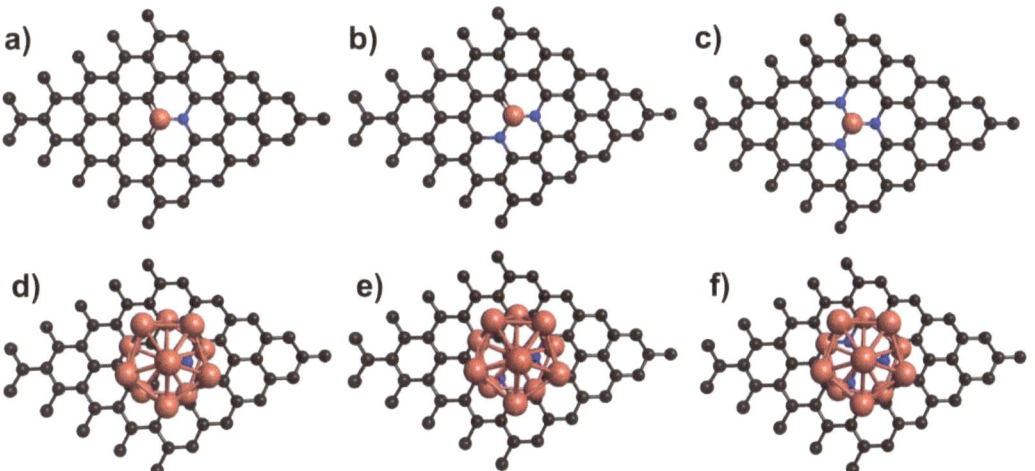

Figure 7. (**a**–**c**) Models of single-atom co-doped graphene; (**d**–**f**) models of cluster and single-atom co-doped graphene.

Table 1. The calculated average adsorption energies (eV/H_2) of H_2 molecules on Sc-decorated N-, 2N-, 3N-doped graphene structures with 1–6 H_2 molecules adsorbed. Reproduced with permission from reference [130].

Number of H_2	1	2	3	4	5	6
Sc-decorated N-doped graphene	0.19	0.18	0.18	0.18	0.16	0.15
Sc-decorated 2N-doped graphene	0.25	0.23	0.22	0.20	0.18	0.17
Sc-decorated 3N-doped graphene	0.34	0.32	0.29	0.27	0.23	0.19

5. Hydrogen Storage on Graphene with Vacancies

Graphene with vacancies exhibits better reactivity than pristine graphene [132,133]. Theoretical studies have shown that different defects can be introduced in the graphene structure to improve its hydrogen storage properties [122,134–136]. For instance, hydrogen storage on different types of vacancies such as Stone–Wales (SW), single vacancy (SV), and three types of double vacancy was theoretically studied; see Figure 8 [134]. Graphene with SV and mixed SW–SV had gravimetric densities of 5.81 and 7.02 wt.%, respectively, for hydrogen storage [134]. A recent study demonstrated hydrogen storage in double-vacancy graphene (DVG) by using the PBE functional [122]. This structure could store up to nine H_2 molecules (Figure 5d). These results show that graphene structures with vacancies are good candidates for hydrogen storage.

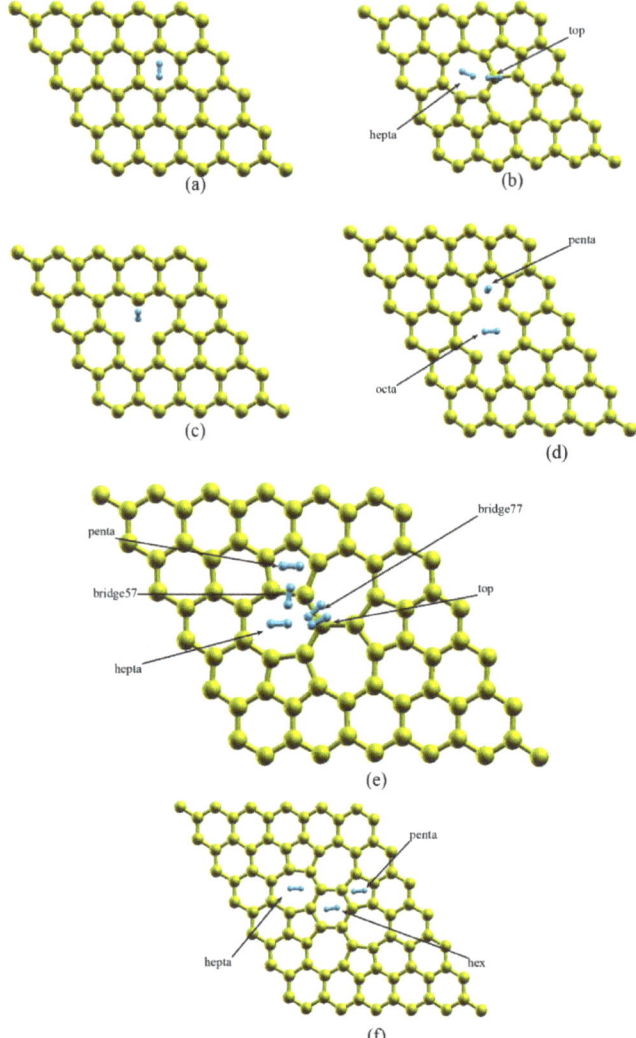

Figure 8. Supercells for hydrogen binding over individual defect systems depicting different initial positions for the adsorption of a hydrogen molecule: (**a**) pristine, (**b**) Stone–Wales, (**c**) single vacancy, (**d**) double vacancy 585, (**e**) double vacancy 555–777, and (**f**) double vacancy 5555–6–7777. Reproduced with permission from reference [134].

6. Hydrogen Storage on Doped-Decorated Graphene

So far, different doped-decorated graphene systems have been studied for hydrogen storage with promising results [54,55,60,91,93,107,126,128,137–145]. In this approach, the doping atoms are embedded in the graphene structure, while the decorating atoms are deposited on the doped graphene sheet. For instance, the use of Mg-decorated B-doped graphene for hydrogen storage was examined by using local-density approximation (LDA) methods [137]. The adsorption of six H_2 molecules on a Mg-decorated B-doped graphene corresponds to a computed adsorption energy of -0.55 eV/H_2, making this material a good candidate for hydrogen storage. In another study, hydrogen adsorption on Ni-, Pd-, and Co-decorated B-doped (BC_5) graphene was investigated using the PW91 functional [139]. When 11 H_2 molecules were adsorbed on Ni-decorated B-doped graphene, the calculated adsorption energy was -0.34 eV/H_2. Recently, hydrogen adsorption on graphene doped with two B atoms and decorated with two Y atoms was investigated employing the Perdew–Wang (PW) functional; see Figure 9 [140]. This system could store 12 H_2 molecules with an adsorption energy of -0.568 eV/H_2. In addition, metal-decorated B-doped (BC_5) graphene was studied for hydrogen storage using the PW91 functional [141]. Up to nine H_2 molecules could be adsorbed on Ni- and Ti-decorated B-doped graphene with an adsorption energy of -0.43 and -0.41 eV/H_2, respectively. Another study examined the use of La-decorated B-doped graphene for hydrogen storage by using the LDA method [142] and showed that up to six H_2 molecules were adsorbed with an adsorption energy of -0.53 eV/H_2. These studies show that decorated-doped graphene systems are good candidates for hydrogen storage.

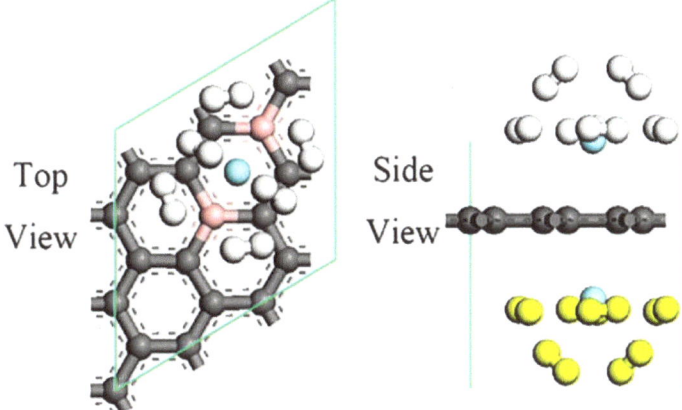

Figure 9. Optimized structures of twelve hydrogen molecules' adsorption on Y coated double-sided graphene with boron doping. Cyan, pink, and dark gray spheres denote Y, boron, and carbon atoms. Light gray and yellow spheres are hydrogen molecules attaching on the top and opposite sides of graphene, respectively. Reproduced with permission from reference [140].

7. Hydrogen Storage on Graphene with Vacancy-Doping

Embedding vacancies-dopants in the graphene structure is another strategy to improve the reactivity of graphene for hydrogen storage. Various doped graphene structures with vacancies have been examined [68,69,93,119,125,143,146–156]. For instance, graphene with SW defects and doped with Li was investigated using a PBE functional with dispersion corrections [68]. This structure can adsorb four H_2 molecules with an optimal adsorption energy for hydrogen storage. In another study, hydrogen adsorption on graphene with double vacancies and doped with Li was investigated using a PBE functional with dispersion correction [125]. This system adsorbed three H_2 molecules with an adsorption energy of -0.20 eV/H_2. Hydrogen storage using DVG and doped with Ti was studied using the PBE approximation [146]. An adsorption energy of -0.21 eV/H_2 was computed for four H_2 molecules on each side of this structure. Recently, DVG (555–777) doped with a Pd_4 cluster was studied using the PBE functional [147]. An adsorption energy of -0.64 eV/H_2 was calculated when five H_2 molecules were adsorbed on this system. In another study, hydrogen storage in DVG doped with 12 metals (Ag, Au, Ca, Li, Mg, Pd, Pt, Sc, Sr, Ti, Y, and Zr) was studied by using the generalized gradient approximation; see Figure 10 [148]. Computations showed that Ca and Sr have the largest capacity and can store up to six H_2 molecules each. More recently, hydrogen storage in graphene structures with double vacancies (585 and 555–777) doped with Ca was studied using the PBE functional with dispersion corrections [149]. These structures can store up to six H_2 molecules each. Also, the capacity of DVG doped with Li for hydrogen storage was computed by using the PW functional [69]. The storage capacity of this structure was 7.26 wt.% when Li was doped on both sides of the defective graphene. These investigations show that graphene structures with vacancy-doping are good candidates for hydrogen storage.

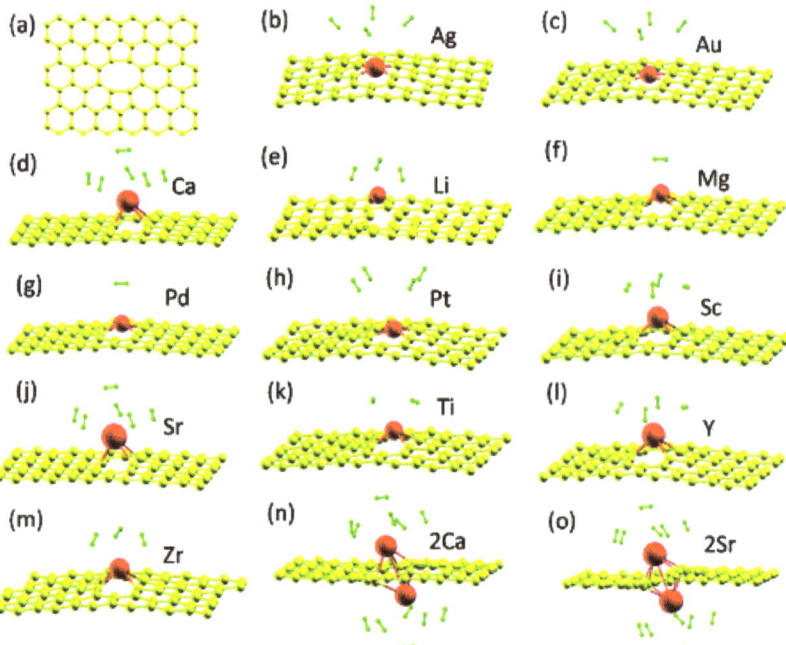

Figure 10. The relaxed atomic geometries for (**a**) a graphene sheet with a DCV, (**b–m**) the 12 different metal adatoms with their maximum hydrogen capacity, and (**n,o**) the Ca and Sr systems with adatoms adsorbed on both sides of the DCV at their maximum H_2 capacities. Reproduced with permission from reference [148].

8. Hydrogen Storage on Graphene with Co-Doping and Vacancies

Adding co-doping and vacancies in the graphene structure is another strategy used to improve the reactivity of graphene for hydrogen storage. To date, several modified graphene structures with co-doping and vacancies have been studied for hydrogen storage [105,119,125,126,128,129,152,153,156]. For instance, Li-B co-doped DVG was studied for hydrogen storage using the PBE functional [125]. This structure can adsorb three H_2 molecules with an adsorption energy like that required by the DOE. In another study, Li-doped pyrrolic N-doped graphene was studied for hydrogen storage employing the PBE functional and considering the van der Waals corrections [126]. This structure can adsorb three H_2 molecules with an adsorption energy of -0.18 eV/H_2. Also, different porphyrin-doped graphene structures were studied for hydrogen storage using the PBE functional [105]. It was computed that Sc-, Ti-, and V-porphyrin-doped graphene can be good candidates for hydrogen storage, since these structures meet the requirements established by the DOE. Recently, Be-porphyrin-doped graphene structure was computed for hydrogen storage employing the PW functional [152]. According to the adsorption energy established by the DOE, a maximum of four H_2 molecules can be adsorbed on Be-porphyrin-doped graphene. These studies show that graphene structures with co-doping and vacancies are good candidates for hydrogen storage via physisorption.

9. Conclusions and Future Directions

This review analyzed the advances in the design of novel graphene-based hydrogen storage materials, highlighting the modifications made to the graphene structure based on DFT studies to improve its hydrogen storage properties. To date, various modified graphene structures, such as decorated graphene, doped graphene, graphene with vacancies, graphene with vacancies-doping, as well as decorated-doped graphene, have been explored to modify the reactivity of pristine graphene. Most of these modified graphene structures are good candidates for hydrogen storage. From this detailed review, the following conclusions and future directions can be suggested:

(a) Graphene structures decorated with single-atoms or atom clusters for hydrogen storage have been examined. The commonly used strategy is to decorate graphene with single atoms. Therefore, more studies on cluster-decorated graphene for hydrogen storage are required. Further, since bimetallic and trimetallic systems are known to have properties very different from those of monometallic systems, it will be interesting to investigate graphene decorated with bimetallic or trimetallic clusters for hydrogen storage. Most graphene systems decorated with clusters or atoms comply with the DOE requirement for hydrogen storage via physisorption. Furthermore, several of the investigated materials, in particular, graphene decorated with Al, Ca, Li, and Ti, had gravimetric capacities higher than the target set by the DOE.

(b) The use of doped graphene for hydrogen storage has been widely investigated. Several strategies, such as single-atom doping, cluster doping, and co-doping, were implemented. These types of doping substantially modify the reactivity of graphene, providing promising materials for hydrogen storage. However, theoretical studies on cluster-doped and co-doped graphene for hydrogen storage are still scarce. Therefore, it is necessary to conduct more detailed research on cluster-doped and co-doped graphene for hydrogen storage.

(c) The use of graphene with vacancies, doped-decorated graphene, and graphene with vacancies-doping are other strategies to modify the reactivity of pristine graphene for hydrogen storage. The existing studies have shown promising results for hydrogen storage. However, comprehensive studies on these systems are necessary.

(d) The graphene structures with co-doping and vacancies have been examined for hydrogen storage. The available studies show that graphene structures with co-doping and vacancies are good candidates for hydrogen storage. However, more studies are required on this type of modified graphene.

(e) Future theoretical studies on modified graphene for hydrogen storage must adopt dispersion corrections. Many existing studies did not include these corrections, limiting the quality of the results. Future studies should also report the gravimetric capacity of the systems as it is an important parameter to determine whether a material is a good candidate for hydrogen storage. Many existing studies only reported the adsorption energy of the H_2 molecule, which is not enough to identify new materials for hydrogen storage.

(f) These theoretical results discussed herein should motivate experimental groups to experimentally validate the theoretical predictions, as many modified graphene systems are shown to be good candidates for hydrogen storage. The knowledge of these systems can be systematized, and the systems can be experimentally evaluated for hydrogen storage.

Author Contributions: Conceptualization, H.C.-M., B.G.-H., F.M.-A., H.R.-C. and E.P.S.-R.; formal analysis, B.G.-H., F.M.-A. and A.G.-V.; data curation, B.G.-H., F.M.-A. and A.G.-V.; writing—original draft preparation, H.C.-M., H.R.-C. and E.P.S.-R.; writing—review and editing, H.C.-M., H.R.-C. and E.P.S.-R.; funding acquisition, B.G.-H. and E.P.S.-R. All authors have read and agreed to the published version of the manuscript.

Funding: This research was funded by Tecnológico Nacional de México through grant number 19057.23-P, and the APC was funded by Tecnologico de Monterrey.

Institutional Review Board Statement: Not applicable.

Informed Consent Statement: Not applicable.

Data Availability Statement: Data are contained within the article.

Conflicts of Interest: The authors declare no conflicts of interest.

References

1. Abdin, Z.; Zafaranloo, A.; Rafiee, A.; Mérida, W.; Lipiński, W.; Khalilpour, K.R. Hydrogen as an energy vector. *Renew. Sustain. Energy Rev.* **2020**, *120*, 109620. [CrossRef]
2. Nazir, H.; Louis, C.; Jose, S.; Prakash, J.; Muthuswamy, N.; Buan, M.E.; Kannan, A.M. Is the H_2 economy realizable in the foreseeable future? Part I: H_2 production methods. *Int. J. Hydrog. Energy* **2020**, *45*, 13777–13788. [CrossRef]
3. Jain, I.P. Hydrogen the fuel for 21st century. *Int. J. Hydrog. Energy* **2009**, *34*, 7368–7378. [CrossRef]
4. Dincer, I.; Acar, C. Review and evaluation of hydrogen production methods for better sustainability. *Int. J. Hydrog. Energy* **2015**, *40*, 11094–11111. [CrossRef]
5. Moradi, R.; Groth, K.M. Hydrogen storage and delivery: Review of the state of the art technologies and risk and reliability analysis. *Int. J. Hydrog. Energy* **2019**, *44*, 12254–12269. [CrossRef]
6. Sharaf, O.Z.; Orhan, M.F. An overview of fuel cell technology: Fundamentals and applications. *Renew. Sustain. Energy Rev.* **2014**, *32*, 810–853. [CrossRef]
7. Nikolaidis, P.; Poullikkas, A. A comparative overview of hydrogen production processes. *Renew. Sustain. Energy Rev.* **2017**, *67*, 597–611. [CrossRef]
8. Da Silva Veras, T.; Mozer, T.S.; da Silva César, A. Hydrogen: Trends, production and characterization of the main process worldwide. *Int. J. Hydrog. Energy* **2017**, *42*, 2018–2033. [CrossRef]
9. Durbin, D.J.; Malardier-Jugroot, C. Review of hydrogen storage techniques for on board vehicle applications. *Int. J. Hydrog. Energy* **2013**, *38*, 14595–14617. [CrossRef]
10. Niaz, S.; Manzoor, T.; Pandith, A.H. Hydrogen storage: Materials, methods and perspectives. *Renew. Sustain. Energy Rev.* **2015**, *50*, 457–469. [CrossRef]
11. Tellez-Cruz, M.M.; Escorihuela, J.; Solorza-Feria, O.; Compañ, V. Proton Exchange Membrane Fuel Cells (PEMFCs): Advances and Challenges. *Polymers* **2021**, *13*, 3064. [CrossRef] [PubMed]
12. Das, V.; Padmanaban, S.; Venkitasamy, K.; Selvamuthukumaran, R.; Blaabjerg, F.; Siano, P. Recent advances and challenges of fuel cell based power system architectures and control—A review. *Renew. Sustain. Energy Rev.* **2017**, *73*, 10–18. [CrossRef]
13. Cruz-Martínez, H.; Guerra-Cabrera, W.; Flores-Rojas, E.; Ruiz-Villalobos, D.; Rojas-Chávez, H.; Peña-Castañeda, Y.A.; Medina, D.I. Pt-Free Metal Nanocatalysts for the Oxygen Reduction Reaction Combining Experiment and Theory: An Overview. *Molecules* **2021**, *26*, 6689. [CrossRef]
14. Ren, J.; Musyoka, N.M.; Langmi, H.W.; Mathe, M.; Liao, S. Current research trends and perspectives on materials-based hydrogen storage solutions: A critical review. *Int. J. Hydrog. Energy* **2017**, *42*, 289–311. [CrossRef]
15. Yang, J.; Sudik, A.; Wolverton, C.; Siegel, D.J. High capacity hydrogen storage materials: Attributes for automotive applications and techniques for materials discovery. *Chem. Soc. Rev.* **2010**, *39*, 656–675. [CrossRef] [PubMed]
16. Kumar, P.; Singh, S.; Hashmi, S.A.R.; Kim, K.H. MXenes: Emerging 2D materials for hydrogen storage. *Nano Energy* **2021**, *85*, 105989. [CrossRef]
17. Gupta, A.; Baron, G.V.; Perreault, P.; Lenaerts, S.; Ciocarlan, R.G.; Cool, P.; Denayer, J.F. Hydrogen clathrates: Next generation hydrogen storage materials. *Energy Storage Mater.* **2021**, *41*, 69–107. [CrossRef]
18. Jena, P. Materials for hydrogen storage: Past, present, and future. *J. Phys. Chem. Lett.* **2011**, *2*, 206–211. [CrossRef]
19. Suh, M.P.; Park, H.J.; Prasad, T.K.; Lim, D.W. Hydrogen storage in metal–organic frameworks. *Chem. Rev.* **2012**, *112*, 782–835. [CrossRef]
20. Yartys, V.A.; Lototskyy, M.V.; Akiba, E.; Albert, R.; Antonov, V.E.; Ares, J.R.; Zhu, M. Magnesium based materials for hydrogen based energy storage: Past, present and future. *Int. J. Hydrog. Energy* **2019**, *44*, 7809–7859. [CrossRef]
21. Jain, I.P.; Jain, P.; Jain, A. Novel hydrogen storage materials: A review of lightweight complex hydrides. *J. Alloy. Compd.* **2010**, *503*, 303–339. [CrossRef]
22. Rusman, N.A.A.; Dahari, M. A review on the current progress of metal hydrides material for solid-state hydrogen storage applications. *Int. J. Hydrog. Energy* **2016**, *41*, 12108–12126. [CrossRef]
23. Akbayrak, S.; Özkar, S. Ammonia borane as hydrogen storage materials. *Int. J. Hydrog. Energy* **2018**, *43*, 18592–18606. [CrossRef]
24. Mohan, M.; Sharma, V.K.; Kumar, E.A.; Gayathri, V. Hydrogen storage in carbon materials—A review. *Energy Storage* **2019**, *1*, e35. [CrossRef]
25. Xia, Y.; Yang, Z.; Zhu, Y. Porous carbon-based materials for hydrogen storage: Advancement and challenges. *J. Mater. Chem. A* **2013**, *1*, 9365–9381. [CrossRef]
26. Cruz-Martínez, H.; Rojas-Chávez, H.; Matadamas-Ortiz, P.T.; Ortiz-Herrera, J.C.; López-Chávez, E.; Solorza-Feria, O.; Medina, D.I. Current progress of Pt-based ORR electrocatalysts for PEMFCs: An integrated view combining theory and experiment. *Mater. Today Phys.* **2021**, *19*, 100406. [CrossRef]

27. Kulkarni, A.; Siahrostami, S.; Patel, A.; Nørskov, J.K. Understanding catalytic activity trends in the oxygen reduction reaction. *Chem. Rev.* **2018**, *118*, 2302–2312. [CrossRef]
28. Wang, Y.; Wang, D.; Li, Y. Rational design of single-atom site electrocatalysts: From theoretical understandings to practical applications. *Adv. Mat.* **2021**, *33*, 2008151. [CrossRef] [PubMed]
29. Cruz-Martínez, H.; Tellez-Cruz, M.M.; Solorza-Feria, O.; Calaminici, P.; Medina, D.I. Catalytic activity trends from pure Pd nanoclusters to M@PdPt (M = Co, Ni, and Cu) core-shell nanoclusters for the oxygen reduction reaction: A first-principles analysis. *Int. J. Hydrog. Energy* **2020**, *45*, 13738–13745. [CrossRef]
30. Muckerman, J.T.; Fujita, E. Theoretical studies of the mechanism of catalytic hydrogen production by a cobaloxime. *Chem. Comm.* **2011**, *47*, 12456–12458. [CrossRef] [PubMed]
31. Jain, A.; Shin, Y.; Persson, K.A. Computational predictions of energy materials using density functional theory. *Nat. Rev. Mater.* **2016**, *1*, 1–13. [CrossRef]
32. Nørskov, J.K.; Bligaard, T.; Rossmeisl, J.; Christensen, C.H. Towards the computational design of solid catalysts. *Nat. Chem.* **2009**, *1*, 37–46. [CrossRef] [PubMed]
33. Curtarolo, S.; Hart, G.L.; Nardelli, M.B.; Mingo, N.; Sanvito, S.; Levy, O. The high-throughput highway to computational materials design. *Nat. Mater.* **2013**, *12*, 191–201. [CrossRef]
34. Kose, A.; Yuksel, N.; Fellah, M.F. Hydrogen adsorption on Ni doped carbon nanocone. *Diam. Relat. Mater.* **2022**, *124*, 108921. [CrossRef]
35. Ganji, M.D.; Hosseini-Khah, S.M.; Amini-Tabar, Z. Theoretical insight into hydrogen adsorption onto graphene: A first-principles B3LYP-D3 study. *Phys. Chem. Chem. Phys.* **2015**, *17*, 2504–2511. [CrossRef]
36. Rangel, E.; Sansores, E. Theoretical study of hydrogen adsorption on nitrogen doped graphene decorated with palladium clusters. *Int. J. Hydrog. Energy* **2014**, *39*, 6558–6566. [CrossRef]
37. Lopez-Corral, I.; de Celis, J.; Juan, A.; Irigoyen, B. DFT study of H_2 adsorption on Pd-decorated single walled carbon nanotubes with C-vacancies. *Int. J. Hydrog. Energy* **2012**, *37*, 10156–10164. [CrossRef]
38. Rodríguez-Quintana, R.; Carbajal-Franco, G.; Rojas-Chávez, H. DFT study of the H_2 molecules adsorption on pristine and Ni doped graphite surfaces. *Mater. Lett.* **2021**, *293*, 129660. [CrossRef]
39. Ren, H.; Cui, C.; Li, X.; Liu, Y. A DFT study of the hydrogen storage potentials and properties of Na-and Li-doped fullerenes. *Int. J. Hydrog. Energy* **2017**, *42*, 312–321. [CrossRef]
40. Lopez-Chavez, E.; Peña-Castañeda, Y.; García-Quiroz, A.; Castillo-Alvarado, F.; Díaz-Gongora, J.; Jimenez-Gonzalez, L. Ti-decorated C_{120} nanotorus: A new molecular structure for hydrogen storage. *Int. J. Hydrog. Energy* **2017**, *42*, 30237–30241. [CrossRef]
41. Akbari, F.; Reisi-Vanani, A.; Darvish Nejad, M.H. DFT study of the electronic and structural properties of single Al and N atoms and Al-N co-doped graphyne toward hydrogen storage. *Appl. Surf. Sci.* **2019**, *488*, 600–610. [CrossRef]
42. Ding, F.; Yakobson, B.I. Challenges in hydrogen adsorptions: From physisorption to chemisorption. *Front. Phys.* **2011**, *6*, 142–150. [CrossRef]
43. Valdés-Madrigal, M.A.; Montejo-Alvaro, F.; Cernas-Ruiz, A.S.; Rojas-Chávez, H.; Román-Doval, R.; Cruz-Martinez, H.; Medina, D.I. Role of defect engineering and surface functionalization in the design of carbon nanotube-based nitrogen oxide sensors. *Int. J. Mol. Sci.* **2021**, *22*, 12968. [CrossRef]
44. Singla, M.; Jaggi, N. Theoretical investigations of hydrogen gas sensing and storage capacity of graphene-based materials: A review. *Sens. Actuator A Phys.* **2021**, *332*, 113118. [CrossRef]
45. Shiraz, H.G.; Tavakoli, O. Investigation of graphene-based systems for hydrogen storage. *Renew. Sustain. Energy Rev.* **2017**, *74*, 104–109. [CrossRef]
46. Cabria, I.; López, M.J.; Alonso, J.A. Searching for DFT-based methods that include dispersion interactions to calculate the physisorption of H_2 on benzene and graphene. *J. Chem. Phys.* **2017**, *146*, 214104. [CrossRef]
47. Meng, S.; Kaxiras, E.; Zhang, Z. Metal− diboride nanotubes as high-capacity hydrogen storage media. *Nano Lett.* **2007**, *7*, 663–667. [CrossRef]
48. Wu, M.; Wang, Q.; Sun, Q.; Jena, P. Functionalized graphitic carbon nitride for efficient energy storage. *J. Phys. Chem. C* **2013**, *117*, 6055–6059. [CrossRef]
49. Jin, X.; Qi, P.; Yang, H.; Zhang, Y.; Li, J.; Chen, H. Enhanced hydrogen adsorption on Li-coated $B_{12}C_6N_6$. *J. Chem. Phys.* **2016**, *145*, 164301. [CrossRef] [PubMed]
50. Ao, Z.; Dou, S.; Xu, Z.; Jiang, Q.; Wang, G. Hydrogen storage in porous graphene with Al decoration. *Int. J. Hydrog. Energy* **2014**, *39*, 16244–16251. [CrossRef]
51. Cui, S.; Zhao, N.; Shi, C.; Feng, C.; He, C.; Li, J.; Liu, E. Effect of hydrogen molecule dissociation on hydrogen storage capacity of graphene with metal atom decorated. *J. Phys. Chem. C* **2014**, *118*, 839–844. [CrossRef]
52. Liu, Y.; Zhou, Y.; Yang, S.; Xu, H.; Lan, Z.; Xiong, J.; Gu, H. A DFT study on enhanced adsorption of H_2 on Be-decorated porous graphene nanosheet and the effects of applied electrical fields. *Int. J. Hydrog. Energy* **2021**, *46*, 5891–5903. [CrossRef]
53. Ataca, C.; Aktürk, E.; Ciraci, S. Hydrogen storage of calcium atoms adsorbed on graphene: First-principles plane wave calculations. *Phys. Rev. B* **2009**, *79*, 041406. [CrossRef]
54. Lee, H.; Ihm, J.; Cohen, M.L.; Louie, S.G. Calcium-decorated graphene-based nanostructures for hydrogen storage. *Nano Lett.* **2010**, *10*, 793–798. [CrossRef]

55. Beheshti, E.; Nojeh, A.; Servati, P. A first-principles study of calcium-decorated, boron-doped graphene for high capacity hydrogen storage. *Carbon* **2011**, *49*, 1561–1567. [CrossRef]
56. Hussain, T.; Pathak, B.; Ramzan, M.; Maark, T.A.; Ahuja, R. Calcium doped graphane as a hydrogen storage material. *Appl. Phys. Lett.* **2012**, *100*, 183902. [CrossRef]
57. Gao, Y.; Zhao, N.; Li, J.; Liu, E.; He, C.; Shi, C. Hydrogen spillover storage on Ca-decorated graphene. *Int. J. Hydrog. Energy* **2012**, *37*, 11835–11841. [CrossRef]
58. Wang, V.; Mizuseki, H.; He, H.P.; Chen, G.; Zhang, S.L.; Kawazoe, Y. Calcium-decorated graphene for hydrogen storage: A van der Waals density functional study. *Comput. Mater. Sci.* **2012**, *55*, 180–185. [CrossRef]
59. Valencia, H.; Gil, A.; Frapper, G. Trends in the hydrogen activation and storage by adsorbed 3d transition metal atoms onto graphene and nanotube surfaces: A DFT study and molecular orbital analysis. *J. Phys. Chem. C* **2015**, *119*, 5506–5522. [CrossRef]
60. Ma, S.; Chen, J.; Wang, L.; Jiao, Z. First-principles insight into hydrogen adsorption over Co_4 anchored on defective graphene. *Appl. Surf. Sci.* **2020**, *504*, 144413. [CrossRef]
61. Choudhary, A.; Malakkal, L.; Siripurapu, R.K.; Szpunar, B.; Szpunar, J. First principles calculations of hydrogen storage on Cu and Pd-decorated graphene. *Int. J. Hydrog. Energy* **2016**, *41*, 17652–17656. [CrossRef]
62. Malček, M.; Bučinský, L. On the hydrogen storage performance of Cu-doped and Cu-decorated graphene quantum dots: A computational study. *Theor. Chem. Acc.* **2020**, *139*, 167. [CrossRef]
63. Liu, W.; Liu, Y.; Wang, R.; Hao, L.; Song, D.; Li, Z. DFT study of hydrogen adsorption on Eu-decorated single-and double-sided graphene. *Phys. Status Solidi B* **2014**, *251*, 229–234. [CrossRef]
64. Ataca, C.; Aktürk, E.; Ciraci, S.A.L.İ.M.; Ustunel, H.A.N.D.E. High-capacity hydrogen storage by metallized graphene. *Appl. Phys. Lett.* **2008**, *93*, 043123. [CrossRef]
65. Zhou, M.; Lu, Y.; Zhang, C.; Feng, Y.P. Strain effects on hydrogen storage capability of metal-decorated graphene: A first-principles study. *Appl. Phys. Lett.* **2010**, *97*, 103109. [CrossRef]
66. Zhou, W.; Zhou, J.; Shen, J.; Ouyang, C.; Shi, S. First-principles study of high-capacity hydrogen storage on graphene with Li atoms. *J. Phys. Chem. Solids* **2012**, *73*, 245–251. [CrossRef]
67. Hussain, T.; De Sarkar, A.; Ahuja, R. Strain induced lithium functionalized graphane as a high capacity hydrogen storage material. *Appl. Phys. Lett.* **2012**, *101*, 103907. [CrossRef]
68. Kim, D.; Lee, S.; Hwang, Y.; Yun, K.H.; Chung, Y.C. Hydrogen storage in Li dispersed graphene with Stone–Wales defects: A first-principles study. *Int. J. Hydrog. Energy* **2014**, *39*, 13189–13194. [CrossRef]
69. Seenithurai, S.; Pandyan, R.K.; Kumar, S.V.; Saranya, C.; Mahendran, M. Li-decorated double vacancy graphene for hydrogen storage application: A first principles study. *Int. J. Hydrog. Energy* **2014**, *39*, 11016–11026. [CrossRef]
70. Wang, F.; Zhang, T.; Hou, X.; Zhang, W.; Tang, S.; Sun, H.; Zhang, J. Li-decorated porous graphene as a high-performance hydrogen storage material: A first-principles study. *Int. J. Hydrog. Energy* **2017**, *42*, 10099–10108. [CrossRef]
71. Tachikawa, H.; Iyama, T. Mechanism of hydrogen storage in the graphene nanoflake–lithium–H2 system. *J. Phys. Chem. C* **2019**, *123*, 8709–8716. [CrossRef]
72. Liu, Y.; Gao, S.; Lu, F.; Yu, A.; Song, S.; Shi, H.; Liao, B. Hydrogen adsorption on Li decorated graphyne-like carbon nanosheet: A density functional theory study. *Int. J. Hydrog. Energy* **2020**, *45*, 24938–24946. [CrossRef]
73. Zheng, N.; Yang, S.; Xu, H.; Lan, Z.; Wang, Z.; Gu, H. A DFT study of the enhanced hydrogen storage performance of the Li-decorated graphene nanoribbons. *Vacuum* **2020**, *171*, 109011. [CrossRef]
74. Ibarra-Rodriguez, M.; Sanchez, M. Lithium clusters on graphene surface and their ability to adsorb hydrogen molecules. *Int. J. Hydrog. Energy* **2021**, *46*, 21984–21993. [CrossRef]
75. Amaniseyed, Z.; Tavangar, Z. Hydrogen storage on uncharged and positively charged Mg-decorated graphene. *Int. J. Hydrog. Energy* **2019**, *44*, 3803–3811. [CrossRef]
76. Sigal, A.; Rojas, M.I.; Leiva, E.P.M. Interferents for hydrogen storage on a graphene sheet decorated with nickel: A DFT study. *Int. J. Hydrog. Energy* **2011**, *36*, 3537–3546. [CrossRef]
77. Cabria, I.; López, M.J.; Fraile, S.; Alonso, J.A. Adsorption and dissociation of molecular hydrogen on palladium clusters supported on graphene. *J. Phys. Chem. C* **2012**, *116*, 21179–21189. [CrossRef]
78. Faye, O.; Szpunar, J.A.; Szpunar, B.; Beye, A.C. Hydrogen adsorption and storage on palladium–functionalized graphene with NH-dopant: A first principles calculation. *Appl. Surf. Sci.* **2017**, *392*, 362–374. [CrossRef]
79. Kishnani, V.; Yadav, A.; Mondal, K.; Gupta, A. Palladium-functionalized graphene for hydrogen sensing performance: Theoretical studies. *Energies* **2021**, *14*, 5738. [CrossRef]
80. Sharma, V.; Kagdada, H.L.; Wang, J.; Jha, P.K. Hydrogen adsorption on pristine and platinum decorated graphene quantum dot: A first principle study. *Int. J. Hydrog. Energy* **2020**, *45*, 23977–23987. [CrossRef]
81. Chen, Y.; Wang, J.; Yuan, L.; Zhang, M.; Zhang, C. Sc-decorated porous graphene for high-capacity hydrogen storage: First-principles calculations. *Materials* **2017**, *10*, 894. [CrossRef]
82. Lebon, A.; Carrete, J.; Gallego, L.J.; Vega, A. Ti-decorated zigzag graphene nanoribbons for hydrogen storage. A van der Waals-corrected density-functional study. *Int. J. Hydrog. Energy* **2015**, *40*, 4960–4968. [CrossRef]
83. Yuan, L.; Kang, L.; Chen, Y.; Wang, D.; Gong, J.; Wang, C.; Wu, X. Hydrogen storage capacity on Ti-decorated porous graphene: First-principles investigation. *Appl. Surf. Sci.* **2018**, *434*, 843–849. [CrossRef]

84. Ghalami, Z.; Ghoulipour, V.; Khanchi, A. Hydrogen and deuterium adsorption on uranium decorated graphene nanosheets: A combined molecular dynamics and density functional theory study. *Curr. Appl. Phys.* **2019**, *19*, 536–541. [CrossRef]
85. Yuan, L.; Wang, D.; Gong, J.; Zhang, C.; Zhang, L.; Zhang, M.; Kang, L. First-principles study of V-decorated porous graphene for hydrogen storage. *Chem. Phys. Lett.* **2019**, *726*, 57–61. [CrossRef]
86. Yuan, L.; Chen, Y.; Kang, L.; Zhang, C.; Wang, D.; Wang, C.; Wu, X. First-principles investigation of hydrogen storage capacity of Y-decorated porous graphene. *Appl. Surf. Sci.* **2017**, *399*, 463–468. [CrossRef]
87. Lebon, A.; Carrete, J.; Longo, R.C.; Vega, A.; Gallego, L.J. Molecular hydrogen uptake by zigzag graphene nanoribbons doped with early 3d transition-metal atoms. *Int. J. Hydrog. Energy* **2013**, *38*, 8872–8880. [CrossRef]
88. Zhang, Y.; Cheng, X. First-principles study of Li decorated coronene graphene. *Int. J. Mod. Phys. B* **2017**, *31*, 1750216. [CrossRef]
89. Liu, Y.; Ren, L.; He, Y.; Cheng, H.P. Titanium-decorated graphene for high-capacity hydrogen storage studied by density functional simulations. *J. Phys. Condens. Matter.* **2010**, *22*, 445301. [CrossRef] [PubMed]
90. Bakhshi, F.; Farhadian, N. Co-doped graphene sheets as a novel adsorbent for hydrogen storage: DFT and DFT-D3 correction dispersion study. *Int. J. Hydrog. Energy* **2018**, *43*, 8355–8364. [CrossRef]
91. Faye, O.; Eduok, U.; Szpunar, J.; Szpunar, B.; Samoura, A.; Beye, A. Hydrogen storage on bare Cu atom and Cu-functionalized boron-doped graphene: A first principles study. *Int. J. Hydrog. Energy* **2017**, *42*, 4233–4243. [CrossRef]
92. Fadlallah, M.M.; Abdelrahman, A.G.; Schwingenschlögl, U.; Maarouf, A.A. Graphene and graphene nanomesh supported nickel clusters: Electronic, magnetic, and hydrogen storage properties. *Nanotechnology* **2019**, *30*, 085709. [CrossRef]
93. Ambrusi, R.E.; Luna, C.R.; Juan, A.; Pronsato, M.E. DFT study of Rh-decorated pristine, B-doped and vacancy defected graphene for hydrogen adsorption. *RSC Adv.* **2016**, *6*, 83926–83941. [CrossRef]
94. Available online: https://www.energy.gov/eere/fuelcells/doe-technical-targets-onboard-hydrogen-storage-light-duty-vehicles (accessed on 5 November 2023).
95. Cruz-Martínez, H.; Rojas-Chávez, H.; Valdés-Madrigal, M.A.; López-Sosa, L.; Calaminici, P. Stability and catalytic properties of Pt–Ni clusters supported on pyridinic N-doped graphene nanoflakes: An auxiliary density functional theory study. *Theor. Chem. Acc.* **2022**, *141*, 46. [CrossRef]
96. Wang, X.; Sun, G.; Routh, P.; Kim, D.H.; Huang, W.; Chen, P. Heteroatom-doped graphene materials: Syntheses, properties and applications. *Chem. Soc. Rev.* **2014**, *43*, 7067–7098. [CrossRef]
97. Duan, J.; Chen, S.; Jaroniec, M.; Qiao, S.Z. Heteroatom-doped graphene-based materials for energy-relevant electrocatalytic processes. *ACS Catalys.* **2015**, *5*, 5207–5234. [CrossRef]
98. Martínez-Vargas, A.; Vásquez-López, A.; Antonio-Ruiz, C.D.; Cruz-Martínez, H.; Medina, D.I.; Montejo-Alvaro, F. Stability, Energetic, and Reactivity Properties of NiPd Alloy Clusters Deposited on Graphene with Defects: A Density Functional Theory Study. *Materials* **2022**, *15*, 4710.
99. Putri, L.K.; Ong, W.J.; Chang, W.S.; Chai, S.P. Heteroatom doped graphene in photocatalysis: A review. *Appl. Surf. Sci.* **2015**, *358*, 2–14. [CrossRef]
100. Sánchez-Rodríguez, E.P.; Vargas-Hernández, C.N.; Cruz-Martínez, H.; Medina, D.I. Stability, magnetic, energetic, and reactivity properties of icosahedral M@Pd$_{12}$ (M = Fe, Co, Ni, and Cu) core-shell nanoparticles supported on pyridinic N$_3$-doped graphene. *Solid State Sci.* **2021**, *112*, 106483. [CrossRef]
101. Carrete, J.; Longo, R.C.; Gallego, L.J.; Vega, A.; Balbás, L.C. Al enhances the H$_2$ storage capacity of graphene at nanoribbon borders but not at central sites: A study using nonlocal van der Waals density functionals. *Phys. Rev. B* **2012**, *85*, 125435. [CrossRef]
102. Zhang, H.P.; Luo, X.G.; Lin, X.Y.; Lu, X.; Leng, Y. Density functional theory calculations of hydrogen adsorption on Ti-, Zn-, Zr-, Al-, and N-doped and intrinsic graphene sheets. *Int. J. Hydrog. Energy* **2013**, *38*, 14269–14275. [CrossRef]
103. Cho, J.H.; Yang, S.J.; Lee, K.; Park, C.R. Si-doping effect on the enhanced hydrogen storage of single walled carbon nanotubes and graphene. *Int. J. Hydrog. Energy* **2011**, *36*, 12286–12295. [CrossRef]
104. Nayyar, I.; Ginovska, B.; Karkamkar, A.; Gennett, T.; Autrey, T. Physi-sorption of H$_2$ on pure and boron–doped graphene monolayers: A dispersion–corrected DFT study. *C* **2020**, *6*, 15. [CrossRef]
105. Choi, W.I.; Jhi, S.H.; Kim, K.; Kim, Y.H. Divacancy-nitrogen-assisted transition metal dispersion and hydrogen adsorption in defective graphene: A first-principles study. *Phys. Rev. B* **2010**, *81*, 085441. [CrossRef]
106. Tabtimsai, C.; Rakrai, W.; Wanno, B. Hydrogen adsorption on graphene sheets doped with group 8B transition metal: A DFT investigation. *Vacuum* **2017**, *139*, 101–108. [CrossRef]
107. Ikot, I.J.; Olagoke, P.O.; Louis, H.; Charlie, D.E.; Magu, T.O.; Owen, A.E. Hydrogen storage capacity of Al, Ca, Mg, Ni, and Zn decorated phosphorus-doped graphene: Insight from theoretical calculations. *Int. J. Hydrog. Energy* **2023**, *48*, 13362–13376. [CrossRef]
108. Singla, M.; Sharma, D.; Jaggi, N. Effect of transition metal (Cu and Pt) doping/co-doping on hydrogen gas sensing capability of graphene: A DFT study. *Int. J. Hydrog. Energy* **2021**, *46*, 16188–16201. [CrossRef]
109. Rangel, E.; Ramirez-Arellano, J.M.; Carrillo, I.; Magana, L.F. Hydrogen adsorption around lithium atoms anchored on graphene vacancies. *Int. J. Hydrog. Energy* **2011**, *36*, 13657–13662. [CrossRef]
110. Yang, S.; Lan, Z.; Xu, H.; Lei, G.; Xie, W.; Gu, Q. A first-principles study on hydrogen sensing properties of pristine and Mo-doped graphene. *J. Nanotechnol.* **2018**, *2018*, 2031805. [CrossRef]
111. Ao, Z.M.; Peeters, F.M. Electric field activated hydrogen dissociative adsorption to nitrogen-doped graphene. *J. Phys. Chem. C* **2010**, *114*, 14503–14509. [CrossRef]

112. Petrushenko, I.K.; Petrushenko, K.B. Hydrogen physisorption on nitrogen-doped graphene and graphene-like boron nitride-carbon heterostructures: A DFT study. *Surf. Interfaces* 2019, *17*, 100355. [CrossRef]
113. Ramos-Castillo, C.M.; Reveles, J.U.; Cifuentes-Quintal, M.E.; Zope, R.R.; De Coss, R. Ti_4-and Ni_4-doped defective graphene nanoplatelets as efficient materials for hydrogen storage. *J. Phys. Chem. C* 2016, *120*, 5001–5009. [CrossRef]
114. Alshareef, B.S. DFT investigation of the hydrogen adsorption on graphene and graphene sheet doped with osmium and tungsten. *J. Phys. Chem.* 2020, *10*, 197–204. [CrossRef]
115. Ramos-Castillo, C.M.; Reveles, J.U.; Zope, R.R.; De Coss, R. Palladium clusters supported on graphene monovacancies for hydrogen storage. *J. Phys. Chem. C* 2015, *119*, 8402–8409. [CrossRef]
116. Granja-DelRio, A.; Alonso, J.A.; Lopez, M.J. Competition between palladium clusters and hydrogen to saturate graphene vacancies. *J. Phys. Chem. C* 2017, *121*, 10843–10850. [CrossRef]
117. Granja-DelRío, A.; Alonso, J.A.; López, M.J. Steric and chemical effects on the hydrogen adsorption and dissociation on free and graphene–supported palladium clusters. *Comput. Theor. Chem.* 2017, *1107*, 23–29. [CrossRef]
118. Liao, J.H.; Zhao, Y.J.; Yang, X.B. Controllable hydrogen adsorption and desorption by strain modulation on Ti decorated defective graphene. *Int. J. Hydrog. Energy* 2015, *40*, 12063–12071. [CrossRef]
119. Zhou, Q.; Wang, C.; Fu, Z.; Yuan, L.; Yang, X.; Tang, Y.; Zhang, H. Hydrogen adsorption on palladium anchored defected graphene with B-doping: A theoretical study. *Int. J. Hydrog. Energy* 2015, *40*, 2473–2483. [CrossRef]
120. Granja-DelRío, A.; Alducin, M.; Juaristi, J.I.; López, M.J.; Alonso, J.A. Absence of spillover of hydrogen adsorbed on small palladium clusters anchored to graphene vacancies. *Appl. Surf. Sci.* 2021, *559*, 149835. [CrossRef]
121. López-Corral, I.; Piriz, S.; Faccio, R.; Juan, A.; Avena, M. A van der Waals DFT study of PtH_2 systems absorbed on pristine and defective graphene. *Appl. Surf. Sci.* 2016, *382*, 80–87. [CrossRef]
122. Cui, H.; Zhang, Y.; Tian, W.; Wang, Y.; Liu, T.; Chen, Y.; Yuan, H. A study on hydrogen storage performance of Ti decorated vacancies graphene structure on the first principle. *RSC Adv.* 2021, *11*, 13912–13918. [CrossRef] [PubMed]
123. Ao, Z.M.; Jiang, Q.; Zhang, R.Q.; Tan, T.T.; Li, S. Al doped graphene: A promising material for hydrogen storage at room temperature. *J. Appl. Phys.* 2009, *105*, 074307. [CrossRef]
124. Xiang, C.; Li, A.; Yang, S.; Lan, Z.; Xie, W.; Tang, Y.; Gu, H. Enhanced hydrogen storage performance of graphene nanoflakes doped with Cr atoms: A DFT study. *RSC Adv.* 2019, *9*, 25690–25696. [CrossRef] [PubMed]
125. Zhou, Y.; Chu, W.; Jing, F.; Zheng, J.; Sun, W.; Xue, Y. Enhanced hydrogen storage on Li-doped defective graphene with B substitution: A DFT study. *Appl. Surf. Sci.* 2017, *410*, 166–176. [CrossRef]
126. Lee, S.; Lee, M.; Chung, Y.C. Enhanced hydrogen storage properties under external electric fields of N-doped graphene with Li decoration. *Phys. Chem. Chem. Phys.* 2013, *15*, 3243–3248. [CrossRef]
127. Kim, D.; Lee, S.; Jo, S.; Chung, Y.C. Strain effects on hydrogen storage in Ti decorated pyridinic N-doped graphene. *Phys. Chem. Chem. Phys.* 2013, *15*, 12757–12761. [CrossRef]
128. Lee, S.; Lee, M.; Choi, H.; Yoo, D.S.; Chung, Y.C. Effect of nitrogen induced defects in Li dispersed graphene on hydrogen storage. *Int. J. Hydrog. Energy* 2013, *38*, 4611–4617. [CrossRef]
129. Rangel, E.; Sansores, E.; Vallejo, E.; Hernández-Hernández, A.; López-Pérez, P.A. Study of the interplay between N-graphene defects and small Pd clusters for enhanced hydrogen storage via a spill-over mechanism. *Phys. Chem. Chem. Phys.* 2016, *18*, 33158–33170. [CrossRef]
130. Luo, Z.; Fan, X.; Pan, R.; An, Y. A first-principles study of Sc-decorated graphene with pyridinic-N defects for hydrogen storage. *Int. J. Hydrog. Energy* 2017, *42*, 3106–3113. [CrossRef]
131. Singla, M.; Jaggi, N. Enhanced hydrogen sensing properties in copper decorated nitrogen doped defective graphene nanoribbons: DFT study. *Phys. E Low Dimens. Syst. Nanostruct.* 2021, *131*, 114756. [CrossRef]
132. Rajasekaran, G.; Narayanan, P.; Parashar, A. Effect of point and line defects on mechanical and thermal properties of graphene: A review. *Crit. Rev. Solid State Mater. Sci.* 2016, *41*, 47–71. [CrossRef]
133. Liu, L.; Qing, M.; Wang, Y.; Chen, S. Defects in graphene: Generation, healing, and their effects on the properties of graphene: A review. *J. Mater. Sci. Technol.* 2015, *31*, 599–606. [CrossRef]
134. Yadav, S.; Zhu, Z.; Singh, C.V. Defect engineering of graphene for effective hydrogen storage. *Int. J. Hydrog. Energy* 2014, *39*, 4981–4995. [CrossRef]
135. Gehringer, D.; Dengg, T.; Popov, M.N.; Holec, D. Interactions between a H_2 molecule and carbon nanostructures: A DFT study. *C* 2020, *6*, 16. [CrossRef]
136. Sunnardianto, G.K.; Bokas, G.; Hussein, A.; Walters, C.; Moultos, O.A.; Dey, P. Efficient hydrogen storage in defective graphene and its mechanical stability: A combined density functional theory and molecular dynamics simulation study. *Int. J. Hydrog. Energy* 2021, *46*, 5485–5494. [CrossRef]
137. Lone, B. Mg Decorated Boron doped Graphene for Hydrogen Storage: A DFT Method. *Int. J. Res. Appl. Sci. Eng. Technol.* 2020, *8*, 109–181. [CrossRef]
138. Wu, H.Y.; Fan, X.; Kuo, J.L.; Deng, W.Q. DFT study of hydrogen storage by spillover on graphene with boron substitution. *J. Phys. Chem. C* 2011, *115*, 9241–9249. [CrossRef]
139. Nachimuthu, S.; Lai, P.J.; Jiang, J.C. Efficient hydrogen storage in boron doped graphene decorated by transition metals–A first-principles study. *Carbon* 2014, *73*, 132–140. [CrossRef]

140. Liu, W.; Liu, Y.; Wang, R. Prediction of hydrogen storage on Y-decorated graphene: A density functional theory study. *Appl. Surf. Sci.* **2014**, *296*, 204–208. [CrossRef]
141. Nachimuthu, S.; Lai, P.J.; Leggesse, E.G.; Jiang, J.C. A first principles study on boron-doped graphene decorated by Ni-Ti-Mg atoms for enhanced hydrogen storage performance. *Sci. Rep.* **2015**, *5*, 16797. [CrossRef]
142. Li, Y.; Mi, Y.; Sun, G. First principles DFT study of hydrogen storage on graphene with La decoration. *J. Mater. Sci. Chem. Eng.* **2015**, *3*, 87. [CrossRef]
143. Ma, L.; Zhang, J.M.; Xu, K.W.; Ji, V. Hydrogen adsorption and storage on palladium-decorated graphene with boron dopants and vacancy defects: A first-principles study. *Phys. E Low Dimens. Syst. Nanostruct.* **2015**, *66*, 40–47. [CrossRef]
144. Zhu, X. First principles calculations of hydrogen storage on calcium-decorated, boron-doped bilayer graphene. *J. Mater. Sci. Chem. Eng.* **2018**, *6*, 1–12. [CrossRef]
145. Wang, J.; Chen, Y.; Yuan, L.; Zhang, M.; Zhang, C. Scandium decoration of boron doped porous graphene for high-capacity hydrogen storage. *Molecules* **2019**, *24*, 2382. [CrossRef]
146. Chu, S.; Hu, L.; Hu, X.; Yang, M.; Deng, J. Titanium-embedded graphene as high-capacity hydrogen-storage media. *Int. J. Hydrog. Energy* **2011**, *36*, 12324–12328. [CrossRef]
147. Sen, D.; Thapa, R.; Chattopadhyay, K.K. Small Pd cluster adsorbed double vacancy defect graphene sheet for hydrogen storage: A first-principles study. *Int. J. Hydrog. Energy* **2013**, *38*, 3041–3049. [CrossRef]
148. Fair, K.M.; Cui, X.Y.; Li, L.; Shieh, C.C.; Zheng, R.K.; Liu, Z.W.; Stampfl, C. Hydrogen adsorption capacity of adatoms on double carbon vacancies of graphene: A trend study from first principles. *Phys. Rev. B* **2013**, *87*, 014102. [CrossRef]
149. Ma, L.; Zhang, J.M.; Xu, K.W.; Ji, V. Hydrogen adsorption and storage of Ca-decorated graphene with topological defects: A first-principles study. *Phys. E Low Dimens. Syst. Nanostruct.* **2014**, *63*, 45–51. [CrossRef]
150. Lotfi, R.; Saboohi, Y. A comparative study on hydrogen interaction with defective graphene structures doped by transition metals. *Phys. E Low Dimens. Syst. Nanostruct.* **2014**, *60*, 104–111. [CrossRef]
151. Zhang, X.; Tang, C.; Jiang, Q. Electric field induced enhancement of hydrogen storage capacity for Li atom decorated graphene with Stone-Wales defects. *Int. J. Hydrog. Energy* **2016**, *41*, 10776–10785. [CrossRef]
152. Mahendran, M.; Rekha, B.; Seenithurai, S.; Kodi Pandyan, R.; Vinodh Kumar, S. Hydrogen storage in Beryllium decorated graphene with double vacancy and porphyrin defect—A first principles study. *Funct. Mater. Lett.* **2017**, *10*, 1750023. [CrossRef]
153. Long, J.; Li, J.; Nan, F.; Yin, S.; Li, J.; Cen, W. Tailoring the thermostability and hydrogen storage capacity of Li decorated carbon materials by heteroatom doping. *Appl. Surf. Sci.* **2018**, *435*, 1065–1071. [CrossRef]
154. Akilan, R.; Vinnarasi, S.; Mohanapriya, S.; Shankar, R. Adsorption of H_2 molecules on B/N-doped defected graphene sheets—A DFT study. *Struct. Chem.* **2020**, *31*, 2413–2434. [CrossRef]
155. Ma, K.; Lv, E.; Zheng, D.; Cui, W.; Dong, S.; Yang, W.; Zhou, Y. A first-principles study on titanium-decorated adsorbent for hydrogen storage. *Energies* **2021**, *14*, 6845. [CrossRef]
156. Singla, M.; Jaggi, N. Synergistic effect of Cu decoration and N doping in divacancy defected graphene nanoribbons on hydrogen gas sensing properties: DFT study. *Mat. Chem. Phys.* **2021**, *273*, 125093. [CrossRef]

Disclaimer/Publisher's Note: The statements, opinions and data contained in all publications are solely those of the individual author(s) and contributor(s) and not of MDPI and/or the editor(s). MDPI and/or the editor(s) disclaim responsibility for any injury to people or property resulting from any ideas, methods, instructions or products referred to in the content.

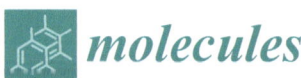

Communication

Waste-Wood-Isolated Cellulose-Based Activated Carbon Paper Electrodes with Graphene Nanoplatelets for Flexible Supercapacitors

Jung Jae Lee [1,†], Su-Hyeong Chae [2,†], Jae Jun Lee [1], Min Sang Lee [1], Wonhyung Yoon [3], Lee Ku Kwac [1], Hong Gun Kim [1] and Hye Kyoung Shin [1,*,†]

[1] Institute of Carbon Technology, Jeonju University, Jeonju 55069, Republic of Korea; darius1028@naver.com (J.J.L.); happyriss@naver.com (J.J.L.); cnfyddl@jj.ac.kr (M.S.L.); kwac29@jj.ac.kr (L.K.K.); hgkim@jj.ac.kr (H.G.K.)
[2] Department of Nano Convergence Engineering, Jeonbuk National University, Jeonju 54896, Republic of Korea; suc_0819@jbnu.ac.kr
[3] Jeonbuk Institute for Regional Program Evaluation, Jeonju 54896, Republic of Korea; yoon126@irpe.or.kr
* Correspondence: jokwanwoo@jj.ac.kr; Fax: +82-63-220-3161
† These authors contributed equally to this work.

Abstract: Waste wood, which has a large amount of cellulose fibers, should be transformed into useful materials for addressing environmental and resource problems. Thus, this study analyzed the application of waste wood as supercapacitor electrode material. First, cellulose fibers were extracted from waste wood and mixed with different contents of graphene nanoplatelets (GnPs) in water. Using a facile filtration method, cellulose papers with GnPs were prepared and converted into carbon papers through carbonization and then to porous activated carbon papers containing GnPs (ACP–GnP) through chemical activation processes. For the morphology of ACP–GnP, activated carbon fibers with abundant pores were formed. The increase in the amount of GnPs attached to the fiber surfaces decreased the number of pores. The Brunauer–Emmett–Teller surface areas and specific capacitance of the ACP–GnP electrodes decreased with an increase in the GnP content. However, the galvanostatic charge–discharge curves of ACPs with higher GnP contents gradually changed into triangular and linear shapes, which are associated with the capacitive performance. For example, ACP with 15 wt% GnP had a low mass transfer resistance and high charge delivery of ions, resulting in the specific capacitance value of 267 Fg^{-1} owing to micropore and mesopore formation during the activation of carbon paper.

Keywords: supercapacitor; waste wood; cellulose fiber; graphene nanoplatelet; activated carbon paper; electrode

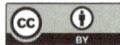

1. Introduction

The continued and enormous energy consumption using fossil fuels has resulted in environmental pollution and resource depletion problems, necessitating the development of energy storage devices [1–6]. Among such devices, supercapacitors storing electrochemical energy changes, have a high power density and long lifecycle, thereby extending the operating time and life of batteries [7–12]. Supercapacitors are primarily composed of two electrodes, electrolytes, and a separation membrane that divides the two electrodes. Electrodes play an important role in supercapacitor charge storage and are categorized as electric double-layer capacitors (EDLCs) and pseudocapacitive supercapacitors based on the electrode materials [13–18]. EDLC electrodes are composed of activated or porous carbon-based materials with large surface areas that allow easy access of electrolyte ions to the electrodes for an increase in charge storage [19,20].

Recently, researchers have investigated agricultural byproducts, such as rice husks [21–24], coconut shells [25–28], or sugarcane bagasse [29–33], as activated carbon precursors in supercapacitor electrodes owing to their renewability, eco-friendliness, and low cost. Agricultural byproducts consist of the composition of cellulose, lignin, hemicellulose, ash, and other substances, which have different characteristic behaviors. Lignin and hemicellulose, which are amorphous structures, function as binders that cling between cellulose fibers. Meanwhile, cellulose, a semi-crystalline linear polymer, is lightweight, renewable, and also has outstanding mechanical properties owing to its high aspect ratio [34–38]. Considering the different characteristics of cellulose, lignin, and hemicellulose, the desired activated carbon materials should be prepared after separating these components. In addition, it is important to separate cellulose fibers as flexible porous materials because they have advantages in producing more flexible paper-shaped electrodes over hemicellulose and lignin-based porous carbon materials as a representative paper-making resource.

For example, Wang et al. [39] studied porous carbon spheres prepared from hemicelluloses discarded during the cellulose fiber extraction process for supercapacitor application. Hemicellulose-based carbon microspheres were prepared via a hydrothermal process and further activated with various activators. Among them, hemicellulose-based activated carbon spheres activated using $ZnCl_2$ showed a specific capacitance of 218 F g^{-1} at 0.2 A g^{-1} in a 6 M KOH solution, but this flexible property has not been reported because they are not paper or mat. Schlee et al. [40] studied microporous carbon fiber mats for freestanding supercapacitors obtained from lignin extracted from eucalyptus. Lignin-based microporous carbon fiber mats exhibited a specific capacitance of 155 F g^{-1} at 0.1 A g^{-1} in a 6 M KOH solution, but this flexible property has not been reported. Kim et al. [24] studied flexible activated carbon paper (ACP)-shaped electrodes with high porosity prepared from cellulose fibers extracted from rice husks. Flexible ACP prepared using only cellulose fibers extracted from rice husks achieved the high specific surface area of 2158.48 m^2 g^{-1} and specific capacitance of 255 F g^{-1} at 1 A g^{-1} in a 1 M KOH solution.

Waste wood comprises a substantial portion of cellulose fibers but has rarely been analyzed as an activated carbon material for supercapacitor electrodes because it contains impurities such as paints, adhesive, and vanishes. Nonetheless, cellulose fibers isolated from waste wood can be converted into useful materials, thereby mitigating the environmental problems caused by waste wood [41–45]. Therefore, activated carbon suitable for a high-capacity supercapacitor electrode from cellulose fibers extracted from waste wood needs to be investigated.

The pore size distribution and electrical conductivity of activated carbon materials are important factors for improving the electrochemical properties of EDLC [46–48]. In this study, cellulose fibers were extracted from waste wood in order to change waste wood into useful materials for addressing environmental and resource problems and mixed with graphene nanoplatelets (GnPs) to enhance the electrical conductivity of the resulting electrode. Subsequently, cellulose papers were prepared with different cellulose fiber and GnP contents via a facile filtration method. These papers were then converted into ACPs through carbonization and chemical activation and, consequently, used as supercapacitor electrode materials. ACPs containing various GnP contents were examined by scanning electron microscopy (SEM), Brunauer–Emmett–Teller (BET) analysis, X-ray diffraction (XRD), and Raman spectral analysis. Moreover, the potential of the results as EDLC materials was analyzed.

2. Results and Discussion

2.1. Morphology of ACP–GnP Samples

Figure 1 shows the SEM images, depicting the morphology of porous ACP containing GnPs. As shown in Figure 1a, the GnP particles are well dispersed and attached to the ACP surfaces, thereby enhancing the electrical conductivity. From the magnified SEM image in Figure 1b, the porous structures of ACP are developed with GnP particles covering and blocking the pores. An increase in the GnP content reduced the porosity of ACP. Nevertheless, the abundant pores on surfaces of the ACP surface can affect the formation of micropores and mesopores to increase the electrochemical capacitance, as shown in Figure 1c.

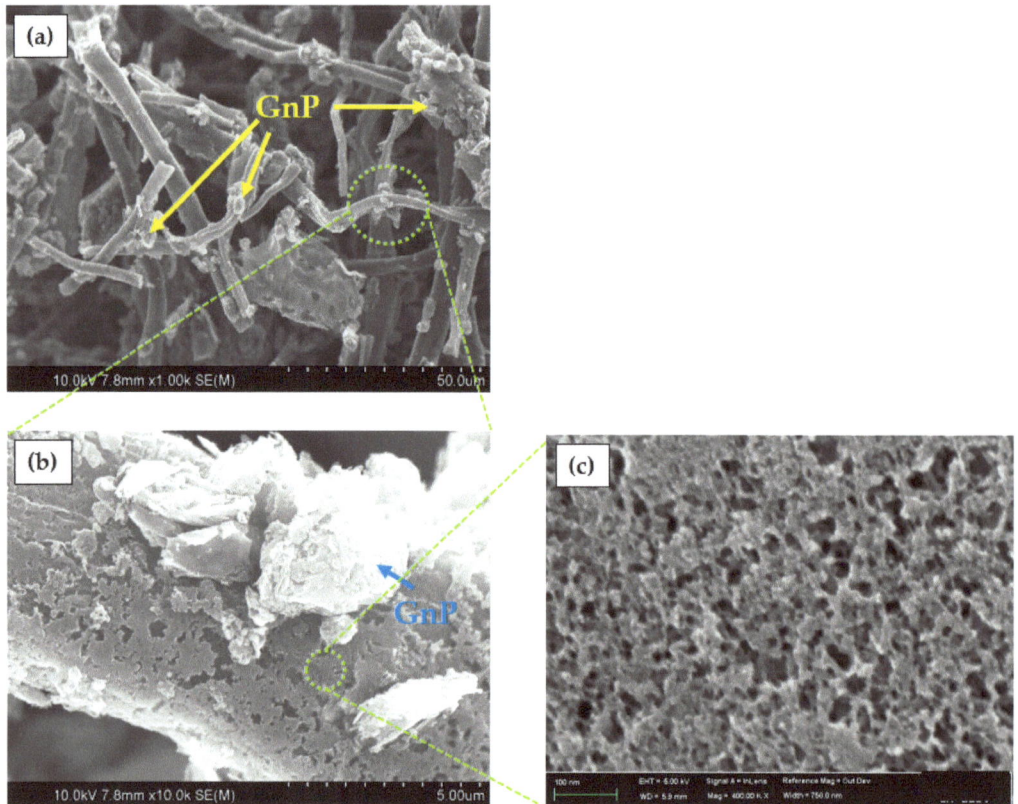

Figure 1. SEM images of ACP–GnP 15 at different magnifications: (**a**) 1000×, (**b**) 10,000×, (**c**) 200,000× ACP–GnP 15.

2.2. Textural Properties of ACP–GnP Samples

Porous ACP was obtained by varying the GnP content using N_2 adsorption–desorption isotherms. As shown in Figure 2, the ACP obtained with different GnP contents comprises a combination of type I and IV isotherms with hysteresis loops according to the BET classification. As shown in Figure 2a, the N_2 adsorption curves at a low relative pressure (p/p_0) of <0.1 for all ACP surfaces drastically increased due to the development of micropores in ACP–GnP. Generally, when p/p_0 approach 0.2, the N_2 in the micropores is completely adsorbed. For $p/p_0 > 0.2$, which is related to the N_2 adsorption in the mesopores and macropores, the volume absorption of N_2 on the ACP–GnP surfaces slowly increased owing to the existence of mesopores. However, the N_2 adsorption curves of the ACP–GnPs decreased as the GnP content increased because the surfaces of the activated carbon cellulose fibers were covered with GnPs, as shown in the SEM images. The BET surface areas of ACP–GnP 0, ACP–GnP 1, ACP–GnP 3, ACP–GnP 5, ACP–GnP 7, and ACP–1100 were 1592.20, 1535.13, 1475.59, 1342.08, 1254. 71, and 921.78 $m^2\ g^{-1}$, respectively.

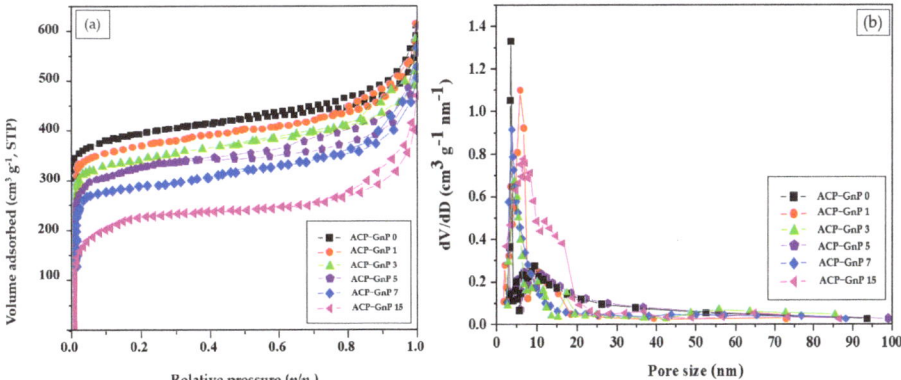

Figure 2. ACP N_2 adsorption and microporosity. (**a**) Experimentally measured adsorption−desorption isotherms and (**b**) computed micropore size distributions.

Figure 2b shows the micropore, mesopore, and macropore distributions for all ACP−GnP samples, which were identified using the Horvath−Kawazoe and Barrett−Joyner−Halenda methods. According to pore size classification (IUPAC), the pores were divided with micropores (diameter, D < 2 nm), mesopores (2 nm ≤ D < 50 nm), and macropores (D > 50 nm). The ACP−GnP samples mostly comprise micropores and mesopores in the size range of 0–40 nm, resulting in a hierarchical pore structure. A specific surface part of ACP is increased to increase the storage capacity of the supercapacitor electrodes. Therefore, pore structures with micropores and mesopores significantly influence the electrical performance. In particular, micropores increase the high surface area, thereby increasing the storage capacity through the formation of electric double layers. Moreover, these allow easy ion transfer pathways. Therefore, the development of microporous and mesoporous structures in ACP−GnP samples plays an important role in enhancing their electrochemical capacity as energy storage materials.

2.3. Crystallinity of ACP−GnP Samples

The XRD patterns of the ACP−GnP samples are shown in Figure 3a, where two representative diffraction peaks appeared at 2θ of approximately 24°–26° corresponding to the (002) of all the ACP−GnP samples, respectively. These peaks are related to the crystalline structures of the carbon materials. In particular, the broad peaks at 2θ = 24–26° are associated with ACP, and the strong and sharp peaks at 26° are related to GnP. All ACPs showed similar full-width at half maximum values and intensities because all waste wood cellulose papers were treated at the same activation and carbonization temperature. Meanwhile, the peak intensities at 2θ of 26° for the GnPs with high crystallinity sharply increased with the increasing GnP content [49,50]. In the Raman spectra in Figure 3b, this characteristic is observed in the two characteristic peaks at 1351 cm^{-1} of the D band, which is related to the disordered or defective graphite structure, and 1610 cm^{-1} of the G band, which is associated with the ordered layered graphite structure. As shown in Figure 3b, the G band intensities increased with the increasing GnP content. The ratio for the intensities of the D and G band (I_G/I_D) were applied to determine the degree of graphitization [51,52]. The I_G/I_D values are 0.97, 1.04, 1.10, 1.15, 1.18, 1.33, and 1.59 for ACP−GnP 0, ACP−GnP 1, ACP−GnP 3, ACP−GnP 5, ACP−GnP 7, and ACP−GnP 15, respectively. An increase in the GnP content increased the degree of crystallinity in ACP, thereby improving the good electrical conductivity and electrochemical performance between the ACP−GnP and electrolyte [53,54].

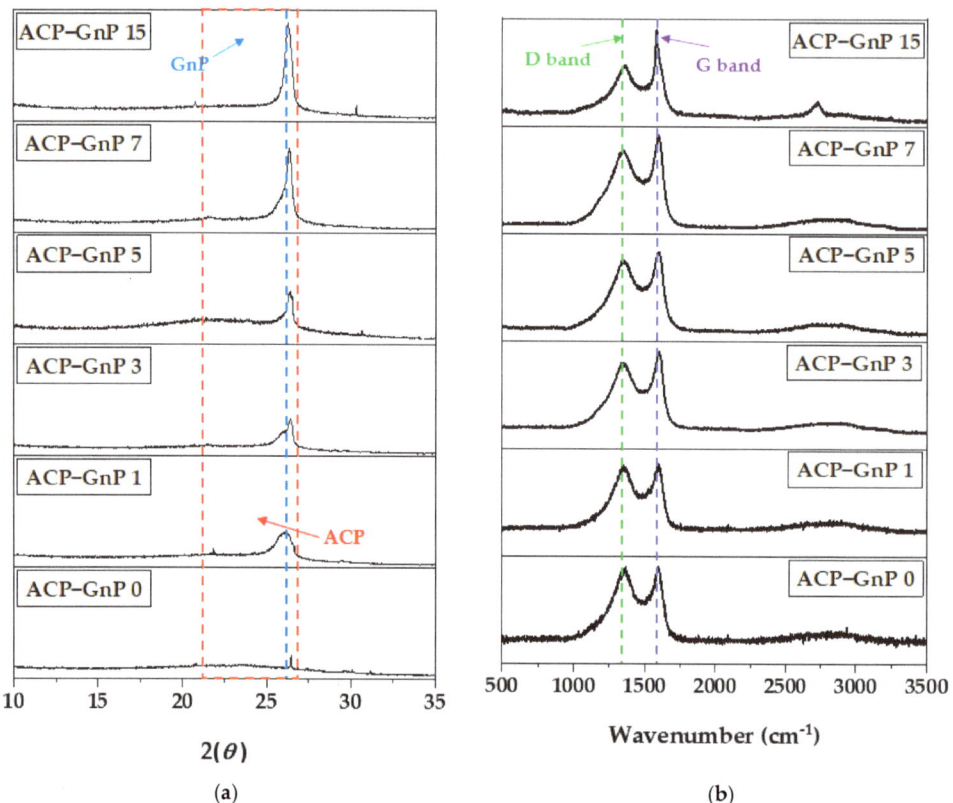

Figure 3. Crystal structure characterization of the ACP–GnP samples. (**a**) XRD patterns and (**b**) Raman spectra.

2.4. Electrochemical Performance of ACPs

The electrochemical performances of the ACPs with various GnP contents as electrodes were evaluated in a three-electrode system using 1 M KOH as the electrolyte. The measurements were conducted within the potential range of −1 V to 0 V at a potential scan rate of 100 mVs^{-1}. The cyclic voltammetry (CV) curves of the ACPs with different GnP contents are shown in Figure 4a. All the curves of the ACPs with different GnP contents showed rice seed-like shapes [55]. As the GnP content increased, the current peaks of the ACPs were increased (in the order of ACP–GnP 15 > ACP–GnP 7 > ACP–GnP 5 > ACP–GnP 3 > ACP–GnP 1 > ACP–GnP 0) owing to the good electrical conductivity of the GnPs. However, the specific capacitance of the ACPs decreased with the increase in the GnP content, as shown in Figure 4b, presenting the galvanostatic charge–discharge (GCD) measurements at a current density of 1 A g^{-1} for the ACP electrodes with different GnP contents. Along with the energy storage performance, the specific capacitance resulted in the GnPs attaching to the fibers and blocking the pores of ACPs. However, the GCD curves of the ACPs with high GnP contents changed into triangular and linear forms with respect to the capacitive performance. The symmetrical and triangular GCD curves demonstrate advisable capacitive conduction and great reversibility, indicating low mass transfer resistance and high charge delivery of ions in the porous ACP–GnP samples. The specific capacitances of the ACP electrodes with various GnP content were obtained using the formula:

$$Cs = \frac{I \triangle t}{m \triangle V}, \qquad (1)$$

where I is the discharge current, Δt is the discharge time, m is the mass of the ACP-GnP electrode, and ΔV is the potential window [24]. At 1 A g^{-1} in 1 M KOH solution, the specific capacitance values of the ACP−GnP 0, ACP−GnP 1, ACP−GnP 3, ACP−GnP 5, ACP−GnP 7, and ACP−GnP 15 electrodes were approximately 425, 411, 398, 3857, 370, and 267 Fg^{-1}.

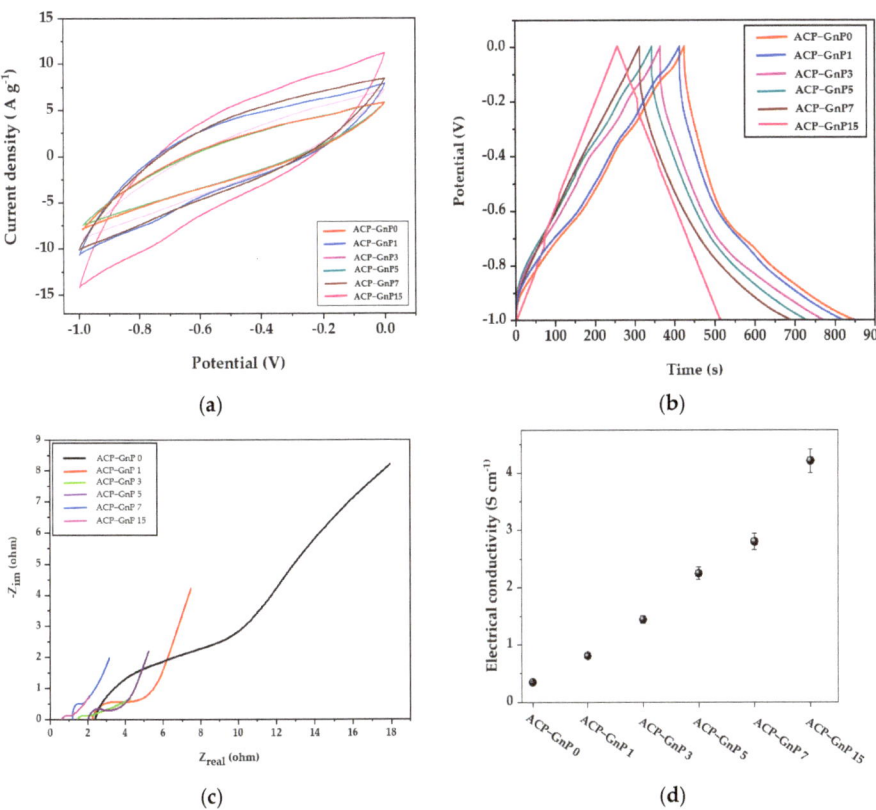

Figure 4. (a) Cyclic voltammograms at a scan rate of 100 mVs^{-1}, (b) GCD profiles at a current density of 1 A g^{-1}, (c) Nyquist plots t in 1 mol L^{-1} KOH, and (d) the electrical conductivities of the ACP electrodes containing various GnP contents.

Figure 4c presented the Nyquist impedance spectrum of the ACP−GnP samples in the frequency range of 0.01–100 kHz. The plots are composed of semicircles in the high-frequency range and slopes in the low-frequency range. The semicircles are related to the resistance of the electrolyte (Rs) and charge-transfer resistance (R$_{ct}$) between the ACP−GnP electrode surfaces and electrolyte. The slopes are attributed to the ion-diffusion resistance in the electrolyte. As shown in Figure 4c,d, as the electrical conductivities increased with an increase in the GnP content, the Rs values of ACP−GnP 0, ACP−GnP 1, ACP−GnP 3, ACP−GnP 5, ACP−GnP 7, and ACP−GnP 15 electrodes decreased as 2.41, 2.24, 1.98, 1.45, 1.21, and 0.62 Ω, respectively. The semicircles shrank, and the slopes increased against the X-axis, resulting in the faster charge transfer of the electrolyte ions into the porous ACP-GnP electrode. Although the increase in the GnP content decreased the specific capacitance of the electrode samples, the GnP content increased the number of the good ion-diffusion pathways and displayed symmetrical and triangular GCD curves. However, the ACP electrode sample with the highest GnP content (15 wt%) displayed a high specific capacitance of 267 Fg^{-1} owing to the development of micropores and mesopores during the activation of carbon paper.

3. Materials and Methods

3.1. Materials

Plywood was sourced from a waste wood treatment plant situated at Jeonju University (Jeonju-si, Republic of Korea). GnP was sourced from Nanografi Nano Technology (Çankaya, Turkey). All chemicals were of analytical grade and used as received.

3.2. Preparation of the Activated Carbon Paper Containing Varying GnP Content

Waste wood chips (5 × 5 cm^2) were alkali-cooked in 15 wt% sodium hydroxide solution for 5 h at 121 °C using an autoclave. After washing using distilled water, alkali-cooked waste woods were first bleached in 2 wt% sodium chlorite and 3 wt% acetic acid solution at 70 °C for 90 min and then bleached a second time in 1.2 wt% sodium hypochlorite solution at room temperature for 60 min. The bleached pulps obtained from a two-step bleaching process were used as cellulose fibers. Waste wood cellulose fibers and GnPs were mixed in water according to the weight percentage. Subsequently, 1 wt% polyacrylamide solution was added as a binder, followed by sonication for 1 h to disperse the GnPs. The papers were prepared by a facile filtration method of the waste wood cellulose fibers and GnP solution with specific weight percentages. The obtained papers were carbonized at 900 °C under a pure N$_2$ (99.999%) atmosphere. The carbon papers were immersed in NiCl$_2$ solution (15 wt%) for 1 h and dried at 80 °C to prepare porous ACPs. High-thermal treatment for activation was carried out at 1000 °C under N$_2$ atmosphere. After the activation, all papers were washed with H$_2$SO$_4$ (0.1 M) to eliminate surplus NiCl$_2$ and neutralized with distilled water. Subsequently, the samples were dried at 80 °C. The ACPs containing the various GnP contents were labeled ACP–GnP 0, ACP–GnP 1, ACP–GnP 3, ACP–GnP 5, ACP–GnP 7, and ACP–GnP 15 according to their GnP content in wt%. Figure 5 displays the schematic of the preparation of ACP-GnP samples from waste wood.

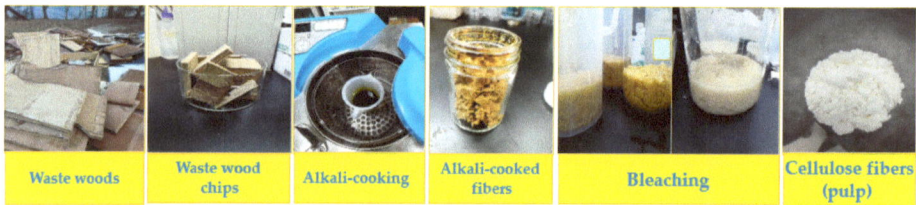

Extraction process of cellulose fibers from waste woods

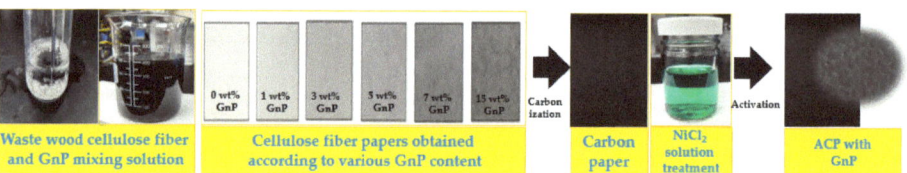

Preparation process of ACP with GnP

Figure 5. Schematic and photographs of the preparation of ACP with GnP.

3.3. Characterization

The morphologies of the ACP-GnP samples were observed by SEM (Hitachi SU-70, Tokyo, Japan). The specific area was evaluated using BET analysis, and the total pore volume was determined from the N_2 adsorption data at p/p_0 of 0.99. Nonlocal density functional theory (NLDFT) was used to estimate the pore size distributions. The crystallinity of the ACP–-GnP samples was estimated by XRD (Rigaku, D/MAX-2500 instrument, Tokyo, Japan), with CuKα radiation at 40 kV and 30 mA, and Raman spectra (Aramis, Horiba Jobin Yvon, Tokyo, Japan) analysis.

3.4. Electrochemical Measurements

CV and GCD measurements of the electrochemical performance of the ACP–GnP electrodes were carried out using a CHI 660E electrochemical workstation (CH Instruments, Inc., Beijing, China). A three-electrode system with a 1 M KOH solution as the electrolyte, ACP-GnP as the electrode, an Ag/AgCl electrode as the reference electrode, and a Pt electrode as the counter electrode was used. The CV curves were obtained in the potential range of −1 to 0 V with the potential scan rates at −100 mV s^{-1} and step size 0.5 mV. GCD tests were conducted with the step-wise increase in the current density by at 1 A g^{-1} in the voltage range of −1 to 0 V vs. Ag/AgCl. Electrochemical impedance spectroscopy was performed in the frequency range of 100 kHz to 0.01 Hz to study the R_s, R_{ct}, and ion-diffusion resistance in the electrolyte.

4. Conclusions

This study demonstrated the conversion of cellulose fibers extracted from waste wood into useful materials. The obtained cellulose fibers were mixed with different GnP contents in water, and the cellulose papers with different GnPs content were obtained by a facile filtration method. Subsequently, porous ACP–GnP samples for application as supercapacitor electrode materials were realized by carbonization and chemical activation. The activated carbon fibers exhibited the formation of abundant pores. An increase in the GnP content attached to the fiber surfaces decreased the number of pores. The BET surface areas and specific capacitance of ACP–GnP electrodes decreased with an increase in the GnP content. However, the GCD curves of ACPs with higher GnP contents gradually changed into triangular and linear shapes, which were associated with their capacitive performance. For example, the GCD curves of ACP–GnP 15 were approximately symmetrical and triangular line, indicating its low mass transfer resistance and high charge delivery. As such, a high specific capacitance of 267 Fg^{-1} was achieved owing to the micropores and mesopores formed during the activation of carbon paper.

Therefore, this work highlighted the use of waste wood as an active carbon source for electrode materials, thereby contributing to addressing resource and environmental problems.

Author Contributions: Conceptualization, H.K.S.; methodology, H.K.S., J.J.L. (Jung Jae Lee) and S.-H.C.; validation, H.K.S., J.J.L. (Jung Jae Lee) and S.-H.C.; formal analysis, H.K.S., J.J.L. (Jung Jae Lee), J.J.L. (Jae Jun Lee) M.S.L., W.Y., L.K.K. and H.G.K.; investigation, H.K.S., J.J.L. (Jung Jae Lee), S.-H.C., J.J.L. (Jae Jun Lee), M.S.L., W.Y., L.K.K. and H.G.K.; resources, H.K.S., J.J.L. (Jae Jun Lee), M.S.L., W.Y., L.K.K. and H.G.K.; data curation, H.K.S., J.J.L. (Jae Jun Lee), S.-H.C., J.J.L. (Jae Jun Lee) and M.S.L.; investigation, H.K.S., J.J.L. (Jae Jun Lee) and S.-H.C.; writing—original draft preparation, H.K.S.; writing—review and editing, H.K.S.; visualization, H.K.S., J.J.L. (Jae Jun Lee) and S.-H.C.; supervision, H.K.S. and H.G.K.; project administration, H.K.S. and H.G.K. All authors have read and agreed to the published version of the manuscript.

Funding: This research was supported by the National Research Council of Science & Technology (NST) grant by the Korea government (MSIT) (No. CPS23091-100), and this research was also supported by the Basic Science Research Program through the National Research Foundation of Korea (NRF) funded by the Ministry of Education (No. 2016R1A6A1A03012069).

Institutional Review Board Statement: Not applicable.

Informed Consent Statement: Not applicable.

Data Availability Statement: Data are contained within the article.

Conflicts of Interest: The authors declare no conflict of interest.

References

1. Deng, J.; Li, M.; Wang, Y. Biomass-derived carbon: Synthesis and applications in energy storage and conversion. *Green Chem.* **2016**, *18*, 4824–4854. [CrossRef]
2. Guo, N.; Li, M.; Sun, X.; Wang, F.; Yang, R. Enzymatic hydrolysis lignin derived hierarchical porous carbon for supercapacitors in ionic liquids with high power and energy densities. *Green Chem.* **2017**, *19*, 2595–2602. [CrossRef]
3. Subramanian, V.; Luo, C.; Stephan, A.M.; Nahm, K.; Thomas, S.; Wei, B. Supercapacitors from activated carbon derived from banana fibers. *J. Phys. Chem. C* **2007**, *111*, 7527–7531. [CrossRef]
4. Peng, S.; Li, L.; Lee, J.K.Y.; Tian, L.; Srinivasan, M.; Adams, S.; Ramakrishna, S. Electrospun carbon nanofibers and their hybrid composites as advanced materials for energy conversion and storage. *Nano Energy* **2016**, *22*, 361–395. [CrossRef]
5. Li, J.; Wang, C.; Zheng, P. Solvothermal preparation of micro/nanostructured TiO_2 with enhanced lithium storage capability. *Mater. Chem. Phys.* **2017**, *190*, 202–208. [CrossRef]
6. Patsidis, A.C.; Kalaitzidou, K.; Psarras, G.C. Dielectric response, functionality and energy storage in epoxy nanocomposites: Barium titanate vs exfoliated graphite nanoplatelets. *Mater. Chem. Phys.* **2012**, *135*, 798–805. [CrossRef]
7. Miller, J.R.; Simon, P. Materials science: Electrochemical capacitors for energy management. *Science* **2008**, *321*, 651–652. [CrossRef]
8. Duy, L.T.; Seo, H. Construction of stretchable supercapacitors using graphene hybrid hydrogels and corrosion-resistant silver nanowire current collectors. *Appl. Surf. Sci.* **2020**, *521*, 146–467. [CrossRef]
9. Dang, F.; Zhao, W.; Tong, W.; Yang, P.; Wang, W.; Liu, Y. Extrinsic design of high-performance programmable supercapacitor with large specific areal capacitance. *Electrochim. Acta* **2023**, *463*, 142845. [CrossRef]
10. Li, G.; Ji, Y.; Zuo, D.; Xu, J.; Zhang, H. Carbon electrodes with double conductive networks for high-performance electrical double-layer capacitors. *Adv. Compos. Hybrid Mater.* **2019**, *2*, 456–461. [CrossRef]
11. Kumar, S.; Saeed, G.; Kim, N.H.; Lee, J.H. Fabrication of Co-Ni-Zn ternary Oxide@NiWO4 core-shell nanowire arrays and Fe2O3-CNTs@GF for ultra-high-performance asymmetric supercapacitor. *Compos. Part B-Eng.* **2019**, *176*, 107223. [CrossRef]
12. Huang, P.; Lethien, C.; Pinaudm, S.; Brousse, K.; Laloo, R.; Turq, V.; Respaud, M.; Demortière, A.; Daffos, B.; Taberna, P.L.; et al. On-chip and freestanding elastic carbon films for micro-supercapacitors. *Science* **2016**, *351*, 691–695. [CrossRef]
13. Chodankar, N.R.; Bagal, I.V.; Ryu, S.W.; Kim, D.H. Hybrid material passivation approach to stabilize the silicon nanowires in aqueous electrolyte for high-energy efficient supercapacitor. *Chem. Eng. J.* **2019**, *362*, 609–618. [CrossRef]
14. Ke, Q.Q.; Guan, C.; Zhang, X.; Zheng, M.R.; Zhang, Y.W.; Cai, Y.Q.; Zhang, H.; Wang, J. Surface-charge-mediated formation of H-TiO2@Ni(OH)2 heterostructures for high performance supercapacitors. *Adv. Mater.* **2017**, *29*, 1604164. [CrossRef]
15. Rodríguez-Rego, J.M.; Carrasco-Amador, J.P.; Mendoza-Cerezo, L.; Marcos-Romero, A.C.; Macías-García, A. Guide for the development and evaluation of supercapacitors with the proposal of novel design to improve their performance. *J. Energy Storage* **2023**, *68*, 107816. [CrossRef]
16. Wang, H.; Feng, H.; Li, J. Graphene and graphene-like layered transition metal review. *Polym. Eng. Sci.* **2022**, *62*, 269–303. [CrossRef]
17. Gao, B.; Li, X.; Ding, K.; Huang, C.; Li, Q.; Chu, P.; Huo, K. Recent progress in nanostructured transition metal nitrides for advanced electrochemical energy storage. *J. Mater. Chem. A* **2019**, *7*, 14–37. [CrossRef]
18. Asghar, A.; Rashid, M.S.; Hussain, S.; Shad, N.A.; Hamza, M.; Chen, Z. Facile hydrothermal synthesis of MoS_2 nano-worms-based aggregate as electrode material for high energy density asymmetric supercapacitor. *Electrochim. Acta* **2023**, *465*, 143011. [CrossRef]
19. Arkhipova, E.A.; Ivanov, A.S.; Maslakov, K.I.; Savilov, S.V. Nitrogen-doped mesoporous graphene nanoflakes for high performance ionic liquid supercapacitors. *Electrochim. Acta* **2020**, *353*, 136463. [CrossRef]
20. Sun, L.; Wang, L.; Tian, C.; Tan, T.; Xie, Y.; Shi, K.; Li, M.; Fu, H. Nitrogen-doped graphene with high nitrogen level via a one-step hydrothermal reaction of graphene oxide with urea for superior capacitive energy storage. *RSC Adv.* **2012**, *2*, 4498–4506. [CrossRef]
21. Arkhipova, E.A.; Novotortsev, R.Y.; Ivanov, A.S.; Maslakov, K.I.; Savilov, S.V. Rice husk-derived activated carbon electrode in redox-active electrolyte—New approach for enhancing supercapacitor performance. *J. Energy Storage* **2022**, *55*, 105699. [CrossRef]
22. Zhang, S.; Zhang, Q.; Zhu, S.; Zhang, H.; Liu, X. Porous carbons derived from desilication treatment and mixed alkali activation of rice husk char for supercapacitors. *Energy Sources A* **2021**, *43*, 282–290. [CrossRef]
23. Chen, J.; Liu, J.; Wu, D.; Bai, X.; Lin, Y.; Wu, T.; Zhang, C.; Chen, D.; Li, H. Improving the supercapcitor performance of activated carbon materials derived from pretreated rice husk. *J. Energy Storage* **2021**, *44*, 103432. [CrossRef]
24. Kim, H.G.; Kim, Y.S.; Kwac, L.K.; Shin, H.K. Characterization of activated carbon paper electrodes prepared by rice husk-isolated cellulose fibers for supercapacitor applications. *Molecules* **2020**, *25*, 3951. [CrossRef] [PubMed]
25. Omokafe, S.M.; Adeniyi, A.A.; Igbafen, E.O.; Oke, S.R.; Olubambi, P.A. Fabrication of activated carbon from coconut shells and its electrochemical properties for supercapacitors. *Int. J. Electrochem. Sci.* **2020**, *15*, 10854–10865. [CrossRef]
26. Jain, A.; Tripathi, S.K. Fabrication and characterization of energy storing supercapacitor devices using coconut shell based activated charcoal electrode. *Mater. Sci. Eng B* **2014**, *183*, 54–60. [CrossRef]

27. Deng, M.; Wang, J.; Zhang, Q. Effect of freezing pretreatment on the performance of activated carbon from coconut shell for supercapacitor application. *Mater. Lett.* **2022**, *306*, 130934. [CrossRef]
28. Medagedara, A.D.T.; Waduge, N.M.; Bandara, T.M.W.J.; Wimalasena, I.G.K.J.; Dissanayake, M.; Tennakone, K.; Rajapakse, R.M.G.; Rupasinghe, C.P.; Kumara, G.R.A. Triethylammonium thiocyanate ionic liquid electrolyte-based supercapacitor fabricated using coconut shell-derived electronically conducting activated charcoal electrode material. *J. Energy Storage* **2022**, *55*, 105628. [CrossRef]
29. Chou, T.C.; Huang, C.; Doong, R. Fabrication of hierarchically ordered porous carbons using sugarcane bagasse as the scaffold for supercapacitor applications. *Synth. Met.* **2014**, *194*, 29–37. [CrossRef]
30. Sarkar, S.; Arya, A.; Gaur, U.K.; Gaur, A. Investigations on porous carbon derived from sugarcane bagasse as an electrode material for supercapacitors. *Biomass Bioenergy* **2020**, *142*, 105730. [CrossRef]
31. Wang, X.; Cao, L.; Lewis, R.; Hreid, T.; Zhang, Z.; Wang, H. Biorefining of sugarcane bagasse to fermentable sugars and surface oxygen group-rich hierarchical porous carbon for supercapacitors. *Renew. Energy* **2020**, *162*, 2306–2317. [CrossRef]
32. Du, B.; Chai, L.; Zhu, H.; Cheng, F.; Wang, X.; Chen, X.; Zhou, J.; Sun, R.C. Effective fractionation strategy of sugarcane bagasse lignin to fabricate quality lignin-based carbon nanofibers supercapacitors. *Inter. J. Biol. Macromol.* **2021**, *184*, 604–6017. [CrossRef] [PubMed]
33. Okonkwo, C.A.; Menkiti, M.C.; Obiora-Okafo, I.A.; Ezenewa, O.N. Controlled pyrolysis of sugarcane bagasse enhanced mesoporous carbon for improving capacitance of supercapacitor electrode. *Biomass Bioenergy* **2021**, *146*, 105996. [CrossRef]
34. Shin, H.K.; Jeun, J.P.; Kim, H.B.; Kang, P.H. Isolation of cellulose fibers from kenaf using electron beam. *Radiat. Phys. Chem.* **2012**, *81*, 936–940. [CrossRef]
35. Yang, H.; Yan, R.; Chen, H.; Lee, D.H.; Zheng, C. Characteristics of hemicellulose, cellulose and lignin pyrolysis. *Fuel* **2007**, *86*, 1781–1788. [CrossRef]
36. Kim, H.G.; Lee, U.S.; Kwac, L.K.; Lee, S.O.; Kim, Y.S.; Shin, H.K. Electron beam irradiation isolates cellulose nanofiber from Korea "Tall Goldenrod" invasive alien plant. *Nanomaterials* **2019**, *9*, 1358. [CrossRef] [PubMed]
37. Bledzki, A.K.; Gassan, J. Composites reinforced with cellulose based fiber. *Prog. Polym. Sci.* **1999**, *24*, 221–274. [CrossRef]
38. Ng, H.M.; Sin, L.T.; Tee, T.T.; Bee, S.T.; Hue, D.; Low, C.Y.; Rahmat, A.R. Extraction of cellulose nanocrystals from plant sources for application as reinforcing agent in polymers. *Compos. Part B* **2015**, *75*, 176–200. [CrossRef]
39. Wang, Y.; Lu, C.; Cao, X.; Wang, Q.; Yang, G.; Chen, J. Porous carbon spheres derived from hemicelluloses for supercapacitor application. *Inter. J. Mol. Sci.* **2022**, *23*, 7101. [CrossRef]
40. Schlee, P.; Hosseinaei, O.; Baker, D.; Landmér, A.; Tomani, P.; Mostazo-López, M.J.; Caxorla-Amorós, D.; Herou, S. From waste to wealth: From kraft lignin to free-standing supercapacitors. *Carbon* **2019**, *145*, 470–480. [CrossRef]
41. Hossain, M.U.; Wang, L.; Iris, K.M.; Tsang, D.S.; Poon, C.S. Environmental and technical feasibility study of upcycling wood waste into cement-bonded particle board. *Constr. Build. Master.* **2018**, *173*, 474–480. [CrossRef]
42. Mancini, M.; Rinnan, Å. Near infrared technique as a tool for the rapid assessment of waste wood quality for energy applications. *Renew. Energy* **2021**, *177*, 113–123. [CrossRef]
43. Tsai, W.-T.; Wu, P.-H. Environmental concerns about carcinogenic air toxics produced from waste woods as alternative energy sources. *Energy Sources A Recover. Util. Environ. Eff.* **2013**, *35*, 725–732. [CrossRef]
44. Humar, M.; Jermer, J.; Peek, R. Regulations in the European Union with emphasis on Germany, Sweden and Slovenia. *Environ. Impacts Treat. Wood* **2006**, *6495*, 37–57. [CrossRef]
45. Ince, C.; Tayançlı, S. Recycling waste wood in cement mortars towards the regeneration of sustainable environment. *Constr. Build. Mater.* **2021**, *299*, 123891. [CrossRef]
46. Zolin, L.; Nair, J.R.; Beneventi, D.; Bella, F.; Destro, M.; Jagdale, P.; Cannavaro, I.; Tagliaferro, A.; Haussy, D.; Geobaldo, F.; et al. A simple route toward next- gen green energy storage concept by nanofibres-based self-supporting electrodes and a solid polymeric design. *Carbon* **2016**, *107*, 811–822. [CrossRef]
47. Reina, M.; Scalia, A.; Auxilia, G.; Fontana, M.; Bella, F.; Ferrero, S.; Lamberti, A. Boosting electric double layer capacitance in laser-induced graphene-based supercapacitors. *Adv. Sustain. Syst.* **2022**, *6*, 100228. [CrossRef]
48. Zhai, Z.; Zhang, L.; Du, T.; Ren, B.; Xu, Y.; Wang, S.; Miao, J.; Liu, Z. A review of carbon materials for supercapacitors. *Mater. Des.* **2022**, *221*, 111017. [CrossRef]
49. Ahmed, J.; Bher, A.; Auras, R.; Al-Zuwayed, S.A.; Joseph, A.; Mulla, M.F.; Alazemi, A. Morphological, thermo-mechanical, and barrier properties of coextruded multilayer polylactide composite films reinforced with graphene nanoplatelets and encapsulated thyme essential oil. *Food Packag. Shelf Life* **2023**, *40*, 101179. [CrossRef]
50. Cheng, S.; Guo, X.; Tan, P.; Lin, M.; Cai, J.; Zhou, Y.; Zhao, D.; Cai, W.; Zhang, Y.; Zhang, X. Aligning graphene nanoplates coplanar in polyvinyl alcohol by using a rotating magnetic field to fabricate thermal interface materials with high through-plane thermal conductivity. *Compos. Part B* **2023**, *264*, 110916. [CrossRef]
51. Sesuk, T.; Tammawat, P.; Jivaganont, P.; Somton, K.; Limthongkul, P.; Kobsiriphat, W. Activated carbon derived from coconut coir pitch as high performance supercapacitor electrode material. *J. Energy Storage* **2019**, *25*, 100910. [CrossRef]
52. Mo, R.J.; Zhao, Y.; Zhao, M.M.; Wu, M.; Wang, C.; Li, J.P.; Kuga, S.; Huang, Y. Graphene-like porous carbon from sheet cellulose as electrodes for supercapacitors. *Chem. Eng. J.* **2018**, *346*, 104–112. [CrossRef]
53. Alcaraz, L.; Fernández, A.L.; Garcíai-Díaz, I.; López, F.A. Preparation and characterization of activated carbons from winemaking wastes and their adsorption of methylene blue. *Adsorpt. Sci. Technol.* **2018**, *36*, 1331–1351. [CrossRef]

54. Darabut, A.M.; Lobko, Y.; Yakovlev, Y.; Rodríguez, M.G.; Veltruská, K.; Šmíd, B.; Kúš, P.; Nováková, J.; Dopita, M.; Vorokhta, M.; et al. Influence of thermal treatment on the structure and electrical conductivity of thermally expanded graphite. *Adv. Powder Technol.* **2022**, *33*, 103884. [CrossRef]
55. Aziz, S.B.; Abdulwahid, R.T.; Sadiq, N.M.; Abdullah, R.M.; Tahir, D.A.; Jameel, D.A.; Hamad, S.M.; Abdullah, O.G. Design of biodegradable polymer blend electrolytes with decoupled ion motion for EDLC device application: Electrical and electrochemical properties. *Results Phys.* **2023**, *51*, 106692. [CrossRef]

Disclaimer/Publisher's Note: The statements, opinions and data contained in all publications are solely those of the individual author(s) and contributor(s) and not of MDPI and/or the editor(s). MDPI and/or the editor(s) disclaim responsibility for any injury to people or property resulting from any ideas, methods, instructions or products referred to in the content.

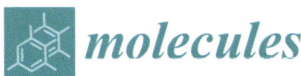

Article

Characterization of Conductive Carbon Nanotubes/Polymer Composites for Stretchable Sensors and Transducers

Laura Fazi [1,2,*], Carla Andreani [1,3], Cadia D'Ottavi [2], Leonardo Duranti [2], Pietro Morales [4], Enrico Preziosi [1,3], Anna Prioriello [2], Giovanni Romanelli [1,3], Valerio Scacco [3], Roberto Senesi [1,3] and Silvia Licoccia [1,2]

1. NAST Centre, University of Rome Tor Vergata, 00133 Rome, Italy
2. Department of Chemical Science and Technologies, University of Rome Tor Vergata, 00133 Rome, Italy
3. Department of Physics, University of Rome Tor Vergata, 00133 Rome, Italy
4. School of Neutron Spectroscopy SONS, University of Rome Tor Vergata, 00133 Rome, Italy
* Correspondence: laura.fazi@uniroma2.it

Abstract: The increasing interest in stretchable conductive composite materials, that can be versatile and suitable for wide-ranging application, has sparked a growing demand for studies of scalable fabrication techniques and specifically tailored geometries. Thanks to the combination of the conductivity and robustness of carbon nanotube (CNT) materials with the viscoelastic properties of polymer films, in particular their stretchability, "surface composites" made of a CNT on polymeric films are a promising way to obtain a low-cost, conductive, elastic, moldable, and patternable material. The use of polymers selected for specific applications, however, requires targeted studies to deeply understand the interface interactions between a CNT and the surface of such polymer films, and in particular the stability and durability of a CNT grafting onto the polymer itself. Here, we present an investigation of the interface properties for a selected group of polymer film substrates with different viscoelastic properties by means of a series of different and complementary experimental techniques. Specifically, we studied the interaction of a single-wall carbon nanotube (SWCNT) deposited on two couples of different polymeric substrates, each one chosen as representative of thermoplastic polymers (i.e., low-density polyethylene (LDPE) and polypropylene (PP)) and thermosetting elastomers (i.e., polyisoprene (PI) and polydimethylsiloxane (PDMS)), respectively. Our results demonstrate that the characteristics of the interface significantly differ for the two classes of polymers with a deeper penetration (up to about 100 μm) into the polymer bulk for the thermosetting substrates. Consequently, the resistance per unit length varies in different ranges, from 1–10 kΩ/cm for typical thermoplastic composite devices (30 μm thick and 2 mm wide) to 0.5–3 MΩ/cm for typical thermosetting elastomer devices (150 μm thick and 2 mm wide). For these reasons, the composites show the different mechanical and electrical responses, therefore suggesting different areas of application of the devices based on such materials.

Keywords: carbon nanotubes; polymer composites; self-assembly; stretchable sensors; stretchable conductors

Citation: Fazi, L.; Andreani, C.; D'Ottavi, C.; Duranti, L.; Morales, P.; Preziosi, E.; Prioriello, A.; Romanelli, G.; Scacco, V.; Senesi, R.; Licoccia, S. Characterization of Conductive Carbon Nanotubes/Polymer Composites for Stretchable Sensors and Transducers. *Molecules* 2023, 28, 1764. https://doi.org/10.3390/molecules28041764

Academic Editors: Luca Tortora and Gianlorenzo Bussetti

Received: 13 December 2022
Revised: 30 January 2023
Accepted: 7 February 2023
Published: 13 February 2023

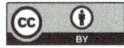

Copyright: © 2023 by the authors. Licensee MDPI, Basel, Switzerland. This article is an open access article distributed under the terms and conditions of the Creative Commons Attribution (CC BY) license (https://creativecommons.org/licenses/by/4.0/).

1. Introduction

The recent advances in the development of composite materials aim at achieving stretchable and flexible materials endowed with tunable electrical properties [1–9]. The development of electromechanical sensors based on such materials, through simple and low-cost procedures, is paramount to optimize manufacturing processes. The process of upgrading to the large-scale production of electromechanical sensors implies in particular the possibility of a wide-ranging extension to biomedical application, aiming at the easy and constant monitoring of patients, and consequently at the improvement in their quality of life. Electrical conductivity varies with the concentration of the conductive component, and it has been reported that it can be made more or less dependent on the strain to fabricate strain sensors with different sensitivities [7,10,11]. Many computational and experimental techniques have been used to study these composites, ranging from numerical simulations to several experimental techniques, the most widely used being scanning electron microscopy (SEM) [12–14] for a surface analysis and confocal Raman microscopy measurements [15–18] for a bulk analysis. The fabrication procedures and subsequent processing have also been reported to significantly affect the composite electromechanical properties [19]. We have previously developed single-wall carbon nanotube (SWCNT, also indicated simply as CNT in the following) polyethylene composite films, combining the thermoplastic properties of the polymer and the conductive and elastic properties of the SWCNT bundles. We have obtained arrays of submillimetric conductive tracks on polyethylene films that have been stretched, shaped, and implanted on the brain cortex of laboratory rats, allowing, for the first time, to successfully probe their electro-corticographic signals for several months [19–21].

In the present work, we have extended the previous study analyzing, by additional techniques, the SWCNT interface with two thermoplastic polymers (low-density polyethylene (LDPE) and polypropylene (PP)) and two thermosetting elastomers (polyisoprene (PI) and polydimethylsiloxane (PDMS)) to gain a deeper understanding of the characteristics of the interwoven polymer chains and carbon nanotube bundles.

We have therefore characterized the SWCNT self-grafting on the surface and the gradient of their penetration inside the polymer films, comparing the two polymeric classes. In addition, we have investigated the consequences of the two different grafting mechanisms on the mechanical and electrical behavior of the prepared composites, with the aim of developing different types of electrical sensing devices for application in medicine and prosthetics as well as in other engineering fields.

2. Results

To have a first insight into the type of grafting of CNTs onto the different polymeric substrates, the first characterization of the self-grafted SWCNT layer was obtained by the optical profilometry of the edge between a conductive track made of CNT bundles deposited by the drop casting of an aqueous suspension of SWCNTs and the polymeric substrates. Figure 1 shows the SWCNT tracks on (a) an LDPE and (b) PP films having a thickness of around about 25 µm (LDPE) and 35 µm (PP). A compact track and a sharp step can be observed for both thermoplastic polymers. Table 1 shows the average step height compared to the root mean square (RMS) roughness of the polymeric substrates after the manual brushing and cleaning performed to remove nonadhering CNT flakes (as described in Materials and Methods). The polished sample obtained by depositing the conducting tracks on polyisoprene shows a negative height due to the removal of the superficial polymer layer together with the surface-grafted CNT.

Images from the optical profilometer complement the previous investigation obtained by scanning electron microscopy (SEM): the tracks, 3 × 30 mm in size, have thickness values which can be varied by increasing the number of drop depositions (2–5 µm per single deposited drop of the nanotube suspension) [19,20]. The SWCNT-deposited layer remains grafted onto the polymer surface, even after the manual brushing performed to remove the residual non-grafted SWCNT flakes. The resulting conductive track sticking onto the polymeric film, stabilized by the penetration of the viscous polymer by capillary forces [19], has a relatively low electrical resistance per unit length, of the order of 1–10 kΩ/cm.

A completely different behavior is observed by optical profilometry for SWCNT tracks deposited on thermosetting elastomers, reported in Figure 1 for the PI (c) and PDMS (d). For this type of polymer, polishing the tracks by mechanical brushing leads to an almost complete removal of the bundles deposited above the surface, but nanotube bundles appear to be anchored deeply into the polymer structure, remaining buried in the polymer bulk. The resulting conductive track, grafted and immersed in the elastomer film, shows a resistance per unit length of the order of 0.5–3 MΩ/cm (about two orders of magnitude higher than on the thermoplastic substrates). Because of the non-uniform volume distribution of the conductive component into the polymer, the electrical characteristics are reported as the resistance per unit length of the conductor rather than the material resistivity.

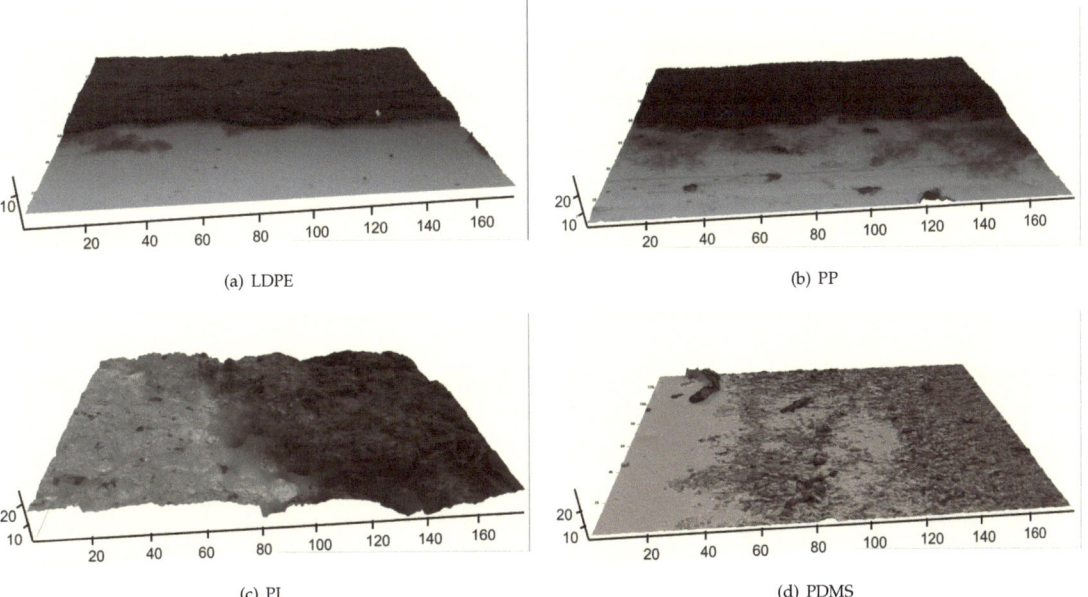

Figure 1. Surface optical profilometry images (all acquired with a 50 × objective) of conductive SWCNT tracks deposited onto different polymer substrates: (**a**) low-density polyethylene (LDPE), (**b**) polypropylene (PP), (**c**) polyisoprene (PI) and (**d**) polydimethylsiloxane (PDMS).

Table 1. RMS roughness of clean polymer substrates and SWCNT tracks and their step heights from optical profilometry. Measurements of nanotube depositions are taken after manual brush polishing.

Polymers	RMS Polymer (µm)	RMS SWCNT Track (µm)	Average Step Height (µm)
LDPE	0.2	0.3	3.0
PP	0.1	0.3	2.0
PI	1.7	3.3	−2.0
PDMS	0.1	0.6	0.7

Figure 2 shows the SEM micrographs of the cross sections of the four samples at different magnifications chosen to highlight the specific characteristics of each sample. The images confirm and explain this different behavior by showing the following:

- For the thermoplastic materials (Figure 2a,b), a fairly well-defined layer of the CNT, where single bundles are easily observed, covers the polymer surface. Looking at the details of the images, one can note the polymer soaking up the CNT layer and accumulating at its surface, thus stabilizing the deposition (see also Appendix A.1 for detail).
- For the elastomeric substrates (Figure 2c,d), the CNT bundles are hardly ever visible in the film section, being immersed in the polymer matrix, and rarely show up as individual "ropes" coated by the polymer, protruding out of the film section.

The penetration gradient of the CNT inside the different polymers was investigated by confocal Raman microscopy. Such a technique allows high-resolution chemical imaging of the samples by a combination of the spectral information acquired through Raman spectroscopy and of the spatial filtering associated with the confocal optical microscope.

The Raman spectral bands derive from the characteristic vibrational modes of the molecules within the samples. When the bands related to these modes are well separated, proper regions of the spectra can be selected to obtain the chemical-physical information on the single components of the materials under investigation. The confocal optics of the microscope allows a volume analysis of the samples by collecting a series of Raman spectra, both on the plane (X, Y) and along the vertical axes (Z). Such a technique can be thus used to obtain the tridimensional information of the composition through the samples. We have thus obtained 3D mapping of the Raman spectroscopic signature of the different materials while scanning the focused laser beam on the plane parallel to the surface of the polymer, for many different planes along its thickness. Carbon nanotubes do not show any significant contribution in the region where the Raman C-H stretching modes due to the polymers appear (2850–2950 cm^{-1}). Such peaks have thus been selected to identify the contribution of the polymeric substrates to the Raman maps. The region related to the Raman G-band (1580–1600 cm^{-1}) was selected to identify the contribution from the CNT in the 3D maps (the details of such spectral signatures are reported in Appendix A.2).

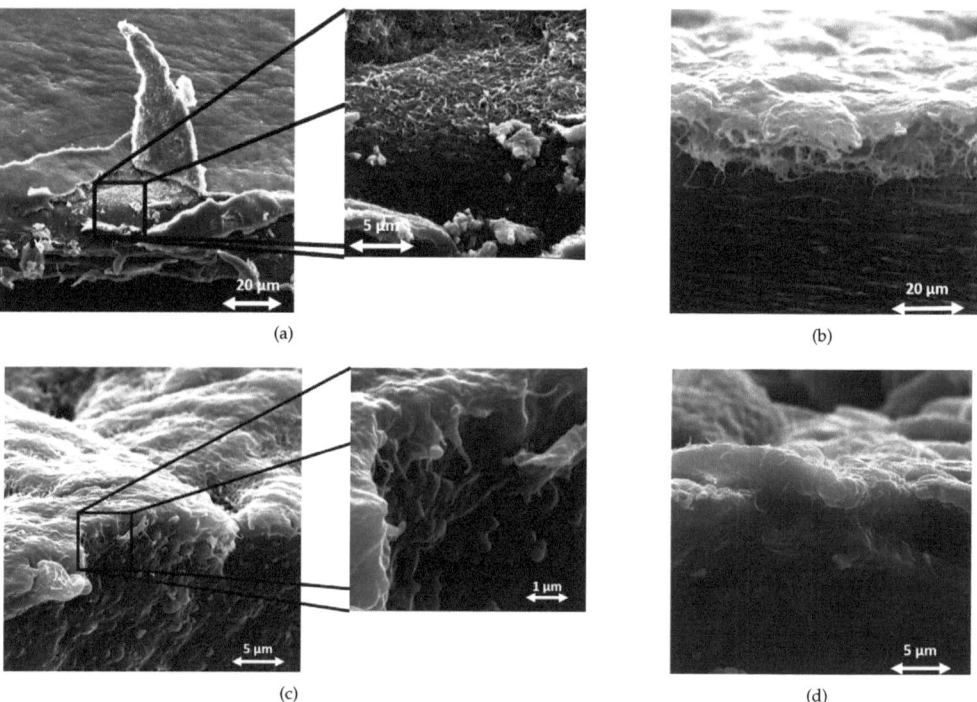

Figure 2. SEM images of SWCNT/polymer composite sections at low angle of incidence. (**a**) LDPE; (**b**) PP; (**c**) PI; (**d**) PDMS.

Figure 3 reports such maps for the different CNT/polymer composites. These maps were acquired by scanning the laser from the pristine polymer face to the CNT-coated side, along planes parallel to the film surface. Such an acquisition procedure allows the laser penetration through the specimen, while otherwise the laser would be absorbed by the CNT layer, without reaching the clean polymer region. Such maps provide an estimate of the maximum depth of the penetration of the SWCNT deposition (the Z coordinate of the plane which first displays a scattering signal from the G-band of SWCNT). As explained in the Materials and Methods section, bright red (green) regions are related to a high CNT (polymer) concentration, as the integral of the Raman contributions related to the CNT (polymer) is high. Yellow and orange regions occur where there is a superposition of both the CNT and polymer contributions (red + green = yellow in the RGB color scheme).

Figure 3a shows the 3D map of a 25 μm thick LDPE film on which the SWCNT was deposited. Nanotubes appear to penetrate up to about 15 μm. This can be assessed from the yellow region that indicates the superposition of the CNT and polymer signals. Figure 3b shows that the SWCNT on a 35 μm thick PP film has a similar behavior, with an average maximum penetration depth of about 25 μm.

Figure 3c refers to a 120 μm thick PI film that, on the contrary, displays a very extended yellow region that proves that CNT bundles penetrate up to about 100 μm. Figure 3d, related to a 250 μm thick PDMS film substrate, shows an SWCNT penetration of up to about 70–80 μm, similar to the case of the PI substrates. Because the laser beam is absorbed by the first layers of the CNT bundles, it was not possible to reconstruct the Raman map along the overall thickness of the specimen, leaving out an unexplored "dark volume".

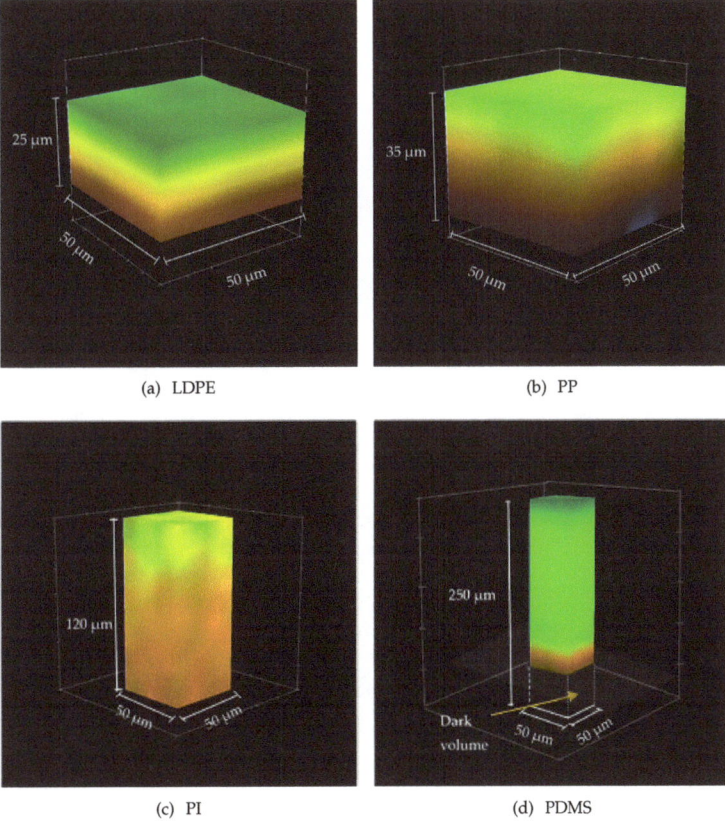

Figure 3. SWCNT penetration obtained from Raman spectral signature of carbon nanotubes (red) and of each polymer (green): (**a**) LDPE; (**b**) PP; (**c**) PI; (**d**) PDMS. Note that the laser beam impinges on the upper side of the 3D maps. In the case of the very thick PDMS substrate (**d**), the volume described as "dark volume" is the region that is not reached by the laser beam due to absorption by the SWCNT gradient.

Two representative electromechanical characterizations for the CNT conductive tracks on the thermoplastic (LDPE) and thermosetting elastomer (PDMS) are reported in Figure 4. They show very different responses: the electrical resistance of the tracks obtained by the same procedure is highly different for the thermoplastic and elastomeric substrates.

Although the electrical resistance of the nanotube bundle tracks deposited on the thermoplastics is fairly low, such resistance increases rapidly, even over the very limited range of the strains explored (up to 20%). Furthermore, such changes in both the resistance and stress are irreversible: as one can see from cycling back the strain to zero, the resistance does not get back to the original value. On the other hand, the resistance values of the CNT tracks on the elastomeric substrates are higher, their relative increase is much slower, the hysteresis of the strain–release cycle is fairly small and the behavior is almost completely reversible.

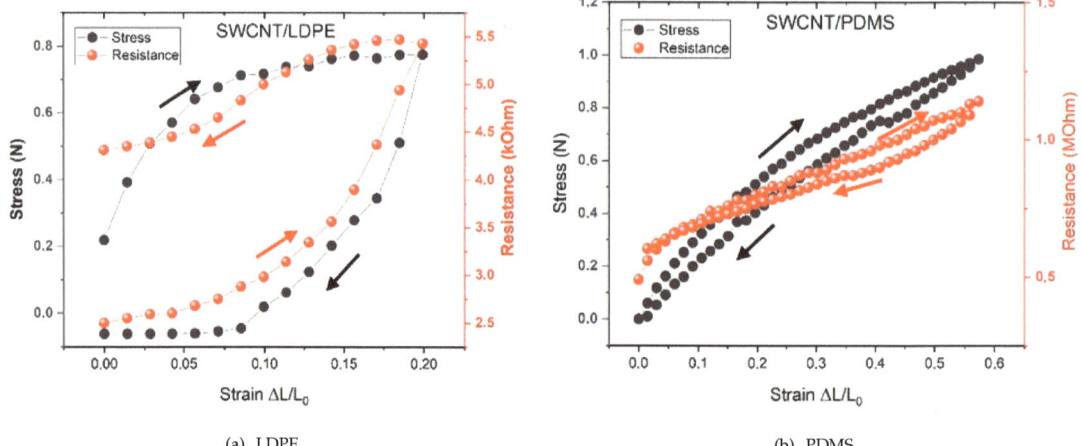

(a) LDPE   (b) PDMS

Figure 4. Mechanical and electrical behavior of self-assembled SWCNT/polymer composite films. Stress–strain and electrical resistance–strain plots for (**a**) thermoplastic (LDPE) and (**b**) thermosetting elastomeric (PDMS) polymer substrates. Resistance versus strain (in red) and stress versus strain (in black) are reported. Note the different y scales and the different shapes of cycles.

The electrical behavior of the different composites appears to be related to their mechanical performance, as shown by the simultaneous recording of the stress–strain and resistance–strain curves on the same specimen. Both types of polymers display hysteresis in both the electrical resistance and the stress due to the relaxation time that the composite structure needs to return to the original configuration once the strain is released. Both hystereses are much larger for the thermoplastic LDPE with respect to the elastomeric PDMS. Possibly, for the 20% strain applied to the LDPE, a permanent plastic deformation of the conductor occurs, associated with a permanent loss of the electrical conductance.

3. Materials and Methods

Self-grafted composites were prepared following the previously reported procedure. Polyester stencils were used to produce arrays of wires and electrodes [19,22]. Purified SWCNT, produced by the HiPCo method [23], were purchased from Carbon Nanotechnologies Inc. The diameter of the individual SWCNT is 0.7 nm, with random chiralities from armchair to zig-zag configuration. SWCNT were grafted on different polymer films by the drop-casting technique. A liquid vector solution was prepared by adding 0.1 mg of Linear Alkylbenzene Sulphonate (LAS) to 10 mg of 10:90 wt.% water/ethanol mixture; 1 mg of SWCNT was then added and dispersed in this solution by combination of the surfactant action of LAS with high-power sonication produced by a Fisherbrand model 120 ultrasonic disintegrator for 60 min. Even after such treatment, the SWCNT dispersion was never completely uniform nor stable for a prolonged period of time. However, by keeping the suspension under continuous sonication in a ultrasonic bath (Elmasonic P) operated at 80 kHz, its homogeneity was maintained high enough to flow through a 200 µm needle for the drop-casting purpose. The vector fluid carrying the SWCNT dispersion was deposited by drop casting on polymeric stencils suitably engineered to define the shape of electrical conductors on polymeric films. The polymeric film substrates were supported and fixed onto a metal plate which was heated to a controlled temperature. While the temperature was kept at approximately 80 °C, the CNT suspension was slowly cast through the needle on the stencil. Evaporation of the water/ethanol solution left a brown/black deposition on the polymer surface. The operation was repeated until the empty spaces within the stencils were completely filled and appeared uniformly black. Irrespective of the hydrophobicity of the polymer surface, the vector droplets drying on the hot polymer caused some inevitable reaggregation of nanotube bundles into small flakes of random geometries. Each CNT track was therefore lightly brushed to remove nonadhering flakes and further cleaned by a jet of purified air. To stabilize the deposition, the temperature was raised to a value only slightly lower than the thermoplastic polymer melting temperature (e.g., 115 °C for our LDPE film, 150 °C for PP films). Samples based on thermosetting elastomers (PDMS and PI) were also heated to 150 °C. All heated samples were maintained at the selected temperature for one minute, then cooled to room temperature to undergo a further step of mechanical brushing. Finally, the stencil was carefully removed and the composite devices thus obtained were used for further characterization.

Surface profilometry measurements were carried out using a KLA Zeta-20 optical profilometer equipped with a 50× objective and a focal step (0.04) μm. The optical scanning and step height measurements have allowed extraction of surface profiles and their roughness; the latter was averaged over 5 profiles collected on representative 100 μm^2 areas from both the pristine polymer and the SWCNT coated portion to assess the thickness of the SWCNT coating and the differences in surface roughness, reported in Table 1. The approximate average thickness of polymer films was measured by a Palmer micrometer, while the optical profilometer supplies more local information on step profiles and roughness, also allowing for 3D surface reconstruction.

SEM scans were obtained by a Tescan Vega (4th Series) electron microscope equipped with a GMU chamber. Secondary electron images were collected in high-vacuum conditions and with beam energies in the 10–20 keV range, selecting the best trade-off in terms of electron penetration and image spatial resolution. To properly study the interface between SWCNTs and the polymers by SEM, the composite films were cut in liquid nitrogen. To obtain a clean section, the samples were soaked in liquid nitrogen to stiffen them, and then they were fractured by means of sharp lancet. Prior to SEM scans, because of their non-conductive nature, the composites were sputter coated with a gold layer of about 10 nm to prevent artifacts due to charge accumulation. The samples were observed by tilting the SEM stage up to 70° angles to find the best position to observe the sides and the edges of the interface layer between the CNT and the polymers, obtaining images as reported in Figure 2.

Confocal Raman microscopy measurements, performed with a Horiba Xplora Plus equipped with a 100 × objective and 638 nm laser excitation, were carried out cutting 2 cm × 2 cm squares from composites that were placed under the microscope, with the naked polymer side facing the objective and the SWCNT layer pointing downward, to reconstruct the tridimensional maps starting from the transparent polymer face. The 3D map was composed of 5 × 5 scanning points (spaced 5 μm) on each of several planes parallel to the surface, corresponding to a number of focal depths (along the Z-axis) with a range depending on the thickness of the polymer. For LDPE, PP, PI and PDMS, the focal depth ranges were 35, 35, 125 and 195 μm, respectively. The z-step for focal distance was approximately 8–10 μm for each composite, with a number of steps depending on the ratio between the depth ranges and the z-step. From the Raman spectra of the composites, two different regions were selected to identify the contributions from SWCNTs and the polymers (see Figure A2). More specifically, to identify the contributions related to SWCNTs, the 1580–1600 cm^{-1} region around the carbon nanotubes Raman G-band (at about 1591 cm^{-1}) was selected, while for the polymers, the C-H Raman stretching mode (around

2850–2950 cm^{-1}) was selected (for further details, see Appendix A.2). The 3D maps in Figure 3 were obtained by a graphical representation of the integrals of the intensities of the Raman spectra in the regions related to CNTs and to polymers as a function of the planar position (X and Y) and focal depth (Z). The red (green) color is associated to the CNTs (polymers), and the higher the value of the integral in the region related to the CNTs (polymer), the brighter the red (green) color becomes.

Electrical resistance–strain data were collected by stretching, via a micrometric slide, conductive tracks made of the different composites, vertically attached to a 120 g metal weight placed on the plate of an analytical balance having 0.1 mg resolution. We then recorded simultaneously the resistance of the conductor and the variation in the gravitational force on the balance. Specimens were modeled in a "dog bone" shape (with construction proportion subject to the conventional ISO 527-1—"Plastics – Determination of the tensile characteristics"). In the case of our stretchable conductive composites, this experimental arrangement also allows for precise simultaneous measurement of the electrical resistance as a function of the strain in the same specimen. Specifically engineered copper clamps provide the necessary electromechanical connection of the specimens. General principles of mechanical characterization were followed, as reported in [24]. Such experimental setup allows a comparison of the mechanical and electrical behavior of the conductive specimens subject to strain, as shown by the plots in Figure 4, relative to the two different representative behaviors of thermoplastic polymers and thermosetting elastomers.

4. Discussion

The experimental evidence supplied by the different techniques employed in this work extends the preliminary analysis [19] on the strong and stable self-grafting of an SWCNT onto polymeric films. The microscopic process of the SWCNT self-grafting onto polymeric substrates is a complex process, strongly affected by fabrication methodologies. The body of results obtained here on composites prepared according to a uniform protocol shows, however, that grafting is very different between the class of thermoplastic substrates and that of elastomers.

More specifically, both the confocal Raman microscopy and SEM data show that the nanotube film grafted on the thermoplastic polymers is compact and thick, penetrating the polymer film up to approximately 20 μm (15 μm in the LDPE and up to 25 μm in the PP). Such depth is sufficient to withstand the brushing procedure devised to remove all the weakly bound CNT flakes. The organic/inorganic materials interact so that many nanotube bundles penetrate the polymer film for several microns, but also the polymer seems to embed the deposited SWCNT layer, contributing to binding it firmly to the substrate and stabilizing the whole layer.

Differently from what was observed with the thermoplastic polymers, in the case of the thermosetting elastomers, the SWCNT layer deposited on the film surface is not soaked by the polymer because of the very high polymer viscosity, which does not decrease significantly during the heating phase of the fabrication. The superficial layer is then easily and almost completely removed by the mechanical brushing. However, both the SEM images and Raman 3D maps show that the nanotubes penetrate deeply (between 70 and 100 μm) into the elastomeric substrates.

This different behavior might be ascribed to the lack of a semi-crystalline phase in strongly cross-linked elastomers. The consequent disordered structure and the density fluctuations, typical of the investigated thermosetting polymers, allow the easier penetration of nanotubes into the polymer structure, even if their viscosity is much higher than for thermoplastic polymers. On the other hand, the lower viscosity of thermoplastics may let these polymer chains drift, by capillary forces, into the layer of the deposited nanotube bundles; these become soaked and stabilized by such a "glueing" effect, which cannot occur in thermosetting elastomers.

The electrical characteristics of the polymers chosen as representative of the two classes (LDPE and PDMS) are strongly dependent on the discussed grafting mechanisms.

The thick layer of the nanotube bundles remaining at the surface of the thermoplastic substrates yields a low electrical resistance, but given the poor elastic behavior of the thermoplastic substrate, it tends to crack at relatively low strains (<20%), thus rapidly and almost irreversibly increasing the conductor resistance. On the other hand, the more uniform dispersion of CNTs into elastomeric substrates causes a higher overall resistivity of the composite. As already noted, while for both types of polymer substrates the electrical behavior reported in Figure 4 seems driven by the corresponding mechanical behavior, the hysteresis is much larger for the thermoplastic substrate, both in stress and in resistance, most likely because of the slower relaxation of the LDPE polymeric chains with respect to the more cross-linked chains of the elastomeric substrate.

It is however interesting to observe in Figure 4 that the initial relaxation of the elastomer, unlike that of the thermoplastic LDPE, leads to a drop in the resistance. This behavior may be related to an increase in the alignment of the CNT bundles driven by the extension of the film, which brings a larger number of CNTs in contact with each other.

Both types of the investigated self-grafted composite types display resistivities in easily accessible ranges. As an example, the resistances of typical conductive tracks, 5 mm wide and 25 mm long, range from a few hundred Ω for thermoplastic substrates to a few MΩ for highly stretched (200–300%) elastomers, where the sensitivity is somewhat higher, reaching values of the gauge factor $\Delta R/R0$ of the order of 5–10. Such a figure is still a factor 10^2 lower than what is reported in the recent literature [8,9], thus limiting their application in the strain sensors field. However, two further needs, in the technology of stretchable conductive composites, are versatility and the ease of engineering [25], characteristics associated with the samples here described. The self-grafting method and the high conductance and elasticity of the as-grown bundled SWCNT ink make the design and development of a variety of different devices extremely easy and inexpensive. The further detailed electromechanical characterization of the investigated self-assembled composites is significant in light of the possible application in several fields all requiring elastic, stretchable and moldable electrical conductors. It is foreseeable that the conductive properties of different types of polymers could be exploited in peculiar environments, such as strongly vibrating systems, or in sensing devices. Moreover, although the systems could be used in individual microsystems, a scale-up toward the mass production of more complex devices is feasible by transferring the nanotube "ink" from stamps rather than drop casting it onto stencils. Some type of particular CNT-polymer electrode arrays for electro-corticographic recordings have already proved to be very successful due to the excellent biocompatibility of polyethylene films and the adaptation of the arrays to the brain shape, and we envisage many other sensing and charge transfer application fields.

5. Conclusions

The interfaces of self-assembled SWCNT/polymer composite regions on polymeric films, both on the surface and in the bulk, have been investigated by several non-destructive techniques.

We have shown that the different grafting behaviors, and the consequent electromechanical responses, follow from the different nature of the polymer (i.e., thermoplastic or thermosetting), possibly because of both the cross-linking of the chains and from the presence or absence of a crystalline phase.

Such differences have important consequences on the electrical behavior of the stretchable conductors. The thick CNT layer, self-grafted on thermoplastic materials, yields a higher conductivity but also a non-constant conductance as a function of the strain, which drops very steeply above a strain of approximately 0.10–0.15, causing the permanent disconnection of the CNT bundles' structures. This is reflected on the high hysteresis on the resistance–strain plot. This limits the application of this type of composite to low-strain devices.

On the other hand, elastomer-based CNT composites have a resistivity about two orders of magnitude higher and penetrate much more deeply into the polymer bulk. These conductors have a more linear behavior of the resistance–strain plot and can be stretched up to three times the original length, returning to the original resistance value with minimal hysteresis. They are thus more suitable for high-strain, heavy-duty devices. Our experimental investigation has thus provided new information on the penetration depth and surface grafting of an SWCNT on different kinds of polymers, together with a better understanding of how the macroscopic mechanical and electrical behavior depend on such grafting mechanisms.

These new findings will contribute to developing more and better performing CNT/polymer composites to improve our stretchable and moldable conductive devices and to associate them to the most appropriate application fields, particularly in the biomedical area, for example, in the technologies associated with prosthetics.

Further studies focused on a more thorough comprehension of the complex microscopic processes of grafting of a CNT on polymeric substrates are currently in progress.

Author Contributions: Conceptualization, L.F., S.L., P.M. and R.S.; investigation, L.F., E.P., A.P., G.R., V.S., C.D., L.D. and P.M.; writing—original draft preparation, L.F., E.P., A.P., G.R. and V.S.; writing—review and editing, P.M., R.S., C.A. and S.L. All authors have read and agreed to the published version of the manuscript.

Funding: This research was funded by POR FESR Lazio 2014-2020-PROGETTI DI GRUPPI DI RICERCA 2020 CUP: E85F21001030002.

Institutional Review Board Statement: Not applicable.

Informed Consent Statement: Not applicable.

Data Availability Statement: Not applicable.

Acknowledgments: The authors gratefully acknowledge the financial support of Regione Lazio (POR FESR Lazio 2014-2020 PROGETTI DI GRUPPI DI RICERCA 2020, Project DIME, Grant Code POR A0375E0084 - CUP: E85F21001030002). Regione Lazio and the University of Rome Tor Vergata are also acknowledged for the financial support to the ISIS@MACH Regional Project (G10795 published by BURL n. 318 69, 27/08/2019) and for the establishment and support of the JRU ISIS@MACH ITALIA, Research Infrastructure hub of ISIS (UK), [MUR official registry U. 0008642.28-05-2020 and U.0013837.04-08-2022].

Conflicts of Interest: The authors declare no conflict of interest. The funders had no role in the design of the study; in the collection, analyses or interpretation of the data; in the writing of the manuscript; or in the decision to publish the results.

Sample Availability: Samples of the compounds SWCNT/LDPE, SWCNT/PP, SWCNT/PI, SWCNT/PDMS composite films are available from the authors.

Abbreviations

The following abbreviations are used in this manuscript:

CNT	Carbon Nanotube
LDPE	Low-Density Polyethylene
PP	Polypropylene
PI	Polyisoprene
PDMS	Polydimethylsiloxane
SWCNT	Single-Wall Carbon Nanotube

Appendix A

Appendix A.1

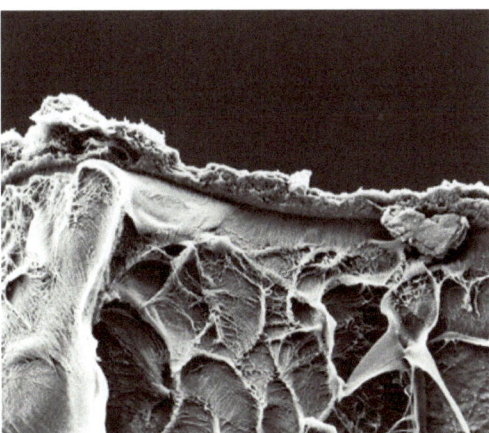

Figure A1. SEM image of SWCNT/LDPE composite sections at low angle of incidence: the compact layer of deposited nanotubes soaked and capped by the polymer is visible along the fracture line.

Appendix A.2

As shown in Figure A2, common features in the Raman spectra of all the polymers investigated are the C-H Raman stretching modes around 2850–2950 cm^{-1}, their proportion and intensity however being different for different polymers. CNTs do not contribute to any peak in the indicated region, which has thus been chosen to characterize the samples. The region of peaks highlighted in green in Figure A2 allowed to identify the contribution from the polymers in the Raman maps reported in the Results section. Conversely, in the region related to the Raman G-band, around 1580–1600 cm^{-1}, the Raman spectra of the polymers do not exhibit any characteristic peak and, in fact, this region (highlighted in red) was used to identify the contribution from the CNTs in the maps.

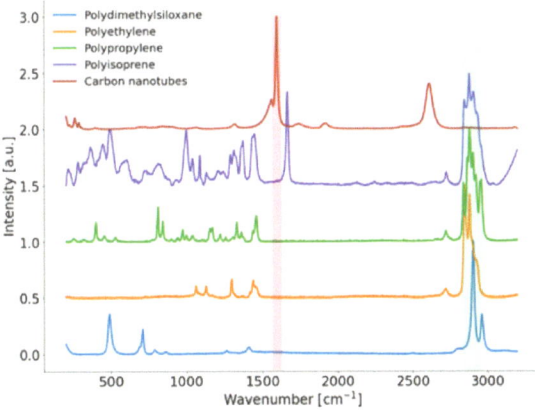

Figure A2. Raman spectra of the composites, highlighting the two different regions selected to identify the contributions from SWCNT and the polymer. The region related to SWCNT at 1580–1600 cm^{-1}, around the carbon nanotubes Raman G-band, is highlighted in red, while for the polymers, the region of the C-H Raman stretching modes (around 2850–2950 cm^{-1}), highlighted in green, has been selected.

References

1. Hu, Y.; Zhao, T.; Zhu, P.; Zhang, Y.; Liang, X.; Sun, R.; Wong, C.P. A low-cost, printable, and stretchable strain sensor based on highly conductive elastic composites with tunable sensitivity for human motion monitoring. *Nano Res.* **2018**, *11*, 1938–1955. [CrossRef]
2. Yang, S.; Li, C.; Cong, T.; Zhao, Y.; Xu, S.; Wang, P.; Pan, L. Sensitivity-Tunable strain sensors based on carbon nanotube@ carbon nanocoil hybrid networks. *Acs Appl. Mater. Interfaces* **2019**, *11*, 38160–38168. [CrossRef] [PubMed]
3. Ji, M.; Deng, H.; Yan, D.; Li, X.; Duan, L.; Fu, Q. Selective localization of multi-walled carbon nanotubes in thermoplastic elastomer blends: An effective method for tunable resistivity–strain sensing behavior. *Compos. Sci. Technol.* **2014**, *92*, 16–26. [CrossRef]
4. Liu, H.; Gao, J.; Huang, W.; Dai, K.; Zheng, G.; Liu, C.; Shen, C.; Yan, X.; Guo, J.; Guo, Z. Electrically conductive strain sensing polyurethane nanocomposites with synergistic carbon nanotubes and graphene bifillers. *Nanoscale* **2016**, *8*, 12977–12989. [CrossRef]
5. Wang, N.; Xu, Z.; Zhan, P.; Dai, K.; Zheng, G.; Liu, C.; Shen, C. A tunable strain sensor based on a carbon nanotubes/electrospun polyamide 6 conductive nanofibrous network embedded into poly (vinyl alcohol) with self-diagnosis capabilities. *J. Mater. Chem.* **2017**, *5*, 4408–4418. [CrossRef]
6. Luo, H.; Zhou, X.; Ma, Y.; Yi, G.; Cheng, X.; Zhu, Y.; Zu, X.; Zhang, N.; Huang, B.; Yu, L. Shape memory-based tunable resistivity of polymer composites. *Appl. Surf. Sci.* **2016**, *363*, 59–65. [CrossRef]
7. Hu, N.; Karube, Y.; Arai, M.; Watanabe, T.; Yan, C.; Li, Y.; Liu, Y.; Fukunaga, H. Investigation on sensitivity of a polymer/carbon nanotube composite strain sensor. *Carbon* **2010**, *48*, 680–687. [CrossRef]
8. Tas, M.O.; Baker, M.A.; Masteghin, M.G.; Bentz, J.; Boxshall, K.; Stolojan, V. Highly stretchable, directionally oriented carbon nanotube/PDMS conductive films with enhanced sensitivity as wearable strain sensors. *ACS Appl. Mater. Interfaces* **2019**, *11*, 39560–39573. [CrossRef]
9. He, Y.; Wu, D.; Zhou, M.; Zheng, Y.; Wang, T.; Lu, C.; Zhang, L.; Liu, H.; Liu, C. Wearable strain sensors based on a porous polydimethylsiloxane hybrid with carbon nanotubes and graphene. *ACS Appl. Mater. Interfaces* **2021**, *13*, 15572–15583. [CrossRef]
10. Liang, L.; Gao, C.; Chen, G.; Guo, C.Y. Large-area, stretchable, super flexible and mechanically stable thermoelectric films of polymer/carbon nanotube composites. *J. Mater. Chem.* **2016**, *4*, 526–532. [CrossRef]
11. Wu, S.; Zhang, J.; Ladani, R.B.; Ravindran, A.R.; Mouritz, A.P.; Kinloch, A.J.; Wang, C.H. Novel electrically conductive porous PDMS/carbon nanofiber composites for deformable strain sensors and conductors. *ACS Appl. Mater. Interfaces* **2017**, *9*, 14207–14215. [CrossRef] [PubMed]
12. Paiva, M.C.; Zhou, B.; Fernando, K.A.S.; Lin, Y.; Kennedy, J.M.; Sun, Y.P. Mechanical and morphological characterization of polymer–carbon nanocomposites from functionalized carbon nanotubes. *Carbon* **2004**, *42*, 2849–2854. [CrossRef]
13. Li, G.Y.; Wang, P.M.; Zhao, X. Mechanical behavior and microstructure of cement composites incorporating surface-treated multi-walled carbon nanotubes. *Carbon* **2005**, *43*, 1239–1245. [CrossRef]
14. Postiglione, G.; Natale, G.; Griffini, G.; Levi, M.; Turri, S. Conductive 3D microstructures by direct 3D printing of polymer/carbon nanotube nanocomposites via liquid deposition modeling. *Compos. Part A Appl. Sci. Manuf.* **2015**, *76*, 110–114. [CrossRef]
15. Zhao, Q.; Wagner, H.D. Raman spectroscopy of carbon–nanotube–based composites. *Philos. Trans. R. Soc. London. Ser. Math. Phys. Eng. Sci.* **2014**, *362*, 2407–2424. [CrossRef]
16. Wood, J.R.; Zhao, Q.; Wagner, H.D. Orientation of carbon nanotubes in polymers and its detection by Raman spectroscopy. *Compos. Part Appl. Sci. Manuf.* **2001**, *32*, 391–399. [CrossRef]
17. Cooper, C.A.; Young, R.J.; Halsall, M. Investigation into the deformation of carbon nanotubes and their composites through the use of Raman spectroscopy. *Compos. Part Appl. Sci. Manuf.* **2001**, *32*, 401–411. [CrossRef]
18. Zhou, W.; Ma, W.; Niu, Z.; Song, L.; Xie, S. Freestanding single-walled carbon nanotube bundle networks: Fabrication, properties and composites. *Chin. Sci. Bull.* **2012**, *57*, 205–224. [CrossRef]
19. Morales, P.; Moyanova, S.; Pavone, L.; Fazi, L.; Mirabile Gattia, D.; Rapone, B.; Gaglione, A.; Senesi, R. Self-grafting carbon nanotubes on polymers for stretchable electronics. *Eur. Phys. J. Plus* **2018**, *133*, 1–11. [CrossRef]
20. Fazi, L.; Gattia, D.M.; Pavone, L.; Prioriello, A.; Scacco, V.; Morales, P.; Federica, M.; Anderson, G.; Slavianka, M.; Senesi, R. Carbon Nanotube-Based Stretchable Hybrid Material Film for Electronic Devices and Applications. *J. Nanosci. Nanotechnol.* **2020**, *20*, 4549–4556. [CrossRef]
21. Pavone, L.; Moyanova, S.; Mastroiacovo, F.; Fazi, L.; Busceti, C.; Gaglione, A.; Martinello, K.; Fucile, S.; Bucci, D.; Senesi, R. Chronic neural interfacing with cerebral cortex using single-walled carbon nanotube-polymer grids. *J. Neural Eng.* **2020**, *17*, 036032. [CrossRef] [PubMed]
22. Fazi, L.; Prioriello, A.; Scacco, V.; Ciccognani, W.; Serra, E.; Gattia, D.M.; Morales, P.; Limiti, E.; Senesi. Stretchable conductors made of single wall carbon nanotubes self-grafted on polymer films. *J. Physics: Conf. Ser.* **2020**, *1548*, 012023. [CrossRef]
23. Dai, H.; Rinzler, A.G.; Nikolaev, P.; Thess, A.; Colbert, D.T.; Smalley, R.E. Single-wall nanotubes produced by metal-catalyzed disproportionation of carbon monoxide. *Chem. Phys. Lett.* **1996**, *260*, 471–475. [CrossRef]

24. ISO 527-5:2009; Plastics-Determination of Tensile Properties. British Standard: Frankfurt am Main, Germany, 1997.
25. Yang, S.; Li, C.; Chen, X.; Zhao, Y.; Zhang, H.; Wen, N.; Fan, Z.; Pan, L. Facile fabrication of high-performance pen ink-decorated textile strain sensors for human motion detection. *Acs Appl. Mater. Interfaces* **2020**, *12*, 19874–19881. [CrossRef]

Disclaimer/Publisher's Note: The statements, opinions and data contained in all publications are solely those of the individual author(s) and contributor(s) and not of MDPI and/or the editor(s). MDPI and/or the editor(s) disclaim responsibility for any injury to people or property resulting from any ideas, methods, instructions or products referred to in the content.

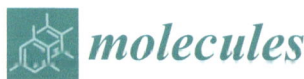

Article

Highly Sensitive Sub-ppm CH₃COOH Detection by Improved Assembly of Sn₃O₄-RGO Nanocomposite

Norazreen Abd Aziz [1,2,*], Mohd Faizol Abdullah [2], Siti Aishah Mohamad Badaruddin [2], Mohd Rofei Mat Hussin [2] and Abdul Manaf Hashim [3]

[1] Faculty of Engineering & Built Environment, Universiti Kebangsaan Malaysia, Bangi 43600, Malaysia
[2] MIMOS Semiconductor (M) Sdn Bhd, Technology Park Malaysia, Kuala Lumpur 57000, Malaysia
[3] Malaysia-Japan International Institute of Technology, Universiti Teknologi Malaysia, Jalan Sultan Yahya Petra, Kuala Lumpur 54100, Malaysia
* Correspondence: norazreen@ukm.edu.my

Abstract: Detection of sub-ppm acetic acid (CH₃COOH) is in demand for environmental gas monitoring. In this article, we propose a CH₃COOH gas sensor based on Sn_3O_4 and reduced graphene oxide (RGO), where the assembly of Sn_3O_4-RGO nanocomposites is dependent on the synthesis method. Three nanocomposites prepared by three different synthesis methods are investigated. The optimum assembly is by hydrothermal reactions of Sn^{4+} salts and pre-reduced RGO (designated as RS nanocomposite). Raman spectra verified the fingerprint of RGO in the synthesized RS nanocomposite. The Sn_3O_4 planes of (111), (210), (130), ($\bar{1}$32) are observed from the X-ray diffractogram, and its average crystallite size is 3.94 nm. X-ray photoelectron spectroscopy on Sn3d and O1s spectra confirm the stoichiometry of Sn_3O_4 with Sn:O ratio = 0.76. Sn_3O_4-RGO-RS exhibits the highest response of 74% and 4% at 2 and 0.3 ppm, respectively. The sensitivity within sub-ppm CH₃COOH is 64%/ppm. Its superior sensing performance is owing to the embedded and uniformly wrapped Sn_3O_4 nanoparticles on RGO sheets. This allows a massive relative change in electron concentration at the Sn_3O_4-RGO heterojunction during the on/off exposure of CH₃COOH. Additionally, the operation is performed at room temperature, possesses good repeatability, and consumes only ~4 μW, and is a step closer to the development of a commercial CH₃COOH sensor.

Keywords: Sn_3O_4 nanoparticles; reduced graphene oxide; heterojunction; CH₃COOH

Citation: Aziz, N.A.; Abdullah, M.F.; Badaruddin, S.A.M.; Hussin, M.R.M.; Hashim, A.M. Highly Sensitive Sub-ppm CH₃COOH Detection by Improved Assembly of Sn₃O₄-RGO Nanocomposite. *Molecules* 2022, 27, 8707. https://doi.org/10.3390/molecules27248707

Academic Editors: Luca Tortora and Gianlorenzo Bussetti

Received: 26 October 2022
Accepted: 29 November 2022
Published: 8 December 2022

Publisher's Note: MDPI stays neutral with regard to jurisdictional claims in published maps and institutional affiliations.

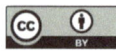

Copyright: © 2022 by the authors. Licensee MDPI, Basel, Switzerland. This article is an open access article distributed under the terms and conditions of the Creative Commons Attribution (CC BY) license (https://creativecommons.org/licenses/by/4.0/).

1. Introduction

Various sensors for detecting and monitoring toxic and harmful gases including volatile organic compounds (VOCs) have been studied to satisfy the regulation of the environmental and gases industry standards. Several significant methods have been used so far to monitor VOCs and other toxic gases including electrochemical sensors [1], acoustic sensors [2], optical sensors [3], and colorimetric sensors [4]. Acetic acid (CH₃COOH), which is one of the most corrosive and highly irritating VOCs, is broadly used in food, plastic, pharmaceutical, and most manufacturing industries [5,6]. There can be many potential health issues including eye and skin irritation, body swelling, particularly the nose, tongue, throat, etc., and respiratory illnesses from prolonged exposure to high concentrations of CH₃COOH. According to guidelines from China and the USA, the maximum allowable concentrations of acetic acid vapor in the workplace are 7.5 ppm (GBZ 2-2002) and 9.3 ppm (D3620-04), respectively [7]. Therefore, developing an ultrasensitive, low limit of detection, low energy consumption, and reliable acetic acid gas sensor is highly desirable for air monitoring in modern industries and workplaces.

Compared to conventional CH₃COOH detection analysis such as gas chromatography and mass spectrometry, chemiresistive metal oxide gas sensors are more suitable for real-time analysis because of their advantages including compact size, easy production, and simple measuring electronics [8–11]. SnO_2, ZnO, and TiO are the most common metal oxide materials which have been extensively used for detecting various kinds of gases due to their high sensitivities, low costs, simple fabrications, and long-term stabilities. In addition to SnO_2 [12–15], other tin oxides with other oxygen stoichiometries such as SnO [16–18], Sn_2O_3 [19], Sn_3O_4 [20–22], and Sn_5O_6 [23], have been widely investigated. Among them, Sn_3O_4, which has a band gap of ~2.9 eV, has attracted significant attention owing to its unique sensing properties. However, these single-material-based gas sensors typically need to be operated at high temperatures to obtain a desirable sensing response, which leads to considerably high power consumption, a scarce lifetime, and poor selectivity of the device [24,25]. Undeniably, there is also a recent work that reported on the successful operation at room temperature of a triethylamine (TEA) gas sensor based on porous SnO_2 films with rich oxygen vacancies [26].

To overcome the above-mentioned drawbacks, the heterostructure that is constructed by incorporating metal oxide semiconductor (MOS) materials with innovative graphene-based materials [27–30] can be a valid alternative. Graphene and its derivatives, especially reduced graphene oxide (RGO) possess several promising features, including a large specific surface area for better adsorption, thermoelectric conductivity, and high carrier mobility at room temperature [31,32]. Generally, RGO under ambient conditions exhibits p-type behavior due to its electron-withdrawing nature, and if the incorporated metal oxide behaves as an n-type semiconductor, the formation of p-n heterostructures may be realized. The p-n heterostructures can modulate the electronic and chemical properties via surface charge transfer and chemical bonding, thus improving the gas sensing performance.

Numerous studies have been conducted to improve the gas sensing characteristics through the formation of metal oxide-RGO nanocomposites including CuO-RGO [33], SnO_2-RGO [34,35], ZnO-RGO [36], TiO_2-RGO [37], and many more. Although the accurate analysis of all the effective parameters is still not clear, the major factors that influence the sensing performance are the assembly of metal oxide nanoparticles with RGO, deoxygenation, and the number of active sites, i.e., oxygen vacancies, O_v and chemisorbed oxygen, O_c available for capturing targeted analytes [38]. From previous work, different microstructures are observed from the family of tin oxide-RGO composites that are prepared by various synthesis techniques, thus leading to different sensing performances [39,40]. To date, only a few studies on metal oxide-RGO-based CH_3COOH sensors have been reported [41,42]. Therefore, we proposed a highly sensitive sub-ppm CH_3COOH sensor based on Sn_3O_4-RGO nanocomposite operating at room temperature.

In this work, we investigate the effect of hydrothermal synthesis conditions on the material microstructures and their sensing performances to CH_3COOH. An exhaustive study on three types of Sn_3O_4-RGO sensing materials that were prepared via (i) hydrothermal reactions of Sn^{4+} salts and pre-reduced RGO (designated as RS nanocomposite) (ii) one-step hydrothermal synthesis from Sn^{4+} and GO (designated as OS nanocomposite), (iii) Sn_3O_4 nanoparticles cast onto RGO nanosheet (designated as CO nanocomposite) to validate the effects of synthesis condition on microstructure and other sensing properties.

2. Materials and Methods
2.1. Materials

The reagents used to synthesize the Sn_3O_4-RGO nanocomposites include a commercial (4 mg/mL) graphene oxide, GO (dispersion in H_2O), and $SnCl_4·5H_2O$ (99%) purchased from Sigma Aldrich. Both were used as received, without any further purification.

2.1.1. Preparation of One-Step Sn_3O_4-RGO Nanocomposite (OS Nanocomposite)

Figure 1a shows the typical one-pot Sn_3O_4-RGO nanocomposite that was synthesized via the facile hydrothermal method. A total of 187.5 µL of (GO) from the bottle and 24 mg of $SnCl_4·5H_2O$ were dissolved in 20 mL of deionized water under magnetic stirring for 1 h to achieve homogenous dispersion. Subsequently, the dispersion was transferred into a 50 mL Teflon-lined stainless-steel autoclave and was heated in the oven at a temperature of 180 °C for 12 h. After cooling down to room temperature, the solution was centrifuged at

4000 rpm for 15 min. At last, the OS nanocomposite was obtained by washing three times with deionized water and one time with ethanol.

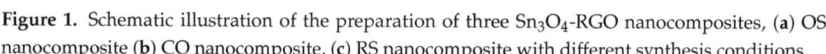

Figure 1. Schematic illustration of the preparation of three Sn_3O_4-RGO nanocomposites, (**a**) OS nanocomposite (**b**) CO nanocomposite, (**c**) RS nanocomposite with different synthesis conditions.

2.1.2. Preparation of Cast-On Sn_3O_4-RGO Nanocomposite (CO Nanocomposite)

CO nanocomposite was obtained by assembling Sn_3O_4 nanoparticles into GO nanosheets through hydrothermal treatment as shown in Figure 1b. Firstly, 24 mg of $SnCl_4·5H_2O$ was dissolved into 20 mL of deionized water with constant magnetic stirring for 1 h. The solution was poured into a 50 mL Teflon-lined stainless-steel autoclave and then heated in the oven at a temperature of 180 °C for 12 h. The resulting Sn_3O_4 nanoparticles were obtained by centrifuge washing four times using deionized water and ethanol. The resulting Sn_3O_4 NPs were poured into 20 mL of deionized water together with 187.5 µL GO and then stirred again for another 1 h. At last, the mixture underwent the same hydrothermal process (180 °C for 12 h) and was washed four times with water and ethanol subsequently to achieve the CO nanocomposite.

2.1.3. Preparation of Pre-Reduced Sn_3O_4-RGO Nanocomposite (RS Nanocomposite)

To achieve RS nanocomposite, a two-step hydrothermal treatment is needed, starting with the thermal reduction of GO as shown in Figure 1c. At first, 187.5 µL of GO was dispersed into 20 mL of deionized water under vigorous stirring for 1 h. Then the mixture was poured into a 50 mL Teflon-lined stainless-steel autoclave for hydrothermal reduction treatment (180 °C for 12 h). The pre-reduced RGO dispersion in deionized water was obtained. Then 24 mg of $SnCl_4 \cdot 5H_2O$ was added to the RGO solution and continued by the same process, i.e., stirring for 1 h and heating at 180 °C for 12 h. Finally, the RS nanocomposite was collected by washing it four times with water and ethanol.

2.2. Material Characterization

The crystal structure and phase composition of each as-prepared sample were evaluated by the X-ray diffraction (XRD) system (PANalytical Empyrean diffractometer with Cu Kα radiation: λ = 1.5418 Å). The oscillation modes of each composite were investigated using 473 nm laser Raman spectroscopy (NTEGRA Spectra MT-MDT). The microstructure and morphology of Sn_3O_4-RGO nanocomposites were inspected by transmission electron microscope (TEM) with an accelerating voltage of 120 kV (Talos, L120C from Thermo Fisher Scientific, Eindhoven, The Netherlands). The composition of S, O, and C were analyzed by X-ray photoemission spectroscopy (XPS) system (NEXSA G2 from Thermo Fisher Scientific) using a monochromated Al Kα source (voltage source: 12 kV, beam size: 100 μm, pass energy survey scan: 200 eV, pass energy narrow scan: 100 eV).

2.3. Sensor Fabrication and Measurement Set-Up

The gas sensor was established by dropping 5 μL aqueous dispersion of different sensing materials prepared previously on a 1 × 1 cm^2 Si/SiO$_2$ substrate where interdigitated electrodes (IDE) were fabricated on it. The Pt/Ti (100/10 nm) IDE geometry consists of 3 pairs of finger electrodes and each electrode has a width and length of 0.1 mm and 2 mm, respectively. The interfinger spacing between electrodes is 0.2 mm. This test structure was constructed using lithography, metallization, and a standard lift-off process. Thus, the coverage of the sensing area was ~6 mm^2. The prepared gas sensing devices were dried overnight in the desiccator. Figure 2 shows a schematic of the measurement setup that was used to investigate the sensing performance of the three different composites towards CH_3COOH. In an enclosed chamber, the sensor was placed on the heater stage and controlled by Nextron Temperature Controller. The temperature was set at room temperature. The flow rates of compressed dry air (CDA) and CH_3COOH were controlled by mass flow controllers of the humidifier system (Cellkraft P-10). The relative humidity was set constant at 5 ± 1% using a closed-loop control system. The testing was performed by applying a direct voltage of 2 V and monitoring changes in the electrical resistance (using source measuring unit Keithley 2410). The sensor response, R_s is quantified by changes in resistance upon exposure to CH_3COOH analytes and air (CDA in this case) as shown in Equation (1).

$$R_s = [(R_g - R_a)/R_a] \times 100\% \tag{1}$$

where R_g is the resistance in the presence of CH_3COOH gas and R_a is the gas sensor's electrical resistance at rest when exposed to CDA. In the meantime, the response time is described as the time needed for the CH_3COOH sensor to respond at 90% of its saturated level and the recovery time is the amount of time required to recover 10% from its initial value when exposed to the air. The sensitivity (unit = %/ppm) of the Sn_3O_4-RGO sensor is calculated from the change of R_s for the varied concentration of acetic acid. To be fair, we set the durations of the on/off flow of acetic acid as constant for all measurements. To record the response and recovery speed, we started to record the measurement as soon as CDA was introduced in the chamber. After 90 s, CDA was automatically shut off and CH_3COOH was released in the chamber immediately.

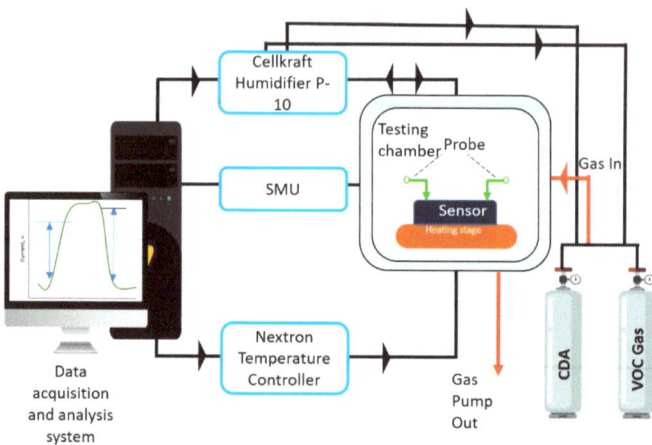

Figure 2. Schematic of illustration CH_3COOH testing setup.

3. Results and Discussion

3.1. Sn_3O_4-RGO Nanocomposites Formation Mechanism

We chose the hydrothermal method to synthesize Sn_3O_4-RGO-based composites as their advantages inhomogeneous distribution and versatile interfacial decorations between RGO and metal oxide. Three kinds of Sn_3O_4-RGO-based nanocomposites were made by changing the preparation condition via a hydrothermal method using GO and $SnCl_4 \cdot 5H_2O$ as precursors. During the synthesis process, there are several reactions that were carried out under the hydrothermal temperature and pressure in the autoclave i.e., (i) the adsorption of Sn^{4+} by GO or RGO, (ii) the reduction of GO into RGO, and (iii) Sn^{4+} decomposing into Sn_3O_4 nanocrystals. The formation chemistry of the Sn_3O_4-RGO nanocomposites is explained as follows:

$$SnCl_4 \cdot 5H_2O \rightarrow Sn^{4+} + Cl^- + 5H^+ + 5OH^- \tag{2}$$

$$Sn^{4+} + 4OH^- \rightarrow Sn(OH)_4 \tag{3}$$

$$3[Sn(OH)_4] \rightarrow Sn_3O_4 + 6H_2O + O_2 \tag{4}$$

Although maintaining the volume of GO and $SnCl_4 \cdot 5H_2O$, the amount of Sn_3O_4 nanostructures, RGO obtained, and also the nanocomposite interfaces may be different due to the tuning of synthesis methods.

3.2. Structural and Morphological Analysis

Figure 3 depicts the XRD patterns ranging from 20° to 60° of all three nanocomposites. Notably, all as-prepared nanocomposites show three strong diffraction peaks at 2θ of 26.41°, 33.82°, and 51.73° which are attributed to (111), (210), (130), and ($\bar{1}32$) planes of triclinic Sn_3O_4 structure (JCPDS Card No 16-0737) [43], indicating the successful formation of the single crystal Sn_3O_4 particles in this work. The full width at half maximum (FWHM) of all peaks is broad, revealing a nanoscale size of Sn_3O_4. The crystallite sizes can be determined by the Debye–Sherrer formula as follows; $D = 0.89\lambda / \beta \cos\theta$, where D is the average crystallite size diameter, λ (Cu Kα) is 0.154 Å, and β is the FWHM of the diffraction curves. The calculated average crystallite size values are 3.91, 3.38, and 3.94 nm for OS, CO, and RS nanocomposites, respectively. The relatively small Sn_3O_4 crystallite size of the CO nanocomposites is because Sn_3O_4 particles underwent two times the hydrothermal treatment as compared to the other method. Thus, the observed XRD results confirm the formation of nanosized Sn_3O_4-RGO nanocomposites. There is no peak observed for the

RGO, which implies that the formation of the RGO plane maybe not be in perfect stacking and needs to be confirmed by Raman analysis.

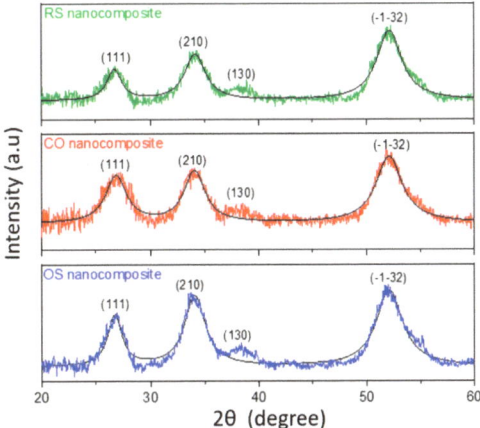

Figure 3. XRD diffractogram of OS, CO, and RS nanocomposites.

The three as-prepared samples were then further characterized by the Raman technique as it is a useful method to characterize the structure of RGO-based materials. Figure 4 shows the Raman spectra of all three OS, CO, and RS nanocomposites. It can be deduced that all samples exhibit two major peaks at ~1300 cm^{-1} and ~1600 cm^{-1}, corresponding to the characteristic D-band (I_D) and G-band (I_G), respectively. The I_D is related to structural defects and partially disordered structure, and the I_G refers to the vibration of sp^2-bonded carbon atoms. The intensity ratio of the D and G bands (I_D/I_G) not only gives information about in-plane crystallite size, L_a, but also indicates the overall degree of disorder within the graphitic carbon [44]. The average value of the I_D/I_G ratio and L_a for all three nanocomposites are 1.07 and 2.93 nm singly. This condition indicates a high disorder of carbon sp^2 atoms leading to high deoxygenation that concludes that GO is successfully reduced by hydrothermal preparation. It is also understood that the rich defects of OS nanocomposite are possibly due to an increase in vacancies, grain boundaries, and amorphous carbon species, as well as the insertion of Sn$_3$O$_4$ nanoparticles into RGO sheets [45]. This Raman scattering analysis demonstrates the existence of RGO in all three Sn$_3$O$_4$-RGO nanocomposites.

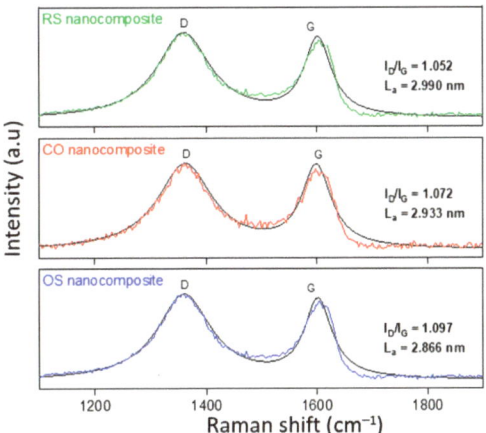

Figure 4. Raman spectra of OS, CO, and RS nanocomposite.

The morphology and surface nature of the as-prepared nanocomposites was characterized by TEM. Figure 5 depicts low-, medium-, and high-magnification TEM images and histograms of the three nanocomposites. From low-magnification TEM images, it can be seen that a huge amount of spherical Sn_3O_4 nanoparticles were formed on massive wrinkled RGO sheets. Most Sn_3O_4 nanoparticles were uniformly dispersed onto RGO sheets but only a small amount of them aggregate at the edge of OS nanocomposite (Figure 5a). Likewise, in the RS nanocomposite, Sn_3O_4 nanoparticles are evenly and densely distributed, only some Sn_3O_4 nanoparticles agglomerate at different spots on RGO sheets (Figure 5j). Meanwhile, a large amount of Sn_3O_4 nanoparticles aggregated on RGO sheets and we also observed the absence of Sn_3O_4 nanoparticles on the edge of CO nanocomposites (Figure 5e). From medium magnification, it is confirmed that there is good dispersity of Sn_3O_4 nanoparticles on the RGO sheet for OS and RS nanocomposites (Figure 5b,j). Meanwhile, for CO nanocomposites, it is confirmed there is an island of aggregated Sn_3O_4 nanoparticles isolated on the edge of some spare place on RGO as shown in Figure 5f. These conditions suggest that OS and RS are the best preparation method for Sn_3O_4-RGO nanocomposites as Sn_3O_4 nanoparticles prefer to grow all over the surface of GO and RGO by pre-adsorbing Sn^{4+} during the hydrothermal synthesis process. High-magnification TEM images as shown in Figure 5c,g,k indicate a clear image of Sn_3O_4 nanoparticles with non-uniform size distribution loading on the surface of RGO sheets. From histogram distribution (Figure 5d,h,l) the average particle sizes of Sn_3O_4 of OS, CO, and RS nanocomposites are 1.81, 1.77, and 1.75 nm, respectively. Thus, they are indicating that single crystal Sn_3O_4 is forming clusters of polycrystalline Sn_3O_4 nanoparticles.

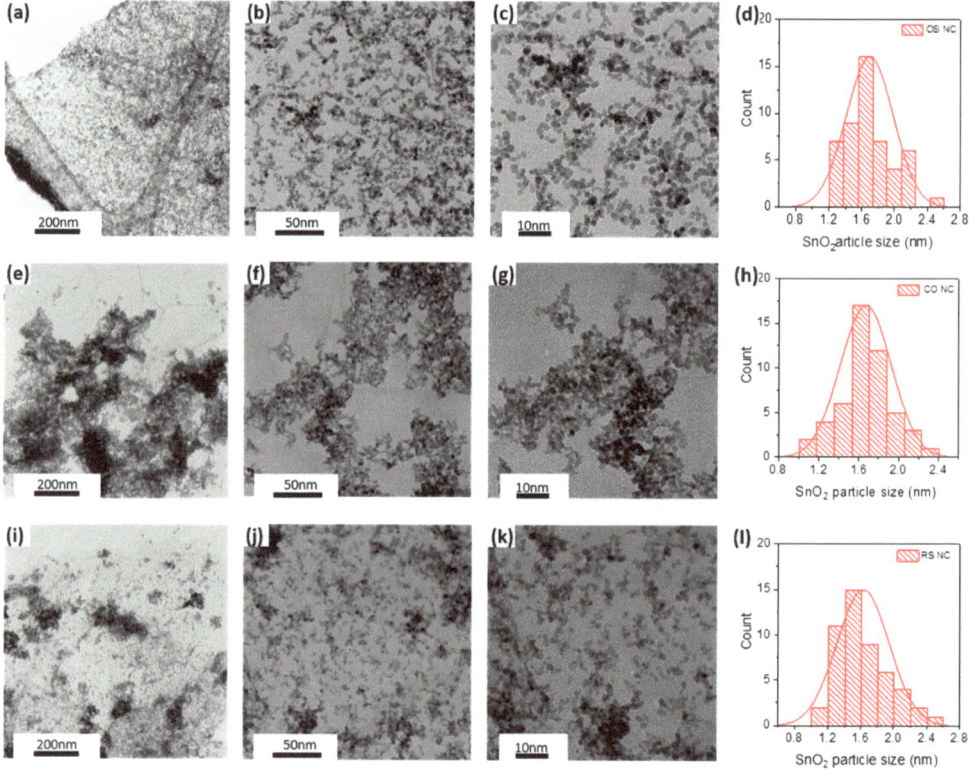

Figure 5. (**a,e,i**) Low magnification, (**b,f,j**) medium magnification, (**c,g,k**) high magnification images, and (**d,h,l**) Particle count histogram of Sn_3O_4 of OS, CO, and RS nanocomposites.

XPS characterization was examined to investigate elements, surface chemistry, and electronic structure of Sn_3O_4-RGO nanocomposites. The survey spectra in Figure 6a indicate the peaks of Sn4d, Sn3d, Sn3p, O1s, and C1s that are observed in the region of 0–1200 eV. Thus, it confirms the presence of three elements of Sn, O, and C in all three nanocomposites. The peaks of Sn and O are much higher than the peak of C, implying the formation of a large amount of Sn_3O_4 nanoparticles. The components of all these elements are tabulated in Table 1. It is found that the ratio of tin and oxygen in these three nanocomposites is around 0.75, revealing the formation of Sn_3O_4 nanoparticles. The ratio of Sn_3O_4:RGO for samples OS, CO, and RS are 2.07, 4.62, and 3.60, respectively. These match with the TEM images in Figure 5, where high values of Sn_3O_4:RGO from samples CO and RS are due to the dispersion of Sn_3O_4 nanoparticles agglomerated onto the RGO sheet. Figure 6b displays the Sn3d spectrum of all three nanocomposites. It is obviously seen that two strong peaks at 487.3 eV and 495.7 eV attribute to the spin–orbit coupling of Sn3d5/2 and Sn3d3/2, respectively.

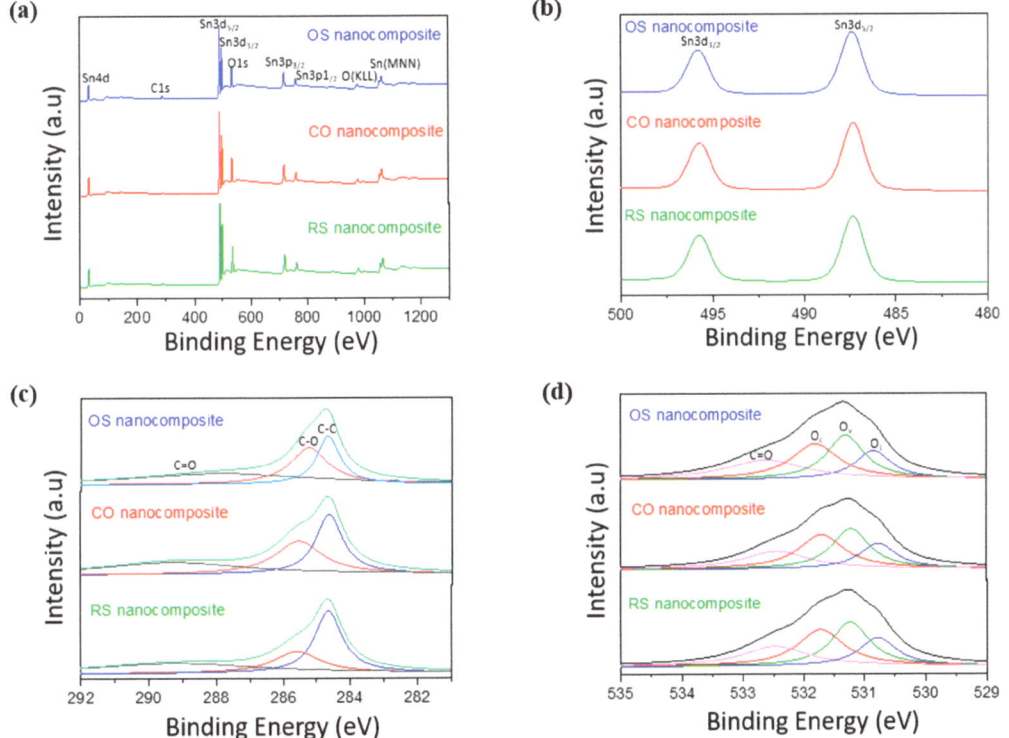

Figure 6. The (**a**) XPS spectra, (**b**) Sn3d XPS spectra, (**c**) C1s XPS spectra, and (**d**) O1s XPS spectra of OS, CO, and RS nanocomposites.

Meanwhile, Figure 6c shows the deconvoluted peaks of the C1s spectrum which exhibits three types of the carbon-associated group including C-C (~284.6 eV), C-O (~285.6 eV), and C=O (~289.2 eV). The components of these band groups are presented in Table 2. Notably, the relative percentage of the C-C band is much higher than that of the C-O and C=O group in both RS and CO nanocomposites, indicating the successful reduction of GO by the hydrothermal process. It can be concluded the reduction degree of RGO in RS nanocomposite is the strongest because the RGO underwent hydrothermal treatment two times. Figure 6d represents the wide and asymmetric feature of O1s which can be divided into four peaks, revealing the presence of four types of O-related species including the Sn-O-Sn lattice O atoms in triclinic Sn_3O_4 (O_L), oxygen vacancies (O_v), chemisorbed oxygen-related species such as hydroxyl groups (O_c), and the C=O band at the binding energies of ~530.8, ~531.2, ~531.7, and ~532.6 eV, respectively. As can be seen from summarized data in Table 3, the atomic percentages of O_c and O_v are considerably high for both RS (O_c = 17.0%, O_v = 16.85%) and CO (O_c = 17.41%, O_v = 18.06%) nanocomposite, which is deemed to enhance the gas sensing response to CH_3COOH. All these observations reveal the successful formation of all three Sn_3O_4-RGO nanocomposites synthesized hydrothermally by three different conditions.

Table 1. The fitting results of the content and content ratio of each atom for OS, CO, and RS nanocomposites.

Samples	Sn (At.%)	C (At.%)	O (At.%)	O* (At.%)	O** (At.%)	Sn:O** [Sn_3O_4]	C:O* [RGO]	Ratio Sn_3O_4:RGO
OS nanocomposite	29.15	19.58	51.27	12.95	38.32	0.76	1.51	2.07
CO nanocomposite	36.1	4.72	59.19	13.07	46.12	0.78	0.36	4.62
RS nanocomposite	33.89	8.88	57.23	12.85	44.38	0.76	0.70	3.60

O* = O atom in RGO (At.%). O** = O in Sn_3O_4 (At.%).

Table 2. The fitting results of C1s XPS spectrum of OS, CO, and RS nanocomposites.

Samples	Carbon Bonding	Binding Energy (eV)	At. (%)	Relative Percentage (%)
OS nanocomposite	C-C	284.6	5.35	27.33
	C-O	285.2	6.67	34.05
	C=O	287.8	7.55	38.60
CO nanocomposite	C-C	284.6	1.68	34.93
	C-O	285.5	1.57	33.25
	C=O	289.2	1.50	31.81
RS nanocomposite	C-C	284.6	3.69	41.61
	C-O	285.6	2.18	24.62
	C=O	289.1	2.99	33.76

Table 3. The fitting results of O1s XPS spectrum of OS, CO, and RS nanocomposites.

Samples	Oxygen Species	Binding Energy (eV)	At (%)	Relative Percentage (%)
OS nanocomposite	O_L (Sn-O)	530.8	8.85	17.26
	O_v (vacancy)	531.3	14.58	28.44
	O_c (chemisorbed)	531.8	14.87	29.01
	C=O	532.6	12.96	25.27
CO nanocomposite	O_L (Sn-O)	530.7	10.65	17.99
	O_v (vacancy)	531.2	17.41	29.41
	O_c (chemisorbed)	531.7	18.06	30.51
	C=O	532.4	13.07	22.07
RS nanocomposite	O_L (Sn-O)	530.7	10.52	18.38
	O_v (vacancy)	531.2	16.85	29.45
	O_c (chemisorbed)	531.7	17.0	29.70
	C=O	532.4	12.85	22.46

3.3. Sensing Response

The sensing properties of the as-prepared nanocomposites sensor were tested for different sub-ppm concentrations of CH_3COOH gas. The gas concentration varied from 0.3 to 6 ppm and the testing was carried out under room temperature at normal atmospheric pressure. Before the gas testing, the current–voltage characteristics of all Sn_3O_4-RGO-based sensors were measured by SMU Keithley 2410. As can be seen in Figure 7a, all three devices showed linear I–V characteristics over the voltage range from 0 to 10 V, which indicated Sn_3O_4-RGO is typical of ohmic electrical contact with electrodes. The corresponding initial resistance and operating power values of devices with CO, OS, and RS sensing materials are 1.24 MΩ, 19.23 kΩ, and 79.5 MΩ, and 3.24 µW, 0.2 mW, and 0.81 µW, respectively. During the sensing, the average power consumption increased to an average of 3.6 µW, 0.25 mW, and 3.9 µW, respectively. Plots for resistance for each device can be found in the Supplementary File. The high conductivity of the CO device is due to enormous Sn_3O_4 nanoparticles which were also confirmed by XPS analysis (Table 1) that could possibly behave similar to metallic wires on RGO sheets.

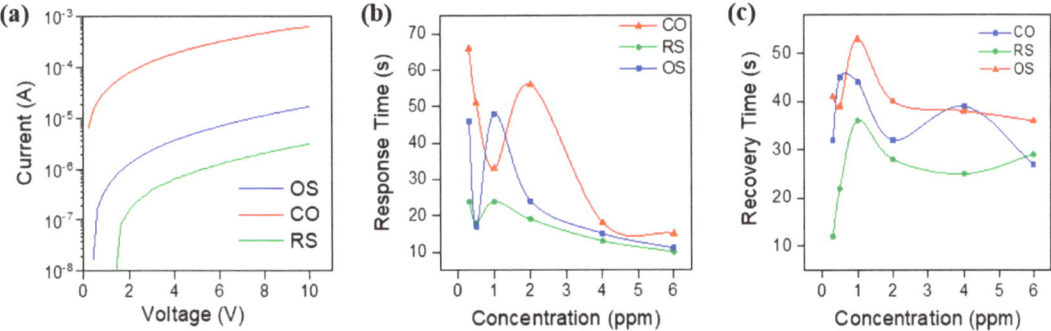

Figure 7. (a) I–V characteristic curve, (b,c) the response and recovery time of the Sn_3O_4-RGO-based sensor to various concentrations CH_3COOH at room temperature.

Figure 7b,c illustrates the response and recovery curves over time for each CH_3COOH concentration. The response and recovery time are defined by the time taken by a sensor to achieve 90% of the total resistance change. From the response curve, it can be clearly observed that generally, all three devices showed faster response with increasing concentration, although at a low concentration of below 1 ppm all three sensors provide a slow response rate. This could be attributed to the lower coverage of CH_3COOH gas molecules to react with adsorbed oxygen ions, hence the change in resistance also takes place slowly. Comparatively, all three sensors could recover to their original condition with a fast recovery rate at a low concentration below 1 ppm. A good sensor should have a high value of response and a fast value for response and recovery time. The Sn_3O_4-RGO-RS sensor presents a more remarkable sensing performance as it exhibits a fast response and shorter recovery time compared to the other two sensors.

Figure 8a–f demonstrates the individual transient response and recovery curves of the three sensors exposed to various CH_3COOH concentrations. Each exposure and recovery cycle is carried out in a 90 s interval under gas exposure followed by a recovery interval of 90 s under dry air conditions. Each cycle is indicated by the white area in the graph marking the start and end. Clearly, the corresponding response values of the lowest concentration 0.3 ppm are about 1.4% (t_{res} = 66 s, t_{rec} = 41 s) and 0.4% (t_{res} = 46 s, t_{rec} = 32 s) detected by OS nanocomposite and CO nanocomposite, respectively. The fluctuating response in Sn_3O_4-RGO-RS (4%) might be due to local carrier annihilations from the recombination of the electron with hole puddles in RGO. On the other hand, it can be clearly observed that the response of the RS nanocomposite sensor is much higher than that of the OS and CO sensors. When the sensor is exposed to the concentrations of 0.5, 1, 2, 4, and 6 ppm, the corresponding response values are about 25.9%, 52%, 72.3%, 73%, and 73.4% respectively.

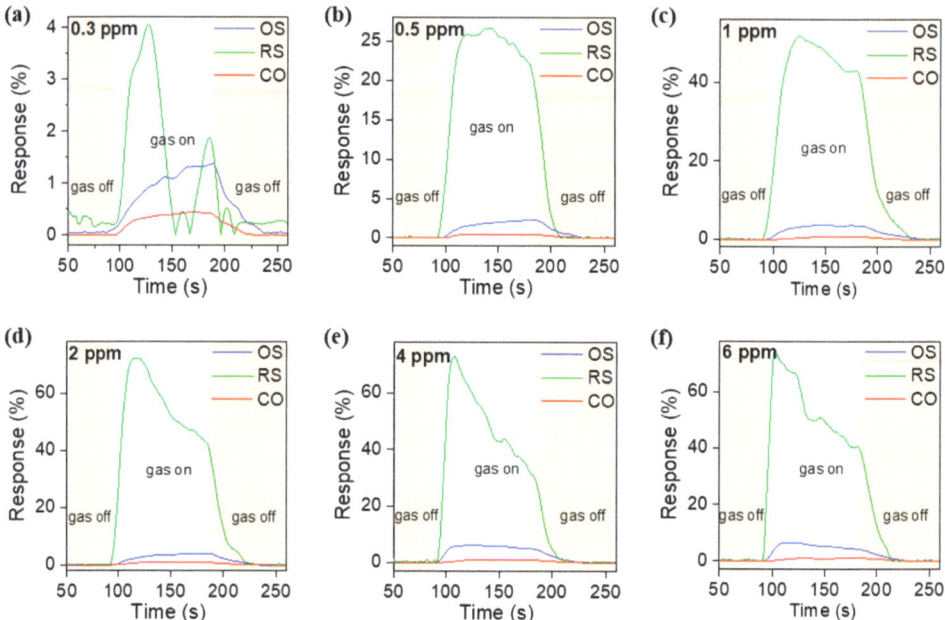

Figure 8. Real-time response–recovery curves of Sn$_3$O$_4$-RGO gas sensors under different CH$_3$COOH concentrations: (**a**) 0.3 ppm, (**b**) 0.5 ppm, (**c**) 1 ppm, (**d**) 2 ppm, (**e**) 4 ppm, and (**f**) 6 ppm.

The response curve of Sn$_3$O$_4$–RGO-based gas sensors to various sub-ppm CH$_3$COOH concentrations was plotted in Figure 9a. Obviously, the response of all three sensors revealed an exponential trend at the beginning and reached saturation at a higher sub-ppm concentration, making 2 ppm the upper limit of detection. Variation of the response as a function of concentration is termed sensitivity, S, which is one of the most important criteria in gas sensing. The RS nanocomposite showed the highest sensitivity of 65.4%/ppm among the other two, OS nanocomposites (S = 3.03%/ppm) and CO nanocomposite (S = 0.45%/ppm). Figure 9b depicts the dynamic transient sensing response of Sn$_3$O$_4$-RGO-RS to 1 ppm CH$_3$COOH. It is unambiguous that the Sn$_3$O$_4$-RGO-RS sensor can maintain consistent response/recovery characteristics during the four cycles of the test, demonstrating good repeatability of the device.

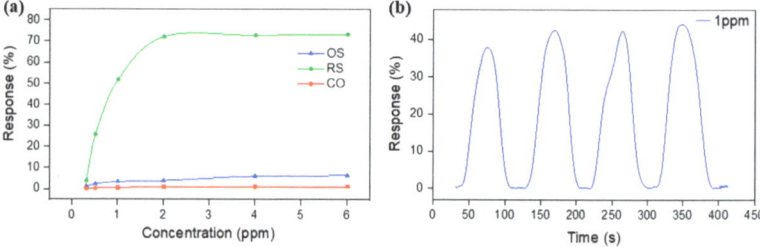

Figure 9. (**a**) Relationship between the sensing response of the Sn$_3$O$_4$-RGO-based sensor and CH$_3$COOH concentration. (**b**) Dynamic transient response curves of the Sn$_3$O$_4$-RGO-RS sensor to 1 ppm CH$_3$COOH during the four cycles of the test.

A comparison of previously reported gas sensors based on sensing materials in terms of their sensing properties toward CH$_3$COOH is summarized in Table 4. In contrast to other materials, our Sn$_3$O$_4$-RGO-based sensor shows excellent CH$_3$COOH sensing performances, including very high response and low limits of detection with acceptable response and recovery rate. Moreover, it provides an effective and simple method for the development of a CH_3COOH gas sensor with good sensitivity and repeatability at room temperature.

Table 4. Summary of CH_3COOH sensors is based on different sensing materials reported in the literature and this work.

Material	Operating Temp. (°C)	Concentration (ppm)	Response (%)	Response Time, t_{res} (s)	Recovery Time, t_{rec} (s)	Ref.
Hierarchical SnO_2 nanoflowers	260	100	47.7	18	11	[46]
Porous flower-like SnO_2	340	20	5.0	11	6	[47]
Mg-doped ZnO/rGO composites	250	100	200	60	35	[48]
Pr-doped ZnO nanofibers	380	400	7.38	51	40	[49]
CdS_xSe_{1-x} nanoribbons	200	100	5.7	80	50	[50]
Mesoporous CuO	200	10	5.6	79	53	[51]
$MgGa_2O_4$/graphene composites	RT	100	363	50	35	[39]
4HQ-rGO/Cu composite	RT	500	1.75	5	5	[40]
Sn_3O_4-RGO-RS nanocomposite	RT	2	74	15	36	This work
Sn_3O_4-RGO-RS nanocomposite	RT	0.3	4	25	11	This work

RT = Room temperature.

3.4. Sensing Mechanism

The above results demonstrated the high-performance CH_3COOH sensing properties of the Sn_3O_4-RGO sensor. As we know, Sn_3O_4 is an n-type semiconductor [41] and RGO nanosheets synthesized using chemical or low thermal treatments exhibit p-type semiconductor characteristics [52]. We proposed two possible sensing mechanisms: (i) the adsorption–desorption pathway on the surface of Sn_3O_4 nanoparticles, and (ii) the formation of Sn_3O_4-RGO heterojunction. Figure 10a illustrates a schematic of the boundary barrier model of Sn_3O_4 grains. When the CH_3COOH sensor is exposed to clean air, the oxygen molecules in the atmosphere are adsorbed onto the surface of the Sn_3O_4 and then capture free conduction electrons creating oxygen anions (O^-, O_2^-) on the surface of the material. This process forms a depletion layer (DL), reduces carrier concentration at the junction, and therefore, displays a high resistance reading. When the sensor is exposed to the targeted gas, the CH_3COOH molecules desorb, or remove the oxygen anions, from the material's surface. As a result, tremendous free electrons are released back into the conduction band of Sn_3O_4, thereby narrowing the electron depletion layer 1 (DL1) and reducing the resistance value.

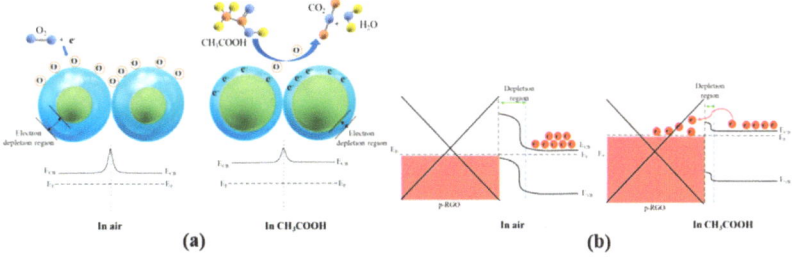

Figure 10. Schematic illustration of sensing mechanism of (a) Sn_3O_4-Sn_3O_4 nanoparticles, (b) Sn_3O_4-RGO nanocomposites.

On another note, based on the TEM image (Figure 5e), most of the Sn_3O_4 nanoparticles are not uniformly distributed on the RGO, and prefer to clump and overlap each other, which is also confirmed by the XPS data where there is an abundant O_v and O_c observed in the CO nanocomposite. However, due to their tendency to clump together, the absorption surface becomes smaller than it should be. This could be the reason for poor contact between RGO and Sn_3O_4 nanoparticles, leading to its poor sensing performances compared to the other two nanocomposites. The possible interaction involved in CH_3COOH gas sensing is as follows [45]:

$$O_2 \text{ (gas)} + 2e^- \rightarrow 2O^- \text{ (ads)} \tag{5}$$

$$CH_3COOH \text{ (ads)} + 4O^- \text{ (ads)} \rightarrow 2CO_2 + 2H_2O + 4e^- \tag{6}$$

Figure 10b reveals another underlying mechanism for the Sn_3O_4-RGO sensor as it introduces a heterojunction between Sn_3O_4 and RGO. Generally, when the sensor is exposed to the air, three types of electron DL could possibly be formed. DL1 formed on the surface of Sn_3O_4 nanoparticles owing to the adsorbed oxygen ions. Meanwhile, the formation of DL2 is by the electrons and transfers from the surface of Sn_3O_4 to the RGO during the formation of heterojunctions. By the third electron depletion, DL3 appears in the area where Sn_3O_4 is embedded in RGO nanosheets and forms the heterojunctions. All these electron depletion layers prevent the migration of electrons, resulting in a high-resistance state of the nanocomposites. When CH_3COOH gas is introduced, the width of all these three DLs will undergo different changes. The trapped electrons in the DL1 will be released back to the Sn_3O_4, decreasing the width of the DL1. DL2 and DL3 are supposed to be narrowed because the reducing CH_3COOH gas molecules may be adsorbed on the surface of RGO and donate the electrons to the RGO lattice, leading to a reduced efficacy of the junction barrier. The Sn_3O_4-RGO-RS nanocomposite exhibited superior sensing properties mainly attributed to its spherical 3D nanostructure and its formation on the RGO sheet. Compared with the other two CO and OS nanocomposites, this sensing film has more embedded and uniformly wrapped Sn_3O_4 nanoparticles on RGO sheets (DL2 and DL3 condition), which is also confirmed by TEM images (Figure 5k) As a result, the magnitude of thermionic emission current is increased during CH_3COOH exposure due to massive relative change in electron concentration.

4. Conclusions

In summary, three Sn_3O_4-RGO nanocomposites were successfully synthesized via three different facile assembly methods. A comparative analysis of nanocomposite assembly was carried out to investigate their performance on CH_3COOH sensing properties. The Sn_3O_4-RGO-RS nanocomposite showed a higher response and sensitivity, faster response, and faster recovery behavior to CH_3COOH compared with another two nanocomposites. The experimental data confirm a clear correlation between surface structures of Sn_3O_4 and distribution of Sn_3O_4 on RGO nanosheets, which influenced their sensing behavior towards CH_3COOH. The present study provides an effective approach that could speed up the development of highly sensitive room temperature CH_3COOH sensors.

Supplementary Materials: The following supporting information can be downloaded at: https://www.mdpi.com/article/10.3390/molecules27248707/s1, Figure S1: Resistance changes measured in the 0.3–6 ppm range of CH_3COOH exposure under (a) OS nanocomposite, (b) CO nanocomposite and (c) RS nanocomposite sensor.

Author Contributions: Conceptualization, N.A.A.; methodology, N.A.A. and S.A.M.B.; validation, N.A.A. and M.F.A.; formal analysis, N.A.A. and M.F.A.; data curation writing—original draft preparation, N.A.A.; writing—review and editing, N.A.A. and M.F.A.; supervision, A.M.H. and M.R.M.H. All authors have read and agreed to the published version of the manuscript.

Funding: This research was funded by Research University Grant UKM (GUP-2019-014) and UTMFR-22H16.

Data Availability Statement: Not applicable.

Acknowledgments: N. A. Aziz thanks the Ministry of Higher Education for the post-doctoral fellowship. This work is financially supported by Research University Grant UKM (GUP-2019-014) and UTMFR-22H16.

Conflicts of Interest: The authors declare no conflict of interest.

References

1. Khan, M.A.H.; Rao, M.V.; Li, Q. Recent Advances in Electrochemical Sensors for Detecting Toxic Gases: NO_2, SO_2 and H_2S. *Sensors* **2019**, *4*, 905. [CrossRef] [PubMed]
2. Kus, F.; Altinkok, C.; Zayim, E.; Erdemir, S.; Tasaltin, C.; Gurol, I. Surface acoustic wave (SAW) sensor for volatile organic compounds (VOCs) detection with calix[4]arene functionalized Gold nanorods (AuNRs) and silver nanocubes (AgNCs). *Sens. Actuators B Chem.* **2021**, *330*, 129402. [CrossRef]
3. Chen, Q.; Liang, L.; Zheng, Q.L.; Zhang, Y.X.; Wen, L. On-chip readout plasmonic mid-IR gas sensor. *Opto-Electron. Adv.* **2020**, *3*, 190040. [CrossRef]
4. Duffy, E.; Cauven, E.; Morrin, A. Colorimetric Sensing of Volatile Organic Compounds Produced from Heated Cooking Oils. *ACS Omega* **2021**, *11*, 7394–7401. [CrossRef] [PubMed]
5. Tao, Y.; Cao, X.; Peng, Y.; Liu, Y.; Zhang, R. Cataluminescence sensor for gaseous acetic acid using a thin film of In_2O_3. *Microchim. Acta* **2012**, *176*, 485–491. [CrossRef]
6. Hosaini, P.N.; Khan, M.F.; Mustaffa, N.I.H.; Amil, N.; Mohamad, N.; Jaafar, S.A.; Nadzir, M.S.M.; Latif, M.T. Concentration and source apportionment of volatile organic compounds (VOCs) in the ambient air of Kuala Lumpur, Malaysia. *Nat. Hazards* **2017**, *85*, 437–452. [CrossRef]
7. Wang, Y.-C.; Sun, Z.-S.; Wang, S.-Z.; Wang, S.-Y.; Cai, S.-X.; Huang, X.-Y.; Li, K.; Chi, Z.-T.; Pan, S.-D.; Xie, W.-F. Sub-ppm acetic acid gas sensor based on In_2O_3 nanofibers. *J. Mater. Sci.* **2019**, *54*, 14055–14063. [CrossRef]
8. Ahmadipour, M.; Pang, A.L.; Ardani, M.R.; Pung, S.-Y.; Ooi, P.C.; Hamzah, A.A.; Wee, M.M.R.; Haniff, M.A.S.M.; Dee, C.F.; Mahmoudi, E.; et al. Detection Of Breath Acetone By Semiconductor Metal Oxide Nanostructures-Based Gas Sensors: A Review. *Mater. Sci. Semicond. Process.* **2022**, *149*, 106897. [CrossRef]
9. Moseley, P.T. Progress in the development of semiconducting metal oxide gas sensors: A review. *Meas. Sci. Technol.* **2017**, *28*, 082001. [CrossRef]
10. Mirzaei, A.; Leonardi, S.G.; Neri, G. Detection of hazardous volatile organic compounds (VOCs) by metal oxide nanostructures-based gas sensors: A review. *Ceram. Int.* **2016**, *42*, 15119–15141. [CrossRef]
11. Tee, T.S.; Hui, T.C.; Yi, C.W.; Chin, Y.C.; Umar, A.A.; Titian, G.R.; Beng, L.H.; Sing, L.K.; Yahaya, M.; Salleh, M.M. Microwave-Assisted Hydrolysis Preparation Of Highly Crystalline Zno Nanorod Array For Room Temperature Photoluminescence-Based Co Gas Sensor. *Sens. Actuators B Chem.* **2016**, *227*, 304–312.
12. Sopiha, K.V.; Oleksandr, I.; Malyi, O.I.; Persson, C.; Wu, P. Chemistry of Oxygen Ionosorption on SnO_2 Surfaces. *ACS Appl. Mater. Interfaces* **2021**, *13*, 33664–33676. [CrossRef] [PubMed]
13. Guo, L.; Wang, Y.; Zeng, H.; Feng, Y.; Yang, X.; Zhang, S.; Xu, Y.; Wang, G.; Wang, Y.; Zhang, Z. Rational Design of SnO_2 Hollow Microspheres Functionalized with Derivatives of Pt Loaded MOFs for Superior Formaldehyde Detection. *Nanomaterials* **2022**, *12*, 1881. [CrossRef]
14. Zhang, R.; Zhou, T.; Wang, L.; Lou, Z.; Deng, J.; Zhang, T. The synthesis and fast ethanol sensing properties of core–shell SnO_2@ZnO composite nanospheres using carbon spheres as templates. *New J. Chem.* **2016**, *40*, 6796–6802. [CrossRef]
15. Zeng, W.; Liu, Y.; Mei, J.; Tang, C.; Luo, K.; Li, S.; Zhan, H.; He, Z. Hierarchical SnO_2–Sn_3O_4 heterostructural gas sensor with high sensitivity and selectivity to NO_2. *Sens. Actuators B Chem.* **2019**, 127010. [CrossRef]
16. Shanmugasundaram, A.; Basak, P.; Satyanarayana, L.; Manorama, S.V. Hierarchical SnO/SnO_2 nanocomposites: Formation of in situ p–n junctions and enhanced H_2 sensing. *Sens. Actuators B Chem.* **2013**, *185*, 265–273. [CrossRef]
17. Li, L.; Zhang, C.; Chen, W. Fabrication of SnO_2-SnO nanocomposites with p-n heterojunctions for the low-temperature sensing of NO_2 gas. *Nanoscale* **2015**, *7*, 12133–12142. [CrossRef]
18. Yu, H.; Yang, T.; Wang, Z.; Li, Z.; Zhao, Q.; Zhang, M. p-N heterostructural sensor with SnO-SnO_2 for fast NO_2 sensing response properties at room temperature. *Sens. Actuators B Chem.* **2018**, *258*, 517–526. [CrossRef]
19. Mäkijaskari, M.A.; Rantala, T.T. Possible structures of nonstoichiometric tin oxide: The composition Sn_2O_3. *Model. Simul. Mat. Sci. Eng.* **2004**, *12*, 33–41. [CrossRef]
20. Berengue, O.M.; Simon, R.A.; Chiquito, A.J.; Dalmaschio, C.J.; Leite, E.R.; Guerreiro, H.A.; Guimarães, F.E.G. Semiconducting Sn_3O_4 nanobelts: Growth and electronic structure. *J. Appl. Phys.* **2010**, *107*, 033717. [CrossRef]
21. Ma, X.; Shen, J.; Hu, D.; Sun, L.; Chen, Y.; Liu, M.; Li, C.; Ruan, S. Preparation of three-dimensional Ce-doped Sn_3O_4 hierarchical microsphere and its application on formaldehyde gas sensor. *J. Alloys Compd.* **2017**, *726*, 1092–1100. [CrossRef]
22. Liu, J.; Wang, C.; Yang, Q.; Gao, Y.; Zhou, X.; Liang, X.; Sun, P.; Lu, G. Hydrothermal synthesis and gas-sensing properties of flower-like Sn_3O_4. *Sens. Actuators B Chem.* **2016**, *224*, 128–133. [CrossRef]
23. Wang, J.; Umezawa, N.; Hosono, H. Mixed Valence Tin Oxides as Novel van der Waals Materials: Theoretical Predictions and Potential Application. *Adv. Energy Mater.* **2016**, *6*, 1501190. [CrossRef]

24. Hoa, N.D.; Duy, N.V.; El-Safty, S.A.; Hieu, N.V. Meso-/Nanoporous semiconducting metal oxides for gas sensor applications. *J. Nanomater.* **2015**, *16*, 186. [CrossRef]
25. Fu, D.C.; Yeop Majlis, B.; Hamzah, A.A.; Choon, O.P.; Mohamed, M.A.; Yaw, T.T. Ultraviolet Light-Assisted Copper Oxide Nanowires Hydrogen Gas Sensor. *Nanoscale Res. Lett.* **2018**, *13*, 150–156.
26. Xu, Y.; Zheng, L.; Yang, C.; Zheng, W.; Liu, X.; Zhang, J. Oxygen Vacancies Enabled Porous SnO_2 Thin Films for Highly Sensitive Detection of Triethylamine at Room Temperature. *ACS Appl. Mater. Interfaces* **2020**, *12*, 20704–20713. [CrossRef]
27. Norizan, M.N.; Abdullah, N.; Halim, N.A.; Demon, S.Z.N.; Mohamad, I.S. Heterojunctions of rGO/Metal Oxide Nanocomposites as Promising Gas-Sensing Materials—A Review. *Nanomaterials* **2022**, *12*, 2278. [CrossRef]
28. Hashtroudi, H.; Yu, A.; Juodkazis, S.; Shafiei, M. Two-Dimensional Dy_2O_3-Pd-PDA/rGO Heterojunction Nanocomposite: Synergistic Effects of Hybridisation, UV Illumination and Relative Humidity on Hydrogen Gas Sensing. *Chemosensors* **2022**, *10*, 78. [CrossRef]
29. Zhang, H.; Guo, Y.; Meng, F. Metal Oxide Semiconductor Sensors for Triethylamine Detection: Sensing Performance and Improvements. *Chemosensors* **2022**, *10*, 231. [CrossRef]
30. Lei, G.; Pan, H.; Mei, H.; Liu, X.; Lu, G.; Lou, C.; Li, Z.; Zhang, J. Emerging single atom catalysts in gas sensors. *Chem. Soc. Rev.* **2022**, *51*, 7260–7280. [CrossRef]
31. Ho, K.C.; Teow, Y.H.; Mohammad, A.W.; Ang, W.L.; Lee, P.H. Development of graphene oxide (GO)/multi-walled carbon nanotubes (MWCNTs) nanocomposite conductive membranes for electrically enhanced fouling mitigation. *J. Membr. Sci.* **2018**, *552*, 189–201. [CrossRef]
32. Allaedini, G.; Mahmoudi, E.; Aminayi, P.; Tasirin, S.M.; Mohammad, A.W. Optical investigation of reduced graphene oxide and reduced graphene oxide/CNTs grown via simple CVD method. *Synth. Met.* **2016**, *220*, 72–77. [CrossRef]
33. Gupta, M.; Hawari, H.F.; Kumar, P.; Burhanudin, Z.A. Copper Oxide/Functionalized Graphene Hybrid Nanostructures for Room Temperature Gas Sensing Applications. *Crystals* **2022**, *12*, 264. [CrossRef]
34. Lee, Z.Y.; Hawari, H.F.B.; Djaswadi, G.W.B.; Kamarudin, K. A Highly Sensitive Room Temperature CO_2 Gas Sensor Based on SnO_2-rGO Hybrid Composite. *Materials* **2021**, *14*, 522. [CrossRef] [PubMed]
35. Jin, L.; Chen, W.; Zhang, H.; Xiao, G.; Yu, C.; Zhou, Q. Characterization of Reduced Graphene Oxide (rGO)-Loaded SnO_2 Nanocomposite and Applications in C_2H_2 Gas Detection. *Appl. Sci.* **2017**, *7*, 19. [CrossRef]
36. Zhang, H.; Cen, Y.; Du, Y.; Ruan, S. Enhanced Acetone Sensing Characteristics of ZnO/Graphene Composites. *Sensors* **2016**, *16*, 1876. [CrossRef]
37. Lee, E.; Lee, D.; Yoon, J.; Yin, Y.; Lee, Y.N.; Uprety, S.; Yoon, Y.S.; Kim, D.-J. Enhanced Gas-Sensing Performance of GO/TiO_2 Composite by Photocatalysis. *Sensors* **2018**, *18*, 3334. [CrossRef]
38. Wang, Z.; Han, T.; Fei, T.; Liu, S.; Zhang, T. Investigation of Microstructure Effect on NO_2 Sensors Based on SnO_2 Nanoparticles/Reduced Graphene Oxide Hybrids. *ACS Appl. Mater. Interfaces* **2018**, *48*, 41773–41783. [CrossRef]
39. Suman, P.H.; Felix, A.A.; Tuller, H.L.; Varela, J.A.; Orlandi, M.O. Comparative gas sensor response of SnO_2, SnO and Sn_3O_4 nanobelts to NO_2 and potential interferents. *Sens. Actuators B Chem.* **2015**, *208*, 122–127. [CrossRef]
40. Suman, P.H.; Longo, E.; Varela, J.A.; Orlandi, M.O. Controlled synthesis of layered Sn_3O_4 nanobelts by carbothermal reduction method and their gas sensor properties. *J. Nanosci. Nanotechnol.* **2014**, *14*, 6662–6668. [CrossRef]
41. He, L.; Gao, C.; Yang, L.; Zhang, K.; Chu, X.; Liang, S.; Zeng, D. Facile synthesis of $MgGa_2O_4$/graphene composites for room temperature acetic acid gas sensing. *Sens. Actuators B Chem.* **2020**, *306*, 127453. [CrossRef]
42. Gong, Y.; Li, H.; Pei, W.; Fan, J.; Umar, A.; Al-Assiri, M.S.; Wang, Y.; Rooija, N.F.; Zhou, G. Assembly with copper(ii) ions and D–π–A molecules on a graphene surface for ultra-fast acetic acid sensing at room temperature. *RSC Adv.* **2019**, *9*, 30432–30438. [CrossRef] [PubMed]
43. Yin, F.; Li, Y.; Yue, W.; Gao, S.; Zhang, C.; Chen, Z. Sn_3O_4/rGO heterostructure as a material for formaldehyde gas sensor with a wide detecting range and low operating temperature. *Sens. Actuators B Chem.* **2020**, *312*, 127954. [CrossRef]
44. Pham, V.T.; Trung, H.L.; Tran, N.K.; Manh, H.C.; Duc, H.N.; Quynh, H.T.T.; Pham, T.H. Hydrothermal synthesis, structure, and photocatalytic properties of SnO_2/rGO nanocomposites with different GO concentrations. *Mater. Res. Express* **2018**, *5*, 095506. [CrossRef]
45. Wang, Z.; Zhang, T.; Han, T.; Fei, T.; Liu, S.; Lu, G. Oxygen vacancy engineering for enhanced sensing performances: A case of SnO_2 nanoparticles-reduced graphene oxide hybrids for ultrasensitive ppb-level room-temperature NO_2 sensing. *Sens. Actuators B Chem.* **2018**, *226*, 812–822. [CrossRef]
46. Jin, W.; Ma, S.; Tie, Z.; Li, W.; Luo, J.; Cheng, L.; Xu, X.; Wang, T.; Jiang, X.; Mao, Y. Synthesis of hierarchical SnO_2 nanoflowers with enhanced acetic acid gas sensing properties. *Appl. Surf. Sci.* **2015**, *353*, 71–78. [CrossRef]
47. Wang, T.T.; Ma, S.Y.; Cheng, L.; Xu, X.L.; Luo, J.; Jiang, X.H.; Li, W.Q.; Jin, W.X.; Sun, X.X. Performance of 3D SnO_2 microstructure with porous nanosheets for acetic acid sensing. *Mater. Lett.* **2015**, *142*, 141–144. [CrossRef]
48. Khorramshahi, V.; Karamdel, J.; Yousefi, R. Acetic acid sensing of Mg-doped ZnO thin films fabricated by the sol–gel method. *J. Mater. Sci. Mater. Electron.* **2018**, *29*, 14679–14688. [CrossRef]
49. Wang, S.; Ma, A.; Sun, R.; Qin, F.; Yang, X.; Li, F.; Li, X.; Yang, X. Characterization of electrospun Pr-doped ZnO nanostructure for acetic acid sensor. *Sens. Actuators B Chem.* **2014**, *193*, 326–333. [CrossRef]
50. Jie, Z.; Fan, L.; Yan, Z.; Sun, J.; Shao, M. Visible-light-enhanced gas sensing of CdS_xSe_{1-x} nanoribbons for acetic acid at room temperature. *Sens. Actuators B Chem.* **2015**, *215*, 497–503.

51. Geng, W.; Ma, Z.; Yang, J.; Duan, L.; Li, F.; Zhang, Q. Pore size dependent acetic acid gas sensing performance of mesoporous CuO. *Sens Actuators B Chem.* **2021**, *334*, 129639. [CrossRef]
52. Abdullah, M.F. Defect Repair of Thermally Reduced Graphene Oxide by Gold Nanoparticles as a p-Type Transparent Conductor. *J. Electron. Mater.* **2021**, *50*, 6795–6803. [CrossRef]

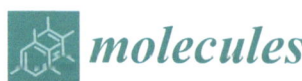 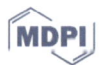

Article

Optical Anisotropy of Porphyrin Nanocrystals Modified by the Electrochemical Dissolution

Rossella Yivlialin *, Claudia Filoni, Francesco Goto, Alberto Calloni, Lamberto Duò, Franco Ciccacci and Gianlorenzo Bussetti

Department of Physics, Politecnico di Milano, p.zza Leonardo da Vinci 32, 20133 Milano, Italy
* Correspondence: rossella.yivlialin@polimi.it

Abstract: Reflectance anisotropy spectroscopy (RAS) coupled to an electrochemical cell represents a powerful tool to correlate changes in the surface optical anisotropy to changes in the electrochemical currents related to electrochemical reactions. The high sensitivity of RAS in the range of the absorption bands of organic systems, such as porphyrins, allows us to directly correlate the variations of the optical anisotropy signal to modifications in the solid-state aggregation of the porphyrin molecules. By combining in situ RAS to electrochemical techniques, we studied the case of vacuum-deposited porphyrin nanocrystals, which have been recently observed dissolving through electrochemical oxidation in diluted sulfuric acid. Specifically, we could identify the first stages of the morphological modifications of the nanocrystals, which we could attribute to the single-electron transfers involved in the oxidation reaction; in this sense, the simultaneous variation of the optical anisotropy with the electron transfer acts as a precursor of the dissolution process of porphyrin nanocrystals.

Keywords: reflectance spectroscopy; porphyrin; dissolution; organic crystals; cyclic voltammetry; AFM

Citation: Yivlialin, R.; Filoni, C.; Goto, F.; Calloni, A.; Duò, L.; Ciccacci, F.; Bussetti, G. Optical Anisotropy of Porphyrin Nanocrystals Modified by the Electrochemical Dissolution. *Molecules* **2022**, *27*, 8010. https://doi.org/10.3390/molecules27228010

Academic Editor: Alberto Pettignano

Received: 12 October 2022
Accepted: 15 November 2022
Published: 18 November 2022

Publisher's Note: MDPI stays neutral with regard to jurisdictional claims in published maps and institutional affiliations.

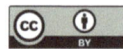

Copyright: © 2022 by the authors. Licensee MDPI, Basel, Switzerland. This article is an open access article distributed under the terms and conditions of the Creative Commons Attribution (CC BY) license (https://creativecommons.org/licenses/by/4.0/).

1. Introduction

Reflectance anisotropy spectroscopy (RAS) has been widely exploited in the past in order to investigate the physical–chemical properties of organic systems featuring different solid phase aggregates and prepared using different growth techniques (Langmuir–Blodgett and Langmuir–Schaefer methods [1,2], physical vapor deposition [3,4], etc.). More specifically, RAS offers the possibility of studying systems that exhibit anisotropies (down to a signal intensity of 10^{-6} [5]) related to the electronic or morphological characteristics of the organic layer, even if it is grown onto an isotropic substrate such as graphite [6]. For instance, this optical spectroscopy has been successfully used to characterize complex 3D nanoarchitectures based on porphyrins layers in order to understand the mechanisms governing their interaction with the environment (i.e., vacuum or vapors), in view of their implementation in organic-based devices and sensors [7–9]. One of the advantages of RAS is the versatility of its experimental configuration, which allows the investigation, in situ, of systems working in different experimental conditions (e.g., UHV, ambient, liquid and gas) [10]. Among the possible environments, liquid media have drawn increasing attention in recent decades, given the increasing interest among the scientific community in the physical processes and chemical/electrochemical reactions occurring specifically at the solid/liquid interfaces [11,12], with the ultimate goal of reproducing or mimicking biological systems. In this respect, successful examples of the application of RAS to inorganic/organic systems studied in an electrochemical cell are the works of Mazine [13], Smith [14], Goletti [15], Barati [16] and Weightman [17]. These works demonstrate that changes in the surface optical anisotropies are strongly correlated with changes in the electrochemical current and that RAS can elucidate details on the atomic and molecular interactions associated with the electrochemical processes.

In the case of porphyrin layers, many studies have focused on the interface using acidic solutions. The morphological/optical evolution of porphyrin layers grown on metal electrodes has been investigated, for instance, by in situ electrochemical atomic force microscopy (EC-AFM) [18,19] and diffuse reflectance spectroscopy, and also *in operando* conditions, i.e., during the activation of electrochemical processes, typically by using cyclic voltammetry (CV) [20]. In particular, some of the authors of the present work recently investigated the particular phenomenon of the dissolution of porphyrin nanocrystals occurring during CVs in acidic solutions [20,21]. There, the possibility of gradually removing porphyrin layers by continuously sweeping the applied EC potential was observed by in situ EC-AFM. However, it was not possible to determine the exact onset of that process by only looking at the morphological evolution of the samples.

In this work, we exploit the coupling between RAS and an EC cell as a powerful tool to precisely determine the early stage of the dissolution process. In fact, by means of the in situ monitoring of the optical anisotropy, we can correlate the oxidation of the porphyrin films to the structural/morphological modifications of the 3D nanocrystals. RAS is used for the direct identification of the EC potential that instantaneously activates modifications in the aggregation state of the molecules in the film, operating as a driving force for the dissolution of the porphyrin nanocrystals.

For this work, a thick layer of porphyrins was vacuum-deposited on a graphite substrate, resulting in the formation of nanocrystals on the surface. This system is well-suited to both RAS and electrochemical techniques for two main reasons: (i) porphyrin nanocrystals in freshly grown samples exhibit a clear anisotropy signal in the Soret-band spectral region [22,23]; (ii) graphite covered with porphyrins behaves as a good working electrode for the electrochemical activities, showing well-defined CV curves [18]. We investigate the oxidation process and the optical/morphological evolution of three types of films, featuring porphyrins with nominally different molecular symmetries: free-base tetraphenylporphyrins (H_2TPP) [24], zinc tetraphenylporphyrins (ZnTPP) [25,26] and iron(tetraphenylporphyrinato) chloride [Fe(TPP)Cl] [27]. These molecules differ one from another in the composition of the inner tetrapyrrolic ring, i.e., due to the presence in the middle of the ring of, respectively, no metal atom, a Zn atom and a Cl-coordinated Fe atom, which potentially influence inter-molecular arrangements and layouts of porphyrin nanocrystals.

2. Results and Discussion

Figure 1 shows the morphology and RAS spectrum of the bare HOPG substrate in air before the vacuum deposition of porphyrin films.

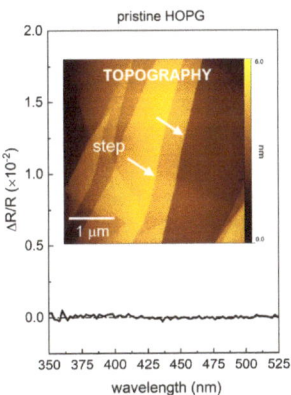

Figure 1. RAS spectrum in the 350–525 nm range of the bare HOPG substrate, acquired in air. The absence of any RAS feature testifies the optical isotropy of HOPG. The AFM image in the inset shows the topography of the HOPG surface in air condition; the white arrows indicate some steps on the surface.

The AFM image shows the typical steps, only a few nm in height, created by the exfoliation of the HOPG surface [28]. The RAS spectrum was acquired as a reference for the subsequent measurement of the porphyrin films, and shows a flat isotropic signal, as expected from the hexagonal symmetry of the HOPG crystal. In the following, we first discuss those samples with a comparable RAS peak line shape: ZnTPP film and H_2TPP films, the latter with a higher peak intensity. Lastly, we consider a Fe(TPP)Cl film, characterized by a different RAS signal.

2.1. ZnTPP Film

After the deposition of the ZnTPP film, the morphology of the sample was checked by AFM in air, before the immersion in the electrolyte. A representative scan is shown in Figure 2a.

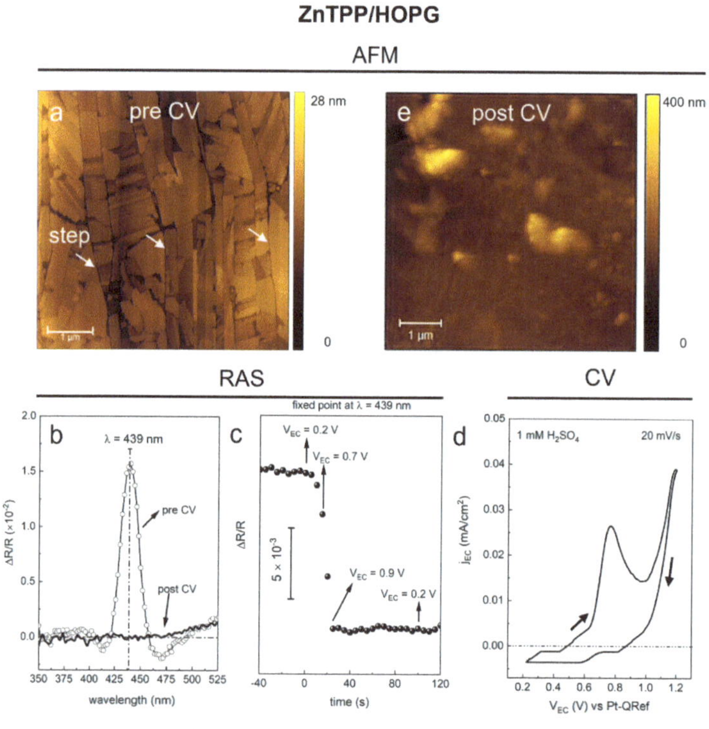

Figure 2. (a) (5 × 5) μm² topographic image of a 6 nm thick ZnTPP/HOPG sample; white arrows points at some steps of the HOPG substrate. The AFM image was acquired ex situ on an as-deposited sample. (b) RAS spectra in the 350–525 nm range, acquired when the sample is in the EC cell filled with a 1 mM H_2SO_4 solution. Spectra acquired before (line + symbol) and after (solid line) the CV are reported. (c) Real-time RAS monitoring of the Soret-related band intensity (λ = 439 nm) during CV in a 1 mM H_2SO_4 solution. The time axis is rescaled to show all the time range covered by the sweep of the EC potentials in the CV; time = 0 s corresponds to the starting point of the CV (V_{EC} = 0.2 V); spectral points are collected every 5 s. The scale of the y-axis is showed by a vertical bar. Arrows and labels indicate the EC potentials reached during the CV. (d) Voltammogram obtained during the CV in a 1 mM H_2SO_4 solution; the potential is swept within the 0.2–1.2 V range, from anodic to cathodic regime (see the black arrows); sweep rate = 20 mV/s; step = 1 mV. (e) (5 × 5) μm² topographic image of the ZnTPP/HOPG sample, acquired ex situ after the EC treatment in a 1 mM H_2SO_4 solution.

For the ZnTPP film, we observe regular 3D porphyrin nanocrystals (about 20 nm high), with sharp edges and angles of almost 90°, laying on a 2D wetting layer [29]. For thick films, the topographic AFM signal gives evidence only of the 3D phase of the sample, due to the extension and high density of the nanocrystals, which hide the 2D wetting layer on the surface.

As extensively discussed by the authors in previous works [22,29], the anisotropy of this kind of samples is maximized when the direction of graphite exfoliation is aligned with the α(β) direction, meaning that ZnTPP nanocrystals are preferentially oriented along the graphite steps. A statistical analysis on all the collected AFM images seems to further confirm this scenario: the image shown in panel *a*, for instance, shows the nanocrystals clearly laying on the graphite terraces, with most of the edges parallel to the steps (see the vertical lines indicated by white arrows).

Since we are interested in the variation of the anisotropy signal when the sample undergoes an electrochemical oxidation in sulfuric acid, the RAS signal was measured on the sample in pristine conditions, as soon as was immersed in the acidic solution and before running the CV. The initial optical anisotropy of the ZnTPP film is clearly visible in the RAS signal (labeled as "pre CV") of Figure 2b, where a main positive RAS peak is observed, centered at 439 nm (FWHM = 20 nm), with an intensity of about 1.6×10^{-2} with respect to the zero line.

This anisotropy arises from the molecular packing in the 3D nanocrystals, since isolated ZnTPP molecules are centrosymmetric, meaning they do not contribute to the overall anisotropy of the sample [22]. A closer inspection of the RAS signal highlights the presence of a negative feature placed at about 470 nm. The overall "pre CV" RAS signal, collected in the Soret-band region, shows the characteristic "derivative-like" shape reported and discussed in the literature [7]. This particular signal behavior directly arises from the superposition of different optical contributions, due to the complex stratified structure of the thin porphyrin films [30,31].

Changes in the RAS signal correlated to chemical processes involving the 3D nanocrystals can be monitored in real-time by following the RAS signal intensity at a fixed wavelength (namely, the one related to the Soret-band at 439 nm) while running the CV. The obtained results are reported in Figure 2c,d.

By comparing panels c and d, we observe that the intensity of the anisotropy signal drastically drops (by about $\frac{1}{4}$ of the initial value) as soon as the EC potential approaches the value of 0.7 V, which corresponds to the onset of the main peak shown in the voltammogram. This peak indicates the presence of an oxidative process, where ZnTPP molecules form radical cation species (V_{EC} = 0.8 V) [20], which anticipates the oxygen evolution reaction (OER) at the sample surface (onset at about V_{EC} = 1.0 V).

Once the V_{EC} = 0.9 V threshold is reached, i.e., after about 25 s from the start of the CV, the RAS anisotropy signal stabilizes around a mean value of zero until the CV is completed (final V_{EC} = 0.2 V, see panel c), with an overall variation of about 1×10^{-2} from the initial value. The disappearance of the optical anisotropy signal from the sample due to the oxidative process is confirmed by the extended RAS spectrum acquired at the end of the CV, as shown in Figure 2b (the spectrum labeled as "post CV"). There, the contrast between the zero signal of the "post CV" spectrum and the sharp peak in the "pre CV" spectrum points out that the EC treatment makes the ZnTPP film, on the macro-scale, optically isotropic in the Soret-band region. As discussed above, the variation of the optical anisotropy of the sample must be related to changes in the morphology or to some removal of the organic layer. In this case, it is likely related to modifications of the 3D nanocrystals. It was already demonstrated by the authors, indeed, that ZnTPP porphyrin nanocrystals undergo some dissolution phenomena during the CVs in acidic solutions [20], while they are stable in static conditions (i.e., when ZnTPP molecules are immersed in the acidic solution, with no EC potential applied) [21].

The morphology shown in Figure 2e confirms the complete loss of crystallinity in the ZnTPP 3D phase of the EC treated sample. The flat paving of the surface created by the dense distribution of regular and oriented nanocrystals, shown in panel a, is replaced by the presence of different agglomerates with irregular shapes and undefined orientations; in addition, graphite steps cannot be distinguished consistently in the case of an amorphous layer covering the substrate [32,33].

2.2. H$_2$TPP Film

A behavior similar to that of ZnTPP was observed for the free base-TPP film. The initial morphology of the H$_2$TPP/HOPG film, observed ex situ on the as-deposited sample, is reported in Figure 3a.

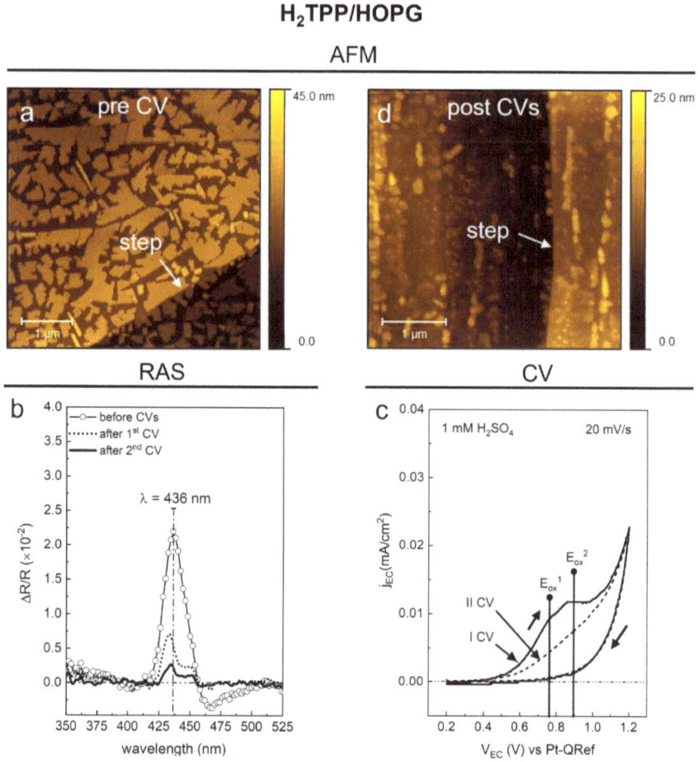

Figure 3. (a) (5 × 5) µm^2 topographic image of the 6 nm thick H$_2$TPP/HOPG sample; the white arrow points at a step of the HOPG substrate. The AFM image was acquired ex situ on the as-deposited sample. (b) RAS spectra in the 350–525 nm range, acquired when the sample is in the EC cell filled with a 1 mM H$_2$SO$_4$ solution. A comparison between three spectra is reported: one acquired before the CVs (line + symbol), a second one after the first CV (dotted line), and a third one after the second CV (solid line). (c) The voltammograms obtained during the two consecutive CVs (labeled as I and II) in a 1 mM H$_2$SO$_4$ solution are shown; range: (0.2–1.2) V, from anodic to cathodic regime; sweep rate = 20 mV/s; step = 1 mV. (d) (3.5 × 3.5) µm^2 topographic image of the H$_2$TPP/HOPG sample, acquired ex situ after the two EC treatments in a 1 mM H$_2$SO$_4$ solution; the white arrow points at one of the steps of the HOPG substrate.

In this figure, 3D porphyrin nanocrystals are shown to be covering the HOPG. In comparison with ZnTPP in Figure 2, nanocrystals look more dendritic, with a lower (about half) surface to volume ratio, calculated by evaluating the bearing area (volume), i.e., the area (volume) of the portion of nanocrystals getting out of the basal plane of the image; the edges and angles are sharp and well-defined, as are the ones observed on the pristine ZnTPP sample. The preferential orientation of the nanocrystals in the exfoliation direction of the HOPG substrate is also confirmed in this case by the RAS azimuthal analysis [29]. The maximum RAS signal is shown in Figure 3b (line + symbol) before the EC treatment.

By comparing it with the "pre CV" spectrum of the ZnTPP sample, we note that the Soret-band shows a similar line shape (FWHM = 20 nm), a blue-shifted spectral position (λ = 436 nm) and a higher intensity of about 2.2×10^{-2}. These small differences in the RAS signal can be reasonably attributed to the different morphology of ZnTPP and H_2TPP nanocrystals.

As for the ZnTPP film, the anisotropy of the thick H_2TPP film originates from the 3D phase of the sample. We point out that, at variance from the ZnTPP case, also the H_2TPP 2D phase shows an intrinsic anisotropy (a RAS feature at about 430 nm with an intensity in the 10^{-3}), created by the alignment the NH-atoms inside the macrocycle of the single molecules along the same direction, as extensively demonstrated by some of the authors [6,22]. However, in the RAS spectrum of Figure 3b, the anisotropy signal coming from the 2D phase is completely hidden by the much more intense signal from the 3D phase (one order of magnitude larger).

The intensity of the Soret-band starts to reduce (evolution not reported here) when the EC potential reaches the value V_{EC} = 0.6 V, during a first CV in a 1 mM H_2SO_4 solution (see "I CV" in Figure 3c). Similar to the ZnTPP case, the anisotropy of the H_2TPP sample is affected by the oxidative process of the molecular film, whose onset is placed at 0.6 V, represented by the appearance of two small anodic features at about V_{EC} = 0.75 V and V_{EC} = 0.9 V in the CV [18]. These features are related to two one-electron oxidation processes (usually called E_{ox}^1, E_{ox}^2) of the H_2TPP molecule which involve the porphine macrocycle and mostly the activity of the inner N atoms [34].

Differently from ZnTPP, the anisotropy of the H_2TPP film is not completely canceled by the EC treatment. In fact, the RAS signal acquired at the end of the first CV (dotted-line, panel b) shows a not-null anisotropy signal where the two main features of the pristine samples are still visible, although with an intensity of about 1/3 of the initial value. A similar line shape is observed, albeit with an even less intense anisotropy signal, after a second CV (full line, panel b); however, the voltammogram of the second CV ("II CV" in panel c) does not clearly show the two one-electron oxidation features observed in the first CV. This behavior suggests that the outer porphyrin layers of the sample, more exposed to the acidic solution, have been fully oxidized or dissolved by the first EC treatment, which modified, without completely removing, the total initial anisotropy of the molecular film. The residual lower anisotropy signal, observed both after the first (dotted-line spectrum) and the second EC treatment (solid line spectrum), indicates that while some H_2TPP layers may have been dissolved during the oxidation, a few layers persist on the HOPG surface [20]. It is worth mentioning that the RAS signal acquired after the second CV shows a shoulder at about 430 nm, with an intensity of about 1.3×10^{-3}. This feature is similar to the anisotropy signal related to the 2D phase observed on thin H_2TPP/HOPG samples, supporting the idea that the EC oxidation causes the dissolution of the uppermost porphyrin layers and the modification of the nanocrystals, making the original thick film closer to a thin H_2TPP film.

An additional note is that the H_2TPP nanocrystals, differently from the ZnTPP ones, are sensitive to the acidic media and undergo etch-pitting phenomena with time, even when they are immersed in a H_2SO_4 solution in static conditions. In the work of ref. [21], it was observed that the etch-pits created on the nanocrystal surface are well-aligned to the crystal edges. Even though the etch-pitting in static conditions is not equivalent to an EC dissolution and is not the focus of the present work, the information gained in our previous work can nevertheless give us an indication of the preferential crystallographic directions involved in the EC dissolution process of the H_2TPP nanocrystals. We speculate that even the dissolution caused by the EC oxidation of the sample starts from the edges of the nanocrystals, thus preserving a certain degree of order in the organic film that we see in the residual anisotropy signals measured after the CV.

The final morphology of the sample, revealed by ex situ AFM, is shown in Figure 3d. As for the ZnTPP 3D phase, the H_2TPP 3D phase after the EC treatment looks quite changed compared to the pristine condition (panel a) and in agreement with previous observations of the morphology of H_2TPP films treated in different kind of acid solutions [18,19]. Differently from the ZnTPP case in Figure 2, here, some form of crystallinity appears to have been preserved and some regular shapes, resembling nanocrystals, are still recognizable; in addition, the prevailing orientation of these 3D structures is still aligned along the HOPG steps. This kind of morphology supports the interpretation of the spectra measured by RAS (Figure 3b), where the residual final anisotropy looks like the convolution of a signal coming from the 2D phase and another one from an electrochemically modified 3D phase.

2.3. Fe(TPP)Cl Film

An example metal-porphyrin with a different molecular symmetry with respect to ZnTPP is represented by Fe(TPP)Cl, the Cl atom being an axial ligand for the Fe atom placed in the middle of the tetrapyrrolic ring. The morphology of the Fe(TPP)Cl/HOPG sample in pristine condition is reported in Figure 4a.

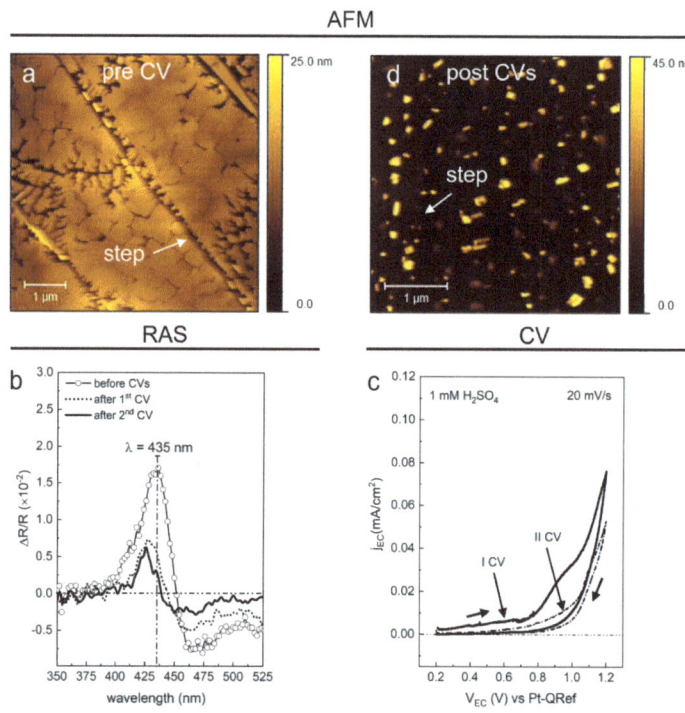

Figure 4. (**a**) (5 × 5) µm² topographic image of the 6 nm thick Fe(TPP)Cl/HOPG sample; the white arrow points at one of the HOPG substrate steps. The AFM image was acquired ex situ on the as-deposited sample. (**b**) RAS spectra in the 350–525 nm range, acquired with the sample in the EC cell filled by a 1 mM H_2SO_4 solution. A comparison between three spectra is reported: one acquired before the CV (line + symbol), a second one after the first CV (dotted line), and a third one after the second CV (solid line). (**c**) Voltammograms obtained during the two consecutive CV (labeled as I and II) in a 1 mM H_2SO_4 solution; range: (0.2–1.2) V, from anodic to cathodic regime; sweep rate = 20 mV/s; step = 1 mV. (**d**) (3.5 × 3.5) µm² topographic image of the Fe(TPP)Cl/HOPG sample acquired ex situ after two EC treatments in a 1 mM H_2SO_4 solution; the white arrow points at one of the steps of the HOPG substrate.

In this case, nanocrystals present different shapes; some of them look like the regular blocks observed on ZnTPP and H_2TPP films, while some others have an irregular and dendritic geometry; again, most of the edges of these structures are aligned to the graphite steps.

The anisotropy signal measured on this sample is labeled as "before CVs" in Figure 4b. As well as for the ZnTPP sample, even for the Fe(TPP)Cl sample, we expect that the main optical anisotropy feature originates from the 3D molecular aggregates. The Soret-band is centered at 435 nm, with an intensity of about 1.7×10^{-2} with respect to the zero line. However, the line shape is more structured than the one observed on the previous samples, presenting a shoulder at 407 nm and a deeper valley at about 470 nm, just before the upcoming Q-bands (not visible in Figure 4b). Interestingly, this result agrees well with the optical spectra measured by Kadish and coworkers on mixed dimeric-monomeric Fe(TPP)Cl systems, where dimers are represented by two porphyrins in the $(Fe^{III}TPP)_2O$ form, held together by a single O ion bridging the metal atoms [35,36]. In our Fe(TPP)Cl sample, the presence of dimeric-monomeric species could be the reason also for the peculiar mixed morphology observed by AFM (see panel a).

The initial RAS signal starts to change during the first CV in sulfuric acid when the EC potential reaches the value of 0.8 V, as we verified by monitoring the Soret-band intensity during the EC process (data not reported here). The voltammogram in panel c shows an anodic feature at about V_{EC} = 0.9 V, just before the OER potential, which corresponds to the single-electron oxidation Fe(III) → Fe(IV) of the middle atom in the porphyrin molecule [36,37]. We speculate that this oxidation proceeds in parallel with a destruction of the porphyrin dimers, leading to variations in the morphology of the Fe(TPP)Cl nanocrystals, as we can argue by looking at the anisotropy signal in the RAS spectrum of panel b labeled "after 1st CV". There, both the intensity and the line shape of the Soret-band were strongly changed, pointing out that a quantitative and qualitative modification of the organic film occurred.

No significant variations of the anisotropy signal, instead, are observed after a second CV ("after 2nd CV" spectrum in panel b), as one could expect by looking at the corresponding featureless voltammogram (dash-dotted line in panel c).

The final morphology of the Fe(TPP)Cl film, as observed by AFM, is reported in Figure 4d. This topographic image shows that the 3D phase was effectively changed from the one we observed in pristine condition. Now, narrower and higher porphyrin aggregates, with almost regular edges, cover the HOPG steps and terraces, and, more interestingly, it is no longer possible to discern the dendritic structures, such as the ones clearly observed in panel a. All these results suggest that the Fe(TPP)Cl dimeric-monomeric system undergoes a structural modification during the oxidation process in sulfuric acid, which implies the disruption of the 3D dendritic phase and the consequent modification of the morphology and optical anisotropy of the porphyrin film.

3. Materials and Methods

3.1. Sample and Solution Preparation

Samples were present in films with a nominal thickness of 6 nm featuring three kinds of tetraphenylporphyrin (TPP) molecules: H_2TPP, ZnTPP and Fe(TPP)Cl (see Scheme 1).

The organic films were deposited in vacuum on highly oriented pyrolytic graphite (HOPG, by Optigraph GmbH, with a mosaic spread of 0.4 degree to ensure a high reflectivity useful for the optical spectroscopy characterization). Before each molecular deposition, HOPG was exfoliated using an adhesive tape always along the same direction, in order to create a preferential orientation for the HOPG steps, thus orienting the porphyrin nanocrystals and ensuring a special direction for the alignment of the RAS apparatus.

The film were grown in an organic molecular beam epitaxy (OMBE) chamber, equipped with heated crucibles for molecular evaporation [38]. The sublimation rate was measured by means of a quartz microbalance and kept at 1 Å/min, corresponding to a sublimation temperature in the range of 260–285 °C for all the molecules. The substrate was kept at RT during the deposition. In these experimental conditions, porphyrins form nanocrystals by following a "layer-plus-island" growth process (i.e., Stranski–Krastanov growth) [23].

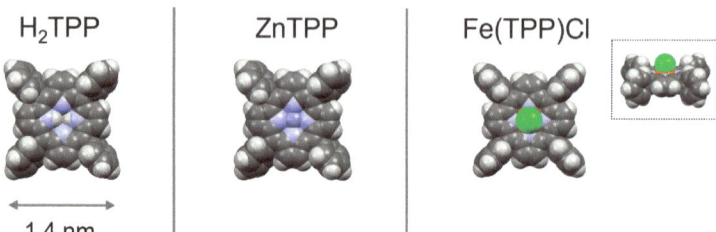

Scheme 1. Sketch of three different porphyrins used in the experiments: dark grey balls = C-atoms; light grey balls = H-atoms; violet balls = N-atoms; dark violet ball = Zn-atom; red ball = Fe-atom; green ball = Cl-atom; the average molecular size is indicated at the bottom. In the Fe(TPP)Cl molecule, the Cl-atom is placed axially on top of the Fe-atom; a side view of the molecule is reported in the inset.

The electrochemical solution consists of 1 mM H_2SO_4 (pH = 3), prepared by diluting in water concentrated H_2SO_4 (95–97% w/w, Merck); the solution was degassed by bubbling pure Ar in a separator funnel for some hours before each experiment.

3.2. RAS Apparatus and EC Cell

The experimental set-up which combines RAS technique to the EC cell is reported in Figure 5.

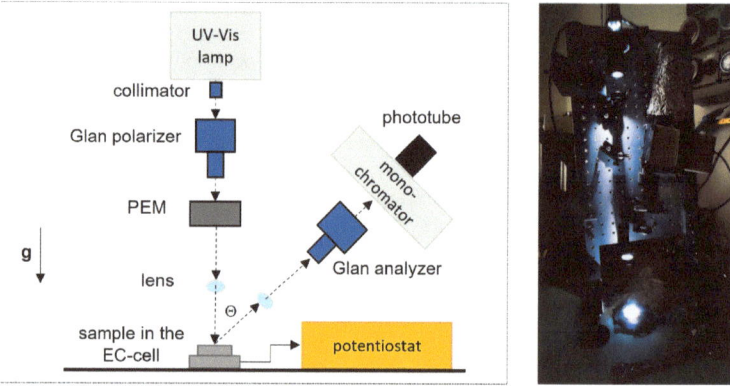

Figure 5. Sketch and picture of the experimental set-up used to couple RAS with the electrochemical measurements. The light beam illuminates the sample from the top-aperture of the EC cell, placed on the table. Reflected light is collected within an angle of about 4° from the impinging beam direction (see the main text for details).

A high-sensitivity homemade RAS apparatus [5] with a light spot diameter of about 5 mm was used to collect the spectra. The light coming from a Xe arc lamp was linearly polarized (α-direction) by a Glan–Thompson optical system and passed through a Photo-Elastic Modulator (PEM), which rotates the light polarization along two mutually orthogonal directions (α and β) at a double frequency with respect to the resonance frequency of 50 kHz. The light beam was properly focused on the sample by a system of lenses and reflected within an angle of few degrees (Θ). Along the reflected light-path, after a second system of lenses, a second Glan polarizer (called analyzer) linearly polarized the light coming from the sample; then, a monochromator and a photomultiplier detector followed.

The RAS signal is defined as the difference in the reflectivity between α and β directions (R_α, R_β) normalized by the total reflectivity ($\overline{R}$):

$$\frac{\Delta R}{\overline{R}} = 2 \frac{R_\alpha(\omega) - R_\beta(\omega)}{R_\alpha(\omega) + R_\beta(\omega)} \tag{1}$$

The anisotropy of the sample is detected by a phase-sensitive lock-in amplifier from EG&G (San Francisco, CA, USA) measuring the signal modulation $\Delta R = R_\alpha - R_\beta$ at the frequency provided by the PEM oscillation.

In the case of thin organic layers, where a complex stratified structure of molecules characterize the film, the reflected light is generally termed as "reflectance", in place of "reflectivity" [39].

It is worth mentioning that the alignment of the sample with respect to the α and β directions of PEM is, *a priori*, unknown; an azimuthal analysis is required to find the maximum of the RAS signal. For the molecular samples analyzed in this work, the maximum value of the anisotropy (in modulus) is reached when the direction of graphite exfoliation is aligned along the α or β direction of PEM (within 10°) [22,29]. RAS measurements were collected in the 330–650 nm wavelength (λ) range; however, in order to focus the discussion on the main porphyrin optical transition, only a shorter range centered on the Soret-transition band at about 436 nm is reported in the text. The evolution of the anisotropy of the samples, which occurs during the EC treatments in solution, was observed by monitoring the variation of the Soret-band intensity while applying different EC potentials to the samples. For this purpose, RAS measurements at fixed λ, corresponding to the spectral position of the Soret-band, were performed by collecting a spectral point every 5 s, according to the sweeping rate used to change the EC potentials during the CV.

To combine the optical spectroscopy with the electrochemistry techniques, in this specific set-up, the RAS apparatus is vertically positioned above the sample. The latter is located inside a home-made three-electrodes EC cell, made of Teflon®, with a top aperture for the light beam. The EC cell is filled by about 1 mL of solution, and the area of the sample surface exposed to the solution is about 20 mm².

The sample represents the working electrode (WE), while two platinum wires are used, respectively, as a counter electrode (CE) and a reference electrode (RE); the latter is a Pt quasi-reference (Pt-QRef) with a stable (within few mV) potential shift of +740 mV vs. a standard hydrogen electrode (SHE) when immersed in acid solution. The EC cell is connected to a potentiostat (PalmSens4) to perform the CV. By running the CV, a linear ramp of potentials is applied to the WE, in the 0.2–1.2 V range, with a sweep rate of 20 mV/s.

3.3. Atomic Force Microscopy

AFM characterizations were collected using a commercial scanning probe microscope (5500 by Keysight Technology, Santa Rosa, CA, USA). The images were acquired in tapping-mode, with silicon tips from NanoSensors, Neuchatel, Switzerland (cantilever force constant: 10–130 N/m; ν_0 = 223 kHz) and typical scan rates of 1.2 line·s^{-1}.

4. Conclusions

We demonstrated that RAS acts as a powerful technique to use in order to detect the first steps of porphyrin nanocrystals dissolution in acidic liquid media. By monitoring the optical anisotropy changes in situ and *in operando* conditions, we confirm that one-electron transfers, occurring at precise EC potentials during the oxidation of ZnTPP/HOPG, H_2TPP/HOPG and Fe(TPP)Cl/HOPG films in sulfuric acid, are responsible for the early stages of structural modifications in porphyrin nanocrystals, in agreement with previous morphological investigations. Interestingly, after the oxidation of the organic film, the 3D phase of ZnTPP films looks completely amorphous, showing a null optical anisotropy signal and a melted-like morphology; conversely, the 3D phase of both H_2TPP and Fe(TPP)Cl films preserves a certain crystallinity, which still gives rise to a peculiar anisotropy signal, representative of a post-oxidation condition. We speculate that the reason for the observed differences in the optical/morphological behavior of the three porphyrin systems could be related to details of the oxidation process of the porphin macrocycle; the identification of the molecular sites involved in the electron transfer processes will be the topic of future investigations using in situ X-ray absorption spectroscopy combined with electrochemistry measurements.

In summary, RAS can be used for real-time monitoring and, from the early stages, modifications of anisotropic organic/inorganic systems which are caused by damaging processes in oxidative/corrosive media or EC conditions.

Author Contributions: Conceptualization, R.Y. and G.B.; methodology, R.Y., F.G. and G.B.; formal analysis, R.Y., C.F. and F.G.; investigation, R.Y. and F.G.; data curation, R.Y.; writing—original draft preparation, R.Y.; writing—review and editing, R.Y., A.C. and G.B.; supervision, G.B., F.C. and L.D.; project administration, G.B.; funding acquisition, G.B. All authors have read and agreed to the published version of the manuscript.

Funding: This research was funded by Fondazione CARIPLO, grant number 2020-0977.

Institutional Review Board Statement: Not applicable.

Informed Consent Statement: Not applicable.

Acknowledgments: The authors are grateful to I. Majumdar and G. Albani for the preparation and growth of the porphyrin samples; L. Ferraro for the home-made RAS set up.

Conflicts of Interest: The authors declare no conflict of interest.

Sample Availability: Samples of the compounds ZnTPP, H_2TPP, Fe(TPP)Cl are available from the authors.

References

1. Goletti, C.; Paolesse, R.; Di Natale, C.; Bussetti, G.; Chiaradia, P.; Froiio, A.; Valli, L.; D'Amico, A. Optical Anisotropy of Porphyrin Langmuir–Blodgett Films. *Surf. Sci.* **2002**, *501*, 31–36. [CrossRef]
2. Goletti, C.; Paolesse, R.; Dalcanale, E.; Berzina, T.; Di Natale, C.; Bussetti, G.; Chiaradia, P.; Froiio, A.; Cristofolini, L.; Costa, M.; et al. Thickness Dependence of the Optical Anisotropy for Porphyrin Octaester Langmuir-Schaefer Films. *Langmuir* **2002**, *18*, 6881–6886. [CrossRef]
3. Goletti, C.; Bussetti, G.; Chiaradia, P.; Sassella, A.; Borghesi, A. The Application of Reflectance Anisotropy Spectroscopy to Organics Deposition. *Org. Electron.* **2004**, *5*, 73–81. [CrossRef]
4. Goletti, C.; Bussetti, G.; Chiaradia, P.; Sassella, A.; Borghesi, A. In Situ Optical Investigation of Oligothiophene Layers Grown by Organic Molecular Beam. *J. Phys. Condens. Matter* **2004**, *16*, S4393. [CrossRef]
5. Bussetti, G.; Ferraro, L.; Bossi, A.; Campione, M.; Duò, L.; Ciccacci, F. A Microprocessor-Aided Platform Enabling Surface Differential Reflectivity and Reflectance Anisotropy Spectroscopy. *Eur. Phys. J. Plus* **2021**, *136*, 421. [CrossRef]
6. Bussetti, G.; Campione, M.; Riva, M.; Picone, A.; Raimondo, L.; Ferraro, L.; Hogan, C.; Palummo, M.; Brambilla, A.; Finazzi, M.; et al. Stable Alignment of Tautomers at Room Temperature in Porphyrin 2D Layers. *Adv. Funct. Mater.* **2014**, *24*, 958–963. [CrossRef]
7. Bussetti, G.; Corradini, C.; Goletti, C.; Chiaradia, P.; Russo, M.; Paolesse, R.; Di Natale, C.; D'Amico, A.; Valli, L. Optical Anisotropy and Gas Sensing Properties of Ordered Porphyrin Films. *Phys. Status Solidi.* **2005**, *242*, 2714–2719. [CrossRef]
8. Bussetti, G.; Cirilli, S.; Violante, A.; Chiaradia, P.; Goletti, C.; Tortora, L.; Paolesse, R.; Martinelli, E.; D'Amico, A.; Di Natale, C.; et al. Optical Anisotropy Readout in Solid-State Porphyrins for the Detection of Volatile Compounds. *Appl. Phys. Lett.* **2009**, *95*, 2007–2010. [CrossRef]
9. Bussetti, G.; Violante, A.; Yivlialin, R.; Cirilli, S.; Bonanni, B.; Chiaradia, P.; Goletti, C.; Tortora, L.; Paolesse, R.; Martinelli, E.; et al. Site-Sensitive Gas Sensing and Analyte Discrimination in Langmuir-Blodgett Porphyrin Films. *J. Phys. Chem. C* **2011**, *115*, 8189–8194. [CrossRef]
10. Weightman, P.; Martin, D.S.; Cole, R.J.; Farrell, T. Reflection Anisotropy Spectroscopy. *Reports Prog. Phys.* **2005**, *68*, 1251. [CrossRef]
11. Wandelt, K. (Ed.) *Encyclopedia of Interfacial Chemistry*, 1st ed.; Elsevier: Amsterdam, The Netherlands, 2018; ISBN 978-0-12-809894-3.
12. De Rosa, S.; Branchini, P.; Yivlialin, R.; Duò, L.; Bussetti, G.; Tortora, L. Disclosing the Graphite Surface Chemistry in Acid Solutions for Anion Intercalation. *ACS Appl. Nano Mater.* **2020**, *3*, 691–698. [CrossRef]
13. Mazine, V.; Borenszstein, Y.; Cagnon, L.; Allongue, P. Optical Reflectance Anisotropy Spectroscopy of the Au(110) Surface in Electrochemical Environment. *Phys. Status Solidi.* **1999**, *175*, 311–316. [CrossRef]
14. Smith, C.I.; Maunder, A.J.; Lucas, C.A.; Nichols, R.J.; Weightman, P. Adsorption of Pyridine on Au(110) as Measured by Reflection Anisotropy Spectroscopy. *J. Electrochem. Soc.* **2003**, *150*, E233. [CrossRef]

15. Goletti, C.; Bussetti, G.; Violante, A.; Bonanni, B.; Di Giovannantonio, M.; Serrano, G.; Breuer, S.; Gentz, K.; Wandelt, K. Cu(110) Surface in Hydrochloric Acid Solution: Potential Dependent Chloride Adsorption and Surface Restructuring. *J. Phys. Chem. C* **2015**, *119*, 1782–1790. [CrossRef]
16. Barati, G.; Solokha, V.; Wandelt, K.; Hingerl, K.; Cobet, C. Chloride-Induced Morphology Transformations of the Cu(110) Surface in Dilute HCl. *Langmuir* **2014**, *30*, 14486–14493. [CrossRef]
17. Weightman, P.; Harrison, P.; Lucas, C.A.; Grunder, Y.; Smith, C.I. The Reflection Anisotropy Spectroscopy of the Au(1 1 0) Surface Structures in Liquid Environments. *J. Phys. Condens. Matter* **2015**, *27*, 475005. [CrossRef]
18. Yivlialin, R.; Bussetti, G.; Penconi, M.; Bossi, A.; Ciccacci, F.; Finazzi, M.; Duò, L. Vacuum-Deposited Porphyrin Protective Films on Graphite: Electrochemical Atomic Force Microscopy Investigation during Anion Intercalation. *ACS Appl. Mater. Interfaces* **2017**, *9*, 4100–4105. [CrossRef]
19. Yivlialin, R.; Penconi, M.; Bussetti, G.; Biroli, A.O.; Finazzi, M.; Duò, L.; Bossi, A. Morphological Changes of Porphine Films on Graphite by Perchloric and Phosphoric Electrolytes: An Electrochemical-AFM Study. *Appl. Surf. Sci.* **2018**, *442*, 501–506. [CrossRef]
20. Bussetti, G.; Filoni, C.; Li Bassi, A.; Bossi, A.; Campione, M.; Orbelli Biroli, A.; Castiglioni, C.; Trabattoni, S.; De Rosa, S.; Tortora, L.; et al. Driving Organic Nanocrystals Dissolution Through Electrochemistry. *Chem. Open* **2021**, *10*, 748–755. [CrossRef]
21. Filoni, C.; Duò, L.; Ciccacci, F.; Li Bassi, A.; Bossi, A.; Campione, M.; Capitani, G.; Denti, I.; Tommasini, M.; Castiglioni, C.; et al. Reactive Dissolution of Organic Nanocrystals at Controlled PH. *ChemNanoMat* **2020**, *6*, 567–575. [CrossRef]
22. Bussetti, G.; Campione, M.; Ferraro, L.; Raimondo, L.; Bonanni, B.; Goletti, C.; Palummo, M.; Hogan, C.; Duò, L.; Finazzi, M.; et al. Probing Two-Dimensional vs Three-Dimensional Molecular Aggregation in Metal-Free Tetraphenylporphyrin Thin Films by Optical Anisotropy. *J. Phys. Chem. C* **2014**, *118*, 15649–15655. [CrossRef]
23. Bussetti, G.; Campione, M.; Raimondo, L.; Yivlialin, R.; Finazzi, M.; Ciccacci, F.; Sassella, A.; Duò, L. Unconventional Post-deposition Chemical Treatment on Ultra-thin H2TPP. *Cryst. Res. Technol.* **2014**, *49*, 581–586. [CrossRef]
24. Kano, K.; Fukuda, K.; Wakami, H.; Nishiyabu, R.; Pasternack, R.F. Factors Influencing Self-Aggregation Tendencies of Cationic Porphyrins in Aqueous Solution. *J. Am. Chem. Soc.* **2000**, *122*, 7494–7502. [CrossRef]
25. Scheidt, W.R.; Mondal, J.U.; Eigenbrot, C.W.; Adler, A.; Radonovich, L.J.; Hoard, J.L. Crystal and Molecular Structure of the Silver(II) and Zinc(II) Derivatives of Meso-Tetraphenylporphyrin. An Exploration of Crystal-Packing Effects on Bond Distance. *Inorg. Chem.* **1986**, *25*, 795–799. [CrossRef]
26. Byrn, M.P.; Curtis, C.J.; Hsiou, Y.; Khan, S.I.; Sawin, P.A.; Tendick, S.K.; Terzis, A.; Strouse, C.E. Porphyrin Sponges: Conservation of Host Structure in over 200 Porphyrin-Based Lattice Clathrates. *J. Am. Chem. Soc.* **1993**, *115*, 9480–9497. [CrossRef]
27. Hunter, S.C.; Smith, B.A.; Hoffmann, C.M.; Wang, X.; Chen, Y.S.; McIntyre, G.J.; Xue, Z.L. Intermolecular Interactions in Solid-State Metalloporphyrins and Their Impacts on Crystal and Molecular Structures. *Inorg. Chem.* **2014**, *53*, 11552–11562. [CrossRef]
28. Bussetti, G.; Yivlialin, R.; Ciccacci, F.; Duò, L.; Gibertini, E.; Accogli, A.; Denti, I.; Magagnin, L.; Micciulla, F.; Cataldo, A.; et al. Electrochemical Scanning Probe Analysis Used as a Benchmark for Carbon Forms Quality Test. *J. Phys. Condens. Matter* **2020**, *33*, 115002. [CrossRef]
29. Bussetti, G.; Campione, M.; Sassella, A.; Duò, L. Optical and Morphological Properties of Ultra-Thin H2TPP, H4TPP and ZnTPP Films. *Phys. Status Solidi Basic Res.* **2015**, *252*, 93857832. [CrossRef]
30. Castillo, C.; Vazquez-Nava, R.A.; Mendoza, B.S. Reflectance Anisotropy for Porphyrin Octaester Langmuir-Schaefer Films. In Proceedings of the Physica Status Solidi C: 5th International Conference on Optics of Surfaces and Interfaces (OSI-V), León, Mexico, 26–30 May 2003; pp. 2971–2975.
31. Mendoza, B.S.; Vázquez-Nava, R.A. Model for Reflectance Anisotropy Spectra of Molecular Layered Systems. *Phys. Rev. B-Condens. Matter Mater. Phys.* **2005**, *72*, 035411. [CrossRef]
32. Ward, S.; Perkins, M.; Zhang, J.; Roberts, C.J.; Madden, C.E.; Luk, S.Y.; Patel, N.; Ebbens, S.J. Identifying and Mapping Surface Amorphous Domains. *Pharm. Res.* **2005**, *22*, 1195–1202. [CrossRef]
33. Raberg, W.; Wandelt, K. Atomically Resolved AFM Investigations of an Amorphous Barium Silicate Surface. *Appl. Phys. A Mater. Sci. Process.* **1998**, *66*, 1143–1146. [CrossRef]
34. Paul-Roth, C.; Rault-Berthelot, J.; Simonneaux, G.; Poriel, C.; Abdalilah, M.; Letessier, J. Electroactive Films of Poly(Tetraphenylporphyrins) with Reduced Bandgap Electroanalytical Chemistry. *J. Electroanal. Chem.* **2006**, *597*, 19–27. [CrossRef]
35. Kadish, K.M.; Larson, G.; Lexa, D.; Momenteau, M. Electrochemical and Spectral Characterization of the Reduction Steps of μ-Oxo-Bis (Iron Tetraphenylporphyrin) Dimer in Dimethylformamide. *J. Am. Chem. Soc.* **1975**, *97*, 282–288. [CrossRef]
36. Kadish, K.M.; Morrison, M.M.; Constant, L.A.; Dickens, L.; Davis, D.G. A Study of Solvent and Substituent Effects on the Redox Potentials and Electron-Transfer Rate Constants of Substituted Iron Meso-Tetraphenylporphyrins. *J. Am. Chem. Soc.* **1976**, *98*, 8387–8390. [CrossRef]
37. Felton, R.H.; Owen, G.S.; Dolphin, D.; Fajer, J. Iron(IV) Porphyrins. *J. Am. Chem. Soc.* **1971**, *2041*, 6332–6334. [CrossRef]
38. Bussetti, G.; Calloni, A.; Celeri, M.; Yivlialin, R.; Finazzi, M.; Bottegoni, F.; Duò, L.; Ciccacci, F. Structure and Electronic Properties of Zn-Tetra-Phenyl-Porphyrin Single- and Multi-Layers Films Grown on Fe(001)-p(1 × 1)O. *Appl. Surf. Sci.* **2016**, *390*, 856–862. [CrossRef]
39. Aspnes, D.E.; Harbison, J.P.; Studna, A.A.; Florez, L.T. Reflectance-Difference Spectroscopy System for Real-Time Measurements of Crystal Growth. *Appl. Phys. Lett.* **1988**, *52*, 957–959. [CrossRef]

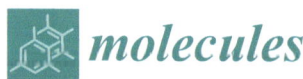 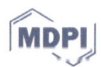

Article

Structure and Dynamics of Adsorbed Dopamine on Solvated Carbon Nanotubes and in a CNT Groove

Qizhang Jia, B. Jill Venton and Kateri H. DuBay *

Department of Chemistry, University of Virginia, Charlottesville, VA 22904, USA; qj3fe@virginia.edu (Q.J.); bjv2n@virginia.edu (B.J.V.)
* Correspondence: dubay@virginia.edu

Abstract: Advanced carbon microelectrodes, including many carbon-nanotube (CNT)-based electrodes, are being developed for the in vivo detection of neurotransmitters such as dopamine (DA). Our prior simulations of DA and dopamine-*o*-quinone (DOQ) on pristine, flat graphene showed rapid surface diffusion for all adsorbed species, but it is not known how CNT surfaces affect dopamine adsorption and surface diffusivity. In this work, we use molecular dynamics simulations to investigate the adsorbed structures and surface diffusion dynamics of DA and DOQ on CNTs of varying curvature and helicity. In addition, we study DA dynamics in a groove between two aligned CNTs to model the spatial constraints at the junctions within CNT assemblies. We find that the adsorbate diffusion on a solvated CNT surface depends upon curvature. However, this effect cannot be attributed to changes in the surface energy roughness because the lateral distributions of the molecular adsorbates are similar across curvatures, diffusivities on zigzag and armchair CNTs are indistinguishable, and the curvature dependence disappears in the absence of solvent. Instead, adsorbate diffusivities correlate with the vertical placement of the adsorbate's moieties, its tilt angle, its orientation along the CNT axis, and the number of waters in its first hydration shell, all of which will influence its effective hydrodynamic radius. Finally, DA diffuses into and remains in the groove between a pair of aligned and solvated CNTs, enhancing diffusivity along the CNT axis. These first studies of surface diffusion on a CNT electrode surface are important for understanding the changes in diffusion dynamics of dopamine on nanostructured carbon electrode surfaces.

Keywords: dopamine diffusion; fast scan cyclic voltammetry; carbon nanotubes; carbon microelectrodes; molecular dynamics; nanomaterials

Citation: Jia, Q.; Venton, B.J.; DuBay, K.H. Structure and Dynamics of Adsorbed Dopamine on Solvated Carbon Nanotubes and in a CNT Groove. *Molecules* **2022**, *27*, 3768. https://doi.org/10.3390/molecules27123768

Academic Editors: Luca Tortora and Gianlorenzo Bussetti

Received: 5 May 2022
Accepted: 6 June 2022
Published: 11 June 2022

Publisher's Note: MDPI stays neutral with regard to jurisdictional claims in published maps and institutional affiliations.

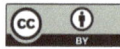

Copyright: © 2022 by the authors. Licensee MDPI, Basel, Switzerland. This article is an open access article distributed under the terms and conditions of the Creative Commons Attribution (CC BY) license (https://creativecommons.org/licenses/by/4.0/).

1. Introduction

Rapid and precise in vivo electroanalytical detection methods have advanced through the development of carbon electrodes with novel micromorphologies, with the functional properties of these aqueous electrochemical interfaces depending on their surface structures [1,2]. In recent years, several carbon microelectrodes have been developed based on carbon nanotubes (CNTs), such as CNT nanoyarns [3], CNT forests [4], and spirally-wrapped CNTs [5]. CNT-based electrodes have been successfully employed to study dopamine (DA), an important neurotransmitter and signaling molecule in neuromodulatory processes [6–8] and a common target analyte for in vivo electroanalytical detection [2,9,10]. CNT-based electrodes have high sensitivity for neurotransmitter detection. CNT yarn electrodes have a limit of detection of 10 nM for dopamine and a linear range up to 25 uM [11]. Their response times are similar to those of carbon-fiber microelectrodes, and the electrochemistry is more reversible, meaning the reduction peak is more evident in the cyclic voltammetry.

Interestingly, scanning electrochemical microscopy (SECM) and scanning electrochemical cell microscopy (SECCM) experiments have shown substantial electrochemical activity on curved CNT surfaces. Pristine CNTs were able to catalytically oxidize and reduce ferrocenyl-methyl-trimethyl-ammonium [12], and the catalytic reduction of heavy transition-metal complexes were observed on pristine CNT sidewalls [13]. A pristine, curved CNT surface greatly enhanced the catalytic reduction of oxygen, as compared to a flat, highly ordered pyrolytic graphite (HOPG) surface [14].

At the same time, localized surface features, such as CNT kinks, oxidized defects, edges, and lattice defects, are all known to enhance electrochemical activity in these materials [2,14,15]. Spatially heterogeneous electrode activity has even been observed on pristine graphene surfaces [16]. Since analyte surface diffusion is much more rapid than adsorption and desorption [17,18], which occurs on the µs to s timescale for these small molecular analytes [19–21], the diffusion timescale of adsorbates between these functionally different locations has been used to explain certain features of electrochemical experiments, such as fast scan cyclic voltammetry (FSCV) scan-rate dependencies [22].

Surface curvature and roughness has been shown to influence adsorbate diffusion on a carbon surface. Shu et al. performed molecular dynamics (MD) simulations to study the surface diffusion of an adatom and found it highly dependent upon the CNT curvature and helicity, suggesting the possible importance of helicity in determining the mass transport of an adsorbate in the axial direction along a CNT [23]. In addition, an atomic force microscope (AFM) study on the clustering process of gold nanoparticles (NPs) on a single layer of graphene placed atop three different substrates—graphite, boronnitride, and SiO_2—demonstrated that rougher carbon surfaces slowed NP diffusion [24].

Surface-dependent solvent dynamics can also play an important role in the diffusion of CNT-adsorbed analytes. Previous research has shown that water's density, mobility, hydrogen-bond networks, and diffusion mechanism in close proximity to a CNT surface are highly dependent upon nanotube geometry [25–27]. The phase behavior and dynamics of water are also known to change under confinement, although these effects may be limited in spaces larger than 15 Å in diameter [27–29]. Interestingly, MD simulations have shown that the diffusion of water in certain regions within a CNT can be faster than in the bulk phase [25,30,31].

Our own prior work used atomistic MD simulations to investigate the diffusion dynamics of DA, its oxidation product, dopamine-o-quinone (DOQ), and their protonated species on the pristine basal plane of flat graphene [18]. The results demonstrated that the rapid adsorption of all species on this defect-free surface occurred even in the absence of a holding potential. In addition, we found that surface solvation has a large effect on adsorbate diffusion, and that adsorbate diffusivity on the solvated surface was similar to that in bulk water. Finally, we found that the protonated species diffused more slowly on the solvated surface, while the oxidized species diffused more rapidly.

In this paper, we extend our previous MD simulations of DA and DOQ on flat graphene to investigate the structures and diffusion dynamics of the same adsorbates on CNT surfaces of differing diameters, helicities, and arrangements. We first describe our model system and simulation techniques and then quantify the diffusivities of DA, DOQ, and their protonated species on various single CNT surfaces, at both the aqueous and vacuum interfaces. We then analyze how the relative populations of various configurations of adsorbed DA and DOQ change on differently curved CNTs, which provides insight into the origin of the observed curvature dependent diffusion. Finally, we discuss our findings regarding the surface diffusion dynamics of DA and DOQ in a CNT groove.

2. Modeling

Atomistic MD simulations were performed within LAMMPS [32] on systems composed of a graphene or CNT surface and a single adsorbate. Most simulations modeled the carbon:water interface, where the surface was solvated with TIP3P water molecules and simulations were conducted within an *NVT* ensemble. Simulations of the carbon:vacuum interface were conducted at fixed *NVE*. To model the interactions in the system, we used the OPLS-AA potential [33], which has been previously validated for use with small organic molecules on graphene surfaces [34,35]. Simulations followed the approach described in our previous study of DA and DOQ diffusion on a pristine flat graphene surface [18]. A detailed discussion of the accuracy of the OPLS-AA potential for these systems and additional details of the equilibration process can be found in that work [18] and the SI.

Although these surfaces operate as electrodes under an external voltage, the full analysis of adsorbate dynamics under a changing potential is remarkably complex and lies outside the scope of this work, which focuses instead on the fundamental influence of the graphene and CNT surfaces on the dynamics of adsorbed DA and DOQ.

2.1. Flat and Curved Pristine Carbon Surfaces

At the microscopic level, many carbon-based microelectrodes are composed of carbon fiber microfilaments and CNT yarns, which consist of disordered graphite and vertically-aligned CNT arrays, respectively [2,3]. To investigate adsorbate dynamics on the pristine carbon versions of these microelectrodes, we created periodic structures of flat graphene and single-walled CNTs of different curvatures and helicities. The surface carbons were immobilized during the simulations, as discussed in our prior work [18] and in keeping with other MD studies on these surfaces [23,26,27,30,31,34,36].

Flat graphene. We modeled a single layer of pristine flat graphene with a lateral box size of 98.2419×97.8420 Å^2, using 3D periodic boundary conditions. A single layer of graphene was used as no differences were observed between adsorbate dynamics on a single and a triple layered fixed carbon surface [18].

Single-walled CNTs. To look at analyte motion on various CNT surfaces, we modeled single-walled CNTs of three diameters and two helicities: armchair and zigzag. Armchair CNTs included $(15, 15)$-CNT, $(22, 22)$-CNT, and $(29, 29)$-CNT, while the zigzag CNTs included $(0, 26)$-CNT, $(0, 38)$-CNT, $(0, 51)$-CNT. Within each set, the radii are approximately 10, 15, and 20 Å, respectively. Details on the CNT diameters, lengths, and helicities are listed in Table S1. In addition, images of the CNTs can been seen in Figure 1. CNTs larger than 20 Å in diameter were chosen to avoid complications arising from significant confinement effects, which are more prominent in CNTs under 15 Å [26,27]. CNTs of of various lengths—ranging from 25 Å to 100 Å—were simulated in order to correct for finite size issues arising from the periodic boundary conditions, as discussed in the SI [18,37–40]. Results are generally presented from 100 Å-long CNTs; however, extrapolations to the infinitely sized systems are included for key cases.

CNT groove. We also placed two $(15, 15)$-CNTs in a parallel alignment along the z-direction to construct a one-dimensional CNT groove. The CNTs are both 100.7 Å long and separated by 3.4 Å, corresponding to the sum of the van der Waals (vdW) radii of the closest carbon atoms on the different CNTs [41].

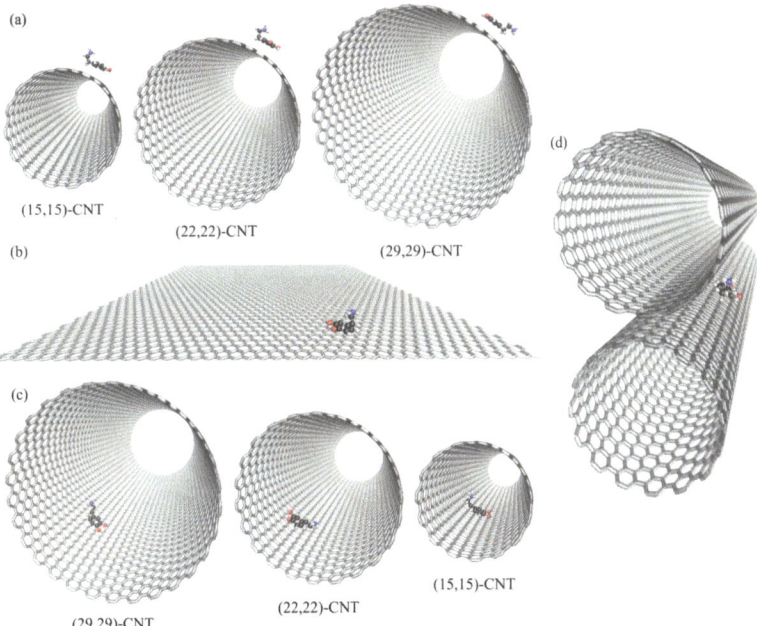

Figure 1. Simulated CNT and graphene surfaces. DA is shown on (**a**) the exterior surfaces of CNTs of varying curvatures, (**b**) flat graphene, and (**c**) the corresponding CNT interiors. In (**d**), DA diffuses along the exterior groove formed by two parallel (15, 15)-CNT nanotubes. The dimensions of the CNTs are listed in Table S1, and the solvating water molecules were omitted here for visual clarity.

2.2. DA and DOQ Adsorbates

We modeled DA and DOQ atomistically, along with their physiologically relevant protonated counterparts, DAH^+ and $DOQH^+$ [42]. A description of the partial charge assignments can be found in [18]. Cl^- ions were added as countercharges for the protonated species. DA and its derivatives contain three key moieties: the side-chain amine, the aromatic ring, and an *ortho*-diol or quinone group [43], see Figure 2. We also modeled the dynamics of a charge neutral atomic adsorbate with the same molar mass as dopamine (153.18 a.u.), which is referred to as "adatom(DA)".

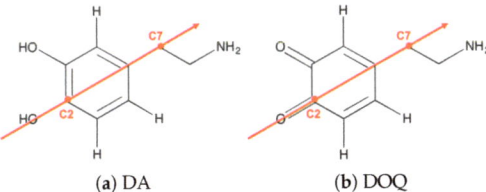

Figure 2. DA and DOQ. The adsorbate structures of DA and DOQ are shown here. The corresponding protonated species, DAH^+ and $DOQH^+$, have an additional hydrogen in their positively charged amine groups. The C2–C7 vectors (red arrows) are used to define the orientation and tilt of the adsorbates above the carbon surface.

3. Results and Discussion

3.1. Solvated Adsorbate Diffusivities Depend on Surface Curvature

Inspired by previous work showing that variations in surface curvature and CNT helicity can alter the diffusional pathways of an atomic adatom on a CNT surface [23], we set out to investigate the motion of DA across a series of solvated CNT surfaces with varying curvatures. The mean squared displacements (MSDs) of the adsorbates along the CNT axis (MSD$_\parallel$) and around its circumference (MSD$_\perp$) are plotted in Figure 3b as a function of time for DA on seven differently curved armchair CNT surfaces: three on the CNT interior, one on flat graphene, and three on the CNT exterior. The 1D diffusivities, $D_\perp$ and $D_\parallel$, and the overall 2D diffusivities, D, are listed in Figure 3c. The diffusion coefficients, D, were computed from the MSDs using the Einstein relation, [26,44] as detailed in the Supplementary Materials.

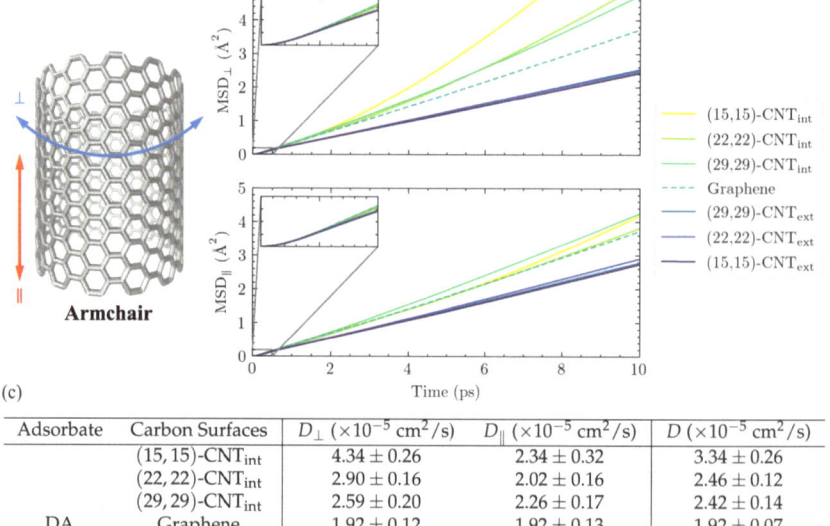

Adsorbate	Carbon Surfaces	$D_\perp$ ($\times 10^{-5}$ cm^2/s)	$D_\parallel$ ($\times 10^{-5}$ cm^2/s)	D ($\times 10^{-5}$ cm^2/s)
	$(15,15)$-CNT$_{int}$	4.34 ± 0.26	2.34 ± 0.32	3.34 ± 0.26
	$(22,22)$-CNT$_{int}$	2.90 ± 0.16	2.02 ± 0.16	2.46 ± 0.12
	$(29,29)$-CNT$_{int}$	2.59 ± 0.20	2.26 ± 0.17	2.42 ± 0.14
DA	Graphene	1.92 ± 0.12	1.92 ± 0.13	1.92 ± 0.07
	$(29,29)$-CNT$_{ext}$	1.24 ± 0.08	1.42 ± 0.10	1.33 ± 0.06
	$(22,22)$-CNT$_{ext}$	1.26 ± 0.09	1.49 ± 0.10	1.37 ± 0.06
	$(15,15)$-CNT$_{ext}$	1.21 ± 0.06	1.39 ± 0.08	1.30 ± 0.04

Figure 3. DA diffusion on differently curved carbon surfaces. Results are shown here for the diffusion of DA on the interior (int) and exterior (ext) surfaces of armchair CNTs of varying diameters and flat graphene. (**a**) The armchair designation [45] refers to the edge morphology of the CNT along the perpendicular direction. Diffusion on the surface in the same direction as the CNT axis is referred to as parallel ($\parallel$), while that around the circumference of the CNT is denoted as perpendicular ($\perp$). All CNTs presented in this table are 100.698 Å along the periodic $\parallel$ direction, and the graphene sheet is 98.2419 × 97.8420 Å^2 in size and periodic in two directions along the surface. (**b**) The MSDs as a function of time are shown in both surface directions: $\perp$ (top panel) and $\parallel$ (bottom panel). (**c**) The diffusion constants $D_\perp$, $D_\parallel$, and the overall 2D D values are computed from linearly fitting the MSD curves in (**b**) using the Einstein relation, Equation (S4), over the 4–10 ps range. In both (**a**,**b**), the carbon surface results are organized from most concave to the most convex.

The observed diffusion constants are smallest on the convex CNT exterior and largest on the concave CNT interior. The largest shifts with curvature are seen in the $D_\perp$ values, in keeping with the direction in which the surface curves. In addition, a clear increase is seen in the $D_\perp$ values among the CNT interior results as the concavity increases from $(29,29)$-CNT$_{int}$ to $(15,15)$-CNT$_{int}$.

In order to compare the resulting diffusion constants to experimental values, we adjust them to correct for an unphysical system size dependence. This known finite-size effect [37–39,46] is discussed in more detail in the Supplementary Materials (see Figure S4 and accompanying text), and the values of the diffusion constants extrapolated to the infinite system size, D_∞, are shown for a subset of the cases in Table 1. In our simulations, the extrapolated 2D diffusion coefficient of DA on flat graphene is 1.3×10^{-5} cm^2/s, while its value ranges from $(1.1–2.5) \times 10^{-5}$ cm^2/s for DA on differently curved CNTs. For comparison, the 3D diffusion coefficient calculated for DA from flow injection experiments is 0.6×10^{-5} cm^2/s [47].

Table 1. Diffusion coefficients extrapolated to the infinite system sizes. For a subset of the carbon surfaces, diffusion constants for the infinite system sizes, D_∞, were extrapolated from a series of differently sized finite simulations. The extrapolation was done to correct for unphysical effects that arise from the necessarily finite simulation sizes, and the D_∞ values thus represent the actual diffusivities expected within the larger physical systems. See SI and Figure S4 for details.

Adsorbate	Carbon Surfaces	$D_{\infty,\perp}$ ($\times 10^{-5}$ cm^2/s)	$D_{\infty,\|}$ ($\times 10^{-5}$ cm^2/s)	D_∞ ($\times 10^{-5}$ cm^2/s)
DA	$(15,15)$-CNT$_{int}$	3.50 ± 0.15	1.41 ± 0.19	2.45 ± 0.13
	Flat Graphene	1.27 ± 0.07	1.22 ± 0.10	1.24 ± 0.06
	$(15,15)$-CNT$_{ext}$	1.17 ± 0.02	1.06 ± 0.05	1.12 ± 0.03

Curvature dependence is observed for DA, DAH$^+$, DOQ, and DOQH$^+$. Table 2 presents the diffusion constants obtained for these four species on both the interior and exterior surfaces of $(15,15)$-CNT, along with the flat graphene results. From these measurements, we find that the curvature-dependence is similar across all four species.

Table 2. 2D diffusion coefficients of DA, DOQ, and their protonated counterparts. The values of the overall 2D diffusion constant, D, were calculated from the MSDs of the adsorbates on the interior of the armchair $(15,15)$-CNT, flat graphene, and the exterior of the armchair $(15,15)$-CNT. Finite system size results are shown here as calculated within the ≈ 100 Å long systems.

D ($\times 10^{-5}$ cm^2/s)	DA	DAH$^+$	DOQ	DOQH$^+$
$(15,15)$-CNT$_{int}$	3.34 ± 0.26	3.24 ± 0.21	3.72 ± 0.29	3.65 ± 0.35
Graphene	1.92 ± 0.07	1.74 ± 0.07	2.29 ± 0.16	1.95 ± 0.14
$(15,15)$-CNT$_{ext}$	1.30 ± 0.04	1.20 ± 0.06	1.53 ± 0.10	1.37 ± 0.05

In addition, across all three curvatures we find that the protonated species, DAH$^+$ and DOQH$^+$, diffuse more slowly than their neutral counterparts, DAH and DOQ, while the oxidized species, DOQ and DOQH$^+$, diffuse more rapidly than their reduced counterparts, DA and DAH$^+$. These trends were previously observed on flat graphene [18] and can be readily explained by differences in the interactions of each species with the solvating water molecules: the positively charged species have increased interactions with the polar solvent, while the oxidized species have reduced interactions with the solvent—their quinone moieties are only able to act as hydrogen bond acceptors, as compared to the reduced diol moieties, which can act as both hydrogen bond donors and acceptors. Increased attractions with the solvent will increase the adsorbate's effective hydrodynamic radius, R_H, which is inversely related to the diffusion constant, D, of a solvated sphere in nonturbulent flow via the Stokes–Einstein equation [36]: $D = \dfrac{k_B T}{c \pi \eta R_H}$, where k_B is the Boltzmann constant, T is temperature, η is solvent viscosity, and c is a constant that describes the boundary conditions at the solvent-sphere interface. The Stokes–Einstein equation cannot be rigorously applied here for these partially solvated, small molecular adsorbates; however, it qualitatively explains the observed trends.

Our simulation results show that DA diffusion clearly depends on placement on the inner or outer surface of the CNT, with enhanced motion on the CNT interior. Overall, this observed curvature dependence is consistent with the general trends observed previously for an atomic adatom [23].

3.2. Dependence Does Not Arise from Curvature-Induced Shifts in Surface Roughness

In the case of the previously studied atomic adatom, the observed reduction of diffusion barriers for the adatom on a surface with negative curvature (the CNT interior) resulted from the smoothing of the carbon energy surface as it changes from convex to flat to concave [23]. However, it is not clear how this effect functions for a molecular adsorbate such as DA, which is larger than the underlying hexagonal carbon structure, flexible, and asymmetric in shape with an uneven charge distribution. In addition, the role of solvent was not considered in the prior work and may mitigate the influence of surface energy roughness. In this section, we probe the role of surface roughness in this system by investigating how the lateral distributions of these adsorbates depend on curvature, how their diffusivities depend on CNT helicity, and how their diffusivities depend on curvature in the absence of solvent.

Lateral distributions of molecular adsorbates are similar across curvatures. In Figure 4, we plot the lateral distributions for the adatom(DA), DA, and its moieties on three differently curved surfaces: the exterior of a $(15,15)$-CNT nanotube, flat graphene, and the interior of a $(15,15)$-CNT nanotube. By comparing these distributions to the underlying hexagonal aromatic ring pattern of the carbon surfaces, we can observe how curvature-induced differences in the energy surface roughness influence the placement of these atomic and molecular adsorbates.

First, we consider the lateral distributions of adatom(DA), an atomic adatom with the same mass as DA. Shown in the first row of Figure 4, these distributions clearly display the characteristic hexagonal pattern that corresponds to the centers of the honeycomb structure of the aromatic carbon surface. As the surface curvature changes from convex to concave, the lateral distribution of adatom(DA) gradually becomes more uniform, as expected from the previously noted smoothing of the surface energy as the curvature becomes more negative [23]. Despite the presence of solvating waters in our simulation, the dependence of adatom(DA)'s lateral distribution on the underlying carbon structure and its curvature persists.

In contrast, the lateral distributions of DA's COM and that of its constituent moieties, as shown in the next four rows of Figure 4, display almost no dependence on the underlying hexagonal carbon structure and we see no clear trend in the distributions with curvature. This lack of structuring and curvature dependence suggests that the underlying surface energy roughness is not a dominant factor in determining the lateral placement of DA, which extends spatially over a region larger than the hexagonal lattice spacing of the underlying carbon surface.

Diffusion coefficients for zigzag and armchair CNTs are indistinguishable. Helicity-dependent diffusion of atomic adsorbates on CNT surfaces has been previously observed in simulations, where different diffusive pathways were observed on armchair and zigzag CNT surfaces due to the surface energy landscapes that emerged upon curving graphene in different directions [23,48]. To probe this effect for our solvated system, we simulated the diffusion of both DA and adatom(DA) on the interior and exterior surfaces of highly curved armchair and zigzag CNTs. Figure 5 shows the two CNT structures with 10 Å radii ($(15,15)$-CNT and $(0,26)$-CNT) as well as the $D_\perp$, $D_\parallel$, and 2D D values obtained from these simulations. The corresponding results on flat graphene are also shown in each case for comparison.

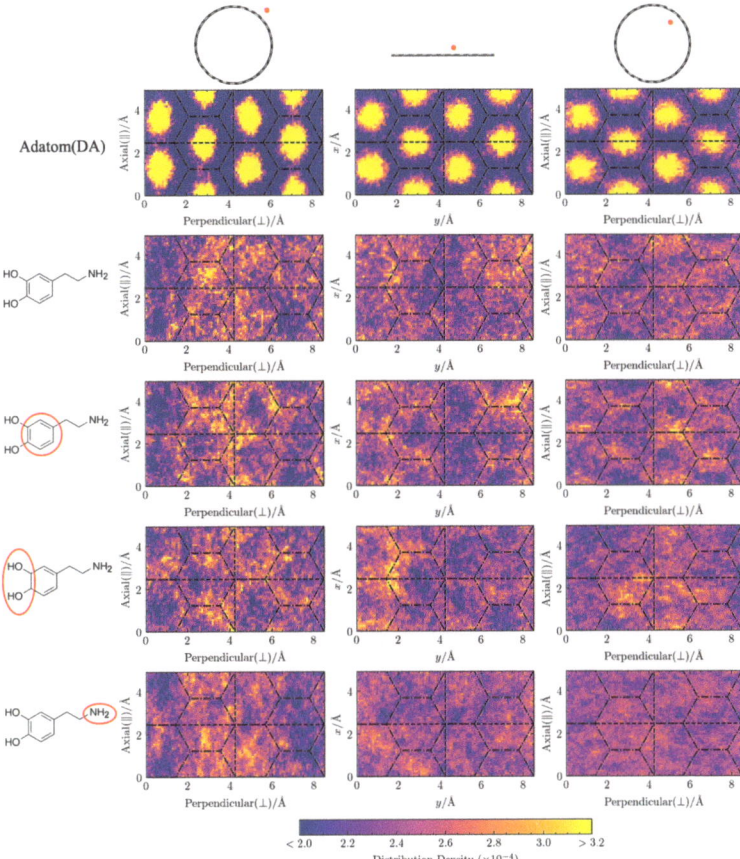

Figure 4. Lateral distributions of adatom(DA) and DA above the CNT and graphene surfaces. The plots show the distribution densities of the adsorbates above the carbon surface. From left to right, the columns show the distributions on the exterior surface of (15, 15)-CNT, on flat graphene, and on the interior surface of (15, 15)-CNT, as indicated with the cartoon images above each column. From top to bottom, the rows show the results for adatom(DA) (an atomic adatom with the mass of DA), the COM of DA, and the three COMs of the red-circled DA moieties. The projected COM coordinates are binned with a spatial resolution of 0.1×0.1 Å^2 and wrapped into 4 unit cells, which are separated by the dashed lines.

We found no significant difference between the armchair and zigzag diffusion constants in our simulations for either the atomic or molecular DA adsorbate. This result is expected for DA itself, given the insensitivity of its lateral distribution to the underlying hexagonal structure in Figure 4. The shift in the lateral distribution for adatom(DA) with curvature, however, suggests that differences between zigzag and armchair diffusivities are possible within our system. Even so, the results for the two cases are statistically indistinguishable, perhaps due to the dominant influence of surface hydration on adsorbate dynamics in these systems which we found in our prior work on flat graphene [18].

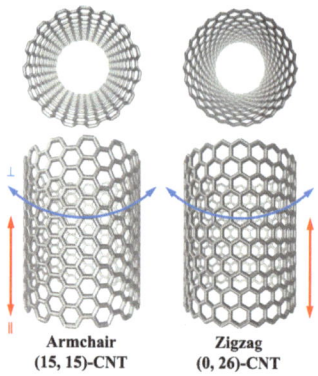

Adsorbate	Carbon Surfaces	$D_\perp$ ($\times 10^{-5}$ cm^2/s)	$D_\parallel$ ($\times 10^{-5}$ cm^2/s)	D ($\times 10^{-5}$ cm^2/s)
DA	$(15,15)$-CNT$_{int}$	4.34 ± 0.26	2.34 ± 0.32	3.34 ± 0.26
	Graphene	1.92 ± 0.12	1.92 ± 0.13	1.92 ± 0.07
	$(15,15)$-CNT$_{ext}$	1.21 ± 0.06	1.39 ± 0.08	1.30 ± 0.04
	$(0,26)$-CNT$_{int}$	4.56 ± 0.44	2.39 ± 0.17	3.48 ± 0.20
	Graphene	1.92 ± 0.13	1.92 ± 0.12	1.92 ± 0.07
	$(0,26)$-CNT$_{ext}$	1.20 ± 0.10	1.42 ± 0.11	1.31 ± 0.08
Adatom(DA)	$(15,15)$-CNT$_{int}$	8.08 ± 0.99	5.14 ± 0.51	6.61 ± 0.52
	Graphene	4.59 ± 0.32	4.71 ± 0.31	4.65 ± 0.29
	$(15,15)$-CNT$_{ext}$	2.95 ± 0.21	3.12 ± 0.27	3.03 ± 0.15
	$(0,26)$-CNT$_{int}$	8.04 ± 0.35	4.71 ± 0.46	6.38 ± 0.32
	Graphene	4.71 ± 0.31	4.59 ± 0.32	4.65 ± 0.29
	$(0,26)$-CNT$_{ext}$	2.96 ± 0.20	3.19 ± 0.16	3.04 ± 0.15

Figure 5. Diffusion coefficients of DA and adatom(DA) on armchair and zigzag CNTs. Armchair and zigzag CNTs are two conformations which describe the carbon atom arrangements along the perpendicular direction. The values of the diffusion constants $D_\perp$, $D_\parallel$ and the overall 2D D were calculated from the MSDs of the adsorbates on the different surfaces. The 1D diffusion constants on the flat graphene surface along the direction with the same chirality as each CNT direction were chosen for the comparison. Finite system size results are shown here as calculated within the 100 Å long systems.

Curvature dependence of D disappears in the absence of solvent. The negligible influence of the carbon surface's hexagonal patterning on DA's lateral distributions in Figure 4 suggests that the differences in D between the CNT surfaces of various curvature in Figure 3 and Table 1 do not actually arise from curvature-mediated changes to the energetic interactions between the adsorbate and the surface. The lack of dependence of DA diffusion on CNT helicity in Figure 5 supports this conclusion.

To isolate the adsorbate–surface interactions and further probe this dependence directly, in Figure 6 we plot MSD$_\parallel$ and MSD$_\perp$ for DA and DOQ on the carbon surfaces in the absence of solvent. Only the neutral species are simulated due to the lack of charge balance under vacuum conditions. The average MSD results for the adsorbates on flat graphene and on the interior and exterior of the $(15,15)$-CNT at the vacuum interface are shown plotted with lines, while the noise on each measurement is indicated by the shaded regions.

The resulting curves are not linear over the time regime plotted, indicating that inertial motion lasts for much longer times at the carbon:vacuum interface than at the carbon:water interface. Since the simulations do not allow for carbon surface fluctuations, which would be expected to significantly reduce the timescale of inertial motion decay in the absence of solvent, these MSD curves are only useful as a way to isolate the direct interactions between the adsorbate and the different carbon surface architectures and test their influence on adsorbate diffusion.

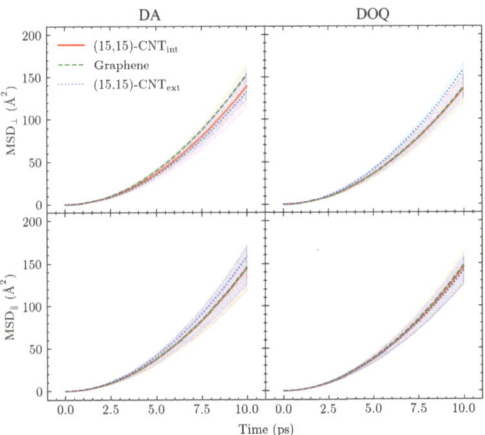

Figure 6. MSDs of DA and DOQ on differently curved carbon:vacuum surfaces. The top and bottom panels show the MSDs as a function of time along two surface directions, $\parallel$ and $\perp$, on graphene and on the interior and exterior of the $(15,15)$-CNT. The left and right panels display the results for adsorbates DA and DOQ, respectively. The lines show the average MSD values, while the shaded regions show the standard deviation in that value across ten trials, with red shading for $(15,15)$-CNT$_{int}$, green shading for flat graphene, and blue shading for $(15,15)$-CNT$_{ext}$.

The results within each panel show significant overlap of the shaded regions and no observable curvature dependence. In addition, the difference between the diffusivities of DA and DOQ disappears, as expected from our conclusions above regarding the importance of solvent and the effective R_H in determining the relative diffusivities of DA, DOQ, and their protonated species [18]. Finally, even the MSD$_\perp$ and MSD$_\parallel$ curves appear identical, indicating that the differences observed in CNT surface diffusion between the axial and perpendicular directions in Figure 3 and Table 1 are also attributable to solvent effects.

Taken together, these results suggest that the curvature dependence that we observe in the diffusion constants for adsorbed DA and DOQ at the carbon:water surface do not actually arise from curvature-induced changes in the energy surface roughness, as was the case in the prior work on an unsolvated atomic adatom [23]. Instead, we conclude that the curvature-dependence of these molecular adsorbates' diffusivities arises from a more complex interplay of surface curvature and surface solvation.

3.3. Adsorbate Structure Depends on Curvature, Charge, and Solvation

In this section, we investigate in detail the adsorbate's configuration on the surface and its dependence on curvature, charge, and solvation. First, we examine the vertical placement of DA and DOQ and its constituent moieties above the different carbon surfaces; in particular, we examine the various configurations available to the amine group. Then, we consider the tilt angle of the aromatic ring above the surface and the adsorbate's orientational alignment with the CNT axis. Finally, we consider how the differently curved surfaces shift the number of water molecules in the first solvation shell around the adsorbate, which will influence the effective hydrodynamic radius, R_H, and, therefore, the diffusivity.

The distance of the adsorbate above the surface depends on curvature, charge, and solvation. The vertical distance, d, is defined as the distance between the COM of a moiety and its closest point on the carbon surface. Figure 7 displays the vertical distributions for the aromatic ring (left column), the diol/quinone (middle column), and the amine group (right column) on the three surfaces. DA and DOQ distributions are shown at both the carbon:water and carbon:vacuum interfaces, while DAH$^+$ and DOQH$^+$ distributions are only shown at the carbon:water interface.

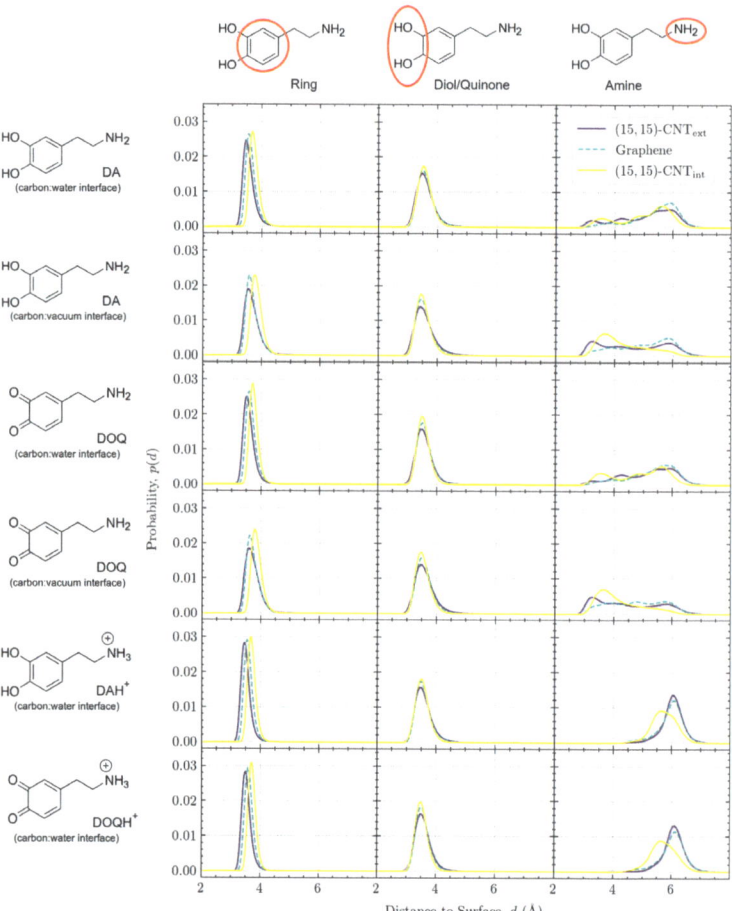

Figure 7. Vertical distributions of DA and DOQ moieties at the carbon:water and carbon:vacuum interfaces. From left to right, three columns show the vertical distributions of the aromatic ring, the diol/quinone moiety, and the amine group, respectively, with d representing the distance between that moiety's COM and the closest point on the surface. From top to bottom, the six rows correspond to DA, DA in vacuum, DOQ, DOQ in vacuum, DAH$^+$, and DOQH$^+$. Colored curves within each subplot indicate the distributions at the flat graphene or the interior and exterior (15,15)-CNT surfaces.

In the left column of Figure 7, the position of the aromatic ring for all solvated species shifts slightly away from the surface as its curvature changes from convex to flat to concave. Due to the ring's structural rigidity, its COM can get closer to the surface when adsorbed on the convex exterior of the CNT than when adsorbed to its concave interior, where interactions with the inward-curving walls shift the center of the ring slightly away from its optimal distance on the flat surface. Interestingly, for the two cases of DA and DOQ at the carbon:vacuum surface, the aromatic ring distributions for both the exterior and interior CNT surfaces shift slightly to the right, as compared to the solvated cases. This shift away from the surface indicates the importance of solvation in determining the optimal vertical position for the CNT-adsorbed aromatic rings.

In contrast, the diol/quinone moiety distributions in the middle column of Figure 7 display no shift with curvature, although the peak narrows slightly in all cases as the curvature of the carbon surface changes from convex to flat to concave. The invariance of these peaks, coupled with their location on the edge of the aromatic ring, provide further evidence that the shift in aromatic ring placement with curvature reflects constraints on the optimal surface ring distance due to the curved surface geometry.

Finally, in the right column of Figure 7, we plot the vertical distributions of the amine tail, which is tethered to the aromatic ring through rotatable bonds and can thus adopt a variety of configurations. Our prior work on flat graphene [18] demonstrated that the vertical distribution of the amine group is sensitive to its protonation state, as the positively charged DAH$^+$ and DOQH$^+$ amines can form additional hydrogen bonds with the bulk phase water molecules. These prior observations showed that the neutral amine vertical distributions have three peaks and span a range of about 3–7 Å from the surface, while the positively charged amines have a narrower distribution around a single peak at $\approx$6 Å from the surface. Similar overall distributions are seen for the CNT exterior and interior surfaces, with a broad, three-peaked distribution for the neutral species and a narrower distribution further from the surface for the charged amines. However, as the curvature changes from the exterior to flat graphene to the interior, the amine distributions are altered, especially for the CNT interior. In addition, we find that the distributions shift closer to the surface for both DA and DOQ at the carbon:vacuum interface as compared to their corresponding distributions at the carbon:water interface.

Amine configurations are highly variable and display significant curvature dependence. Given the complex variation observed in the amine vertical distributions, in Figure 8, we investigate in more detail these distributions for DA at the carbon:water interface. The three peaks for the CNT$_{ext}$, flat graphene, and CNT$_{int}$ distributions have been marked with letters in Figure 8a, their positions are listed in the table shown in Figure 8b, and a sample configuration at the characteristic distance within each peak is shown in Figure 8c.

The peaks closest to the surface in Figure 8a(*i, iv, vii*) correspond to configurations in which the amine group is in close contact with the surface. These first amine distribution peaks are observed at 3.1–3.7 Å (see Figure 8b) on all three surfaces, which is close to the sum of the van der Waals (vdW) radii, 3.27 Å, of a carbon with a nitrogen in the OPLS-AA force field [33]. The amine groups in these configurations are closest to the water molecules in the first layer near the surface, as can be seen in the corresponding sample structures in Figure 8c. The first and the second peaks in the density profile of water are observed at $\approx$3.3 Å and $\approx$6.2 Å, respectively (see Figure S5). The second set of peaks in the amine distribution (*ii, v, viii*) are observed at 4.2–5.2 Å. The amine groups in these configurations are therefore likely to form hydrogen bonds with both the first and second layers of water molecules, as shown in the sample structures in Figure 8c. Last, the third set of peaks (*iii, vi, ix*) are seen at 5.6–5.9 Å, which is closest to the water molecules in the second layer. The sample configurations for these peaks in Figure 8c show the amine tail stretching up toward the bulk water.

Although the presence of these three peaks persist across the curvatures, their locations shift with curvature, as can be seen in Figure 8a. When the curvature changes from convex (purple) to flat (teal), all three peaks shift rightwards. When the curvature changes from flat to concave (yellow), these three peaks shift back toward the left but to a lesser degree.

To understand the trend in the peak closest to the surface, we consider the three structures shown on the left in Figure 8c. "Tentlike" configurations similar to (*i*) are more likely on the convex surface, where the amine group reaches down toward the carbon surface. Even though the center of the aromatic ring is slightly tilted away from the surface, it remains closer to the surface than it would in a similar configuration on a flat or concave surface. The position of the amine as it points down toward the surface corresponds to the leftmost peak in Figure 8a, at 3.19 Å. The structures (*iv*) and (*vii*) also contain amines quite close to the surface, but given the mismatch between the surface curvature and the tentlike structures of (*i*), they are not able to get as close, showing a peak distance of 3.68 Å on the flat graphene surface and of 3.57 Å on the convex surface (see Figure 8b).

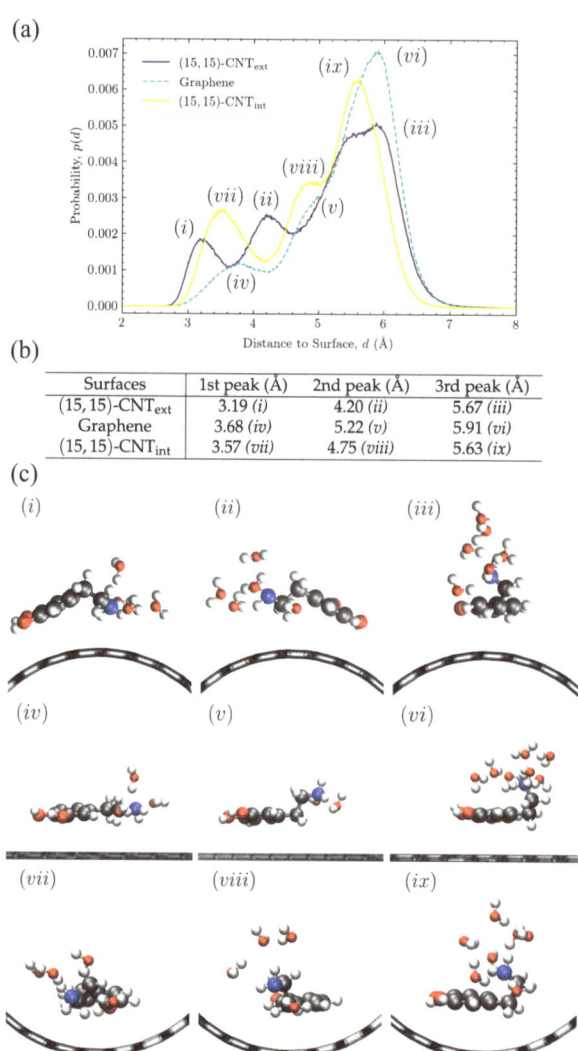

Figure 8. Vertical distributions and configurations of DA at the carbon:water interface. Panel (**a**) shows the vertical distributions of the amine group of DA on flat graphene and on the exterior and interior of a (15, 15)-CNT. The three peaks in each distribution are labeled and correspond to the distances shown in panel (**b**) and the sample conformations shown in panel (**c**). Peak positions in (**b**) were obtained from curve-fitting using Gaussian functions. In panel (**c**), only water molecules within 3 Å radius of the nitrogen in the amine group are displayed.

For the middle peaks, (*ii, v, viii*), represented by the corresponding structures in the middle column of Figure 8c, the leftward shift is even stronger for DA on the convex surface (*ii*) and represents another version of the "tentlike" structures—one with the same tilted aromatic ring but with the amine group pointing back toward the solvent as in structure (*ii*) in Figure 8c. In the next section, we discuss the distributions of these aromatic tilt angles and their curvature dependence. On the flat and concave surfaces, the middle peak corresponds to structures where aromatic ring is parallel to the surface and the amine group is rotated away from the surface by one carbon bond in the linker, as in structures *(v)* and *(viii)*.

The third peak from the surface represents the most probably configuration for all curvatures. In these structures, the two linker bonds that connect the plane of the aromatic ring to the amine group are both oriented to extend the amine out away from the surface (see structures *(iii, vi, ix)* in Figure 8c). The location of this third peak displays the smallest curvature dependency, as can be seen in the relatively small range in the most probable distances listed in Figure 8b, third column. Although the structures shown in Figure 8c only include the neutral DA species, this third peak is the only one observed for the positively charged species, DAH$^+$ and DOQH$^+$ (see the last two rows of Figure 7, right-most column). This result indicates that, when protonated, the amine group remains fully extended into the solvent for all curvatures, similar to structures *(iii, vi, ix)*. These structures also aid in the interpretation of the amine distributions for DA and DOQ at the carbon:vacuum interface in Figure 7 as well. As compared to the same amine distance distributions at the carbon:water interface, the peak locations remain unchanged, but the relative peak heights shift, indicating that configurations with the amine extending away from the surface are significantly less probable in the absence of solvent.

The aromatic ring's tilt angle above the surface depends on curvature, charge, and solvation. The distributions of the tilt angle between the aromatic ring and the surface are shown in Figure 9 for DA on differently curved carbon surfaces at both the carbon:water (Figure 9c) and carbon:vacuum (Figure 9d) interfaces. In addition, the tilt distributions of DA, DOQ, and their protonated species are shown for flat graphene at the aqueous interface in Figure 9e.

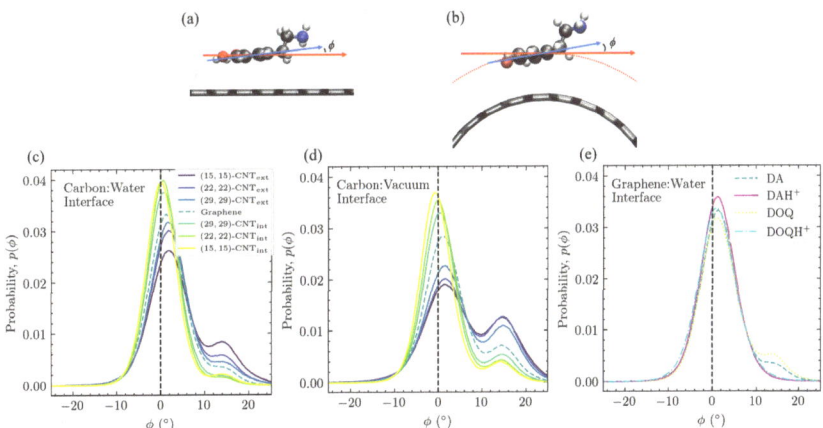

Figure 9. Tilt angle distributions of DA and other adsorbates on differently curved and solvated CNT and graphene surfaces. The tilt angle ϕ is defined as shown in (**a,b**) between the C2–C7 vector (blue arrows) and a vector tangent to the surface at the midpoint of the C2–C7 vector (red arrows). ϕ distributions for DA on differently curved surfaces, plotted as histograms with a binwidth of 0.36°, are shown in (**c**) at the carbon:water interface and in (**d**) at the carbon:vacuum interface. The results for DA, DOQ, and their protonated counterparts are shown in (**e**) on solvated flat graphene.

When adsorbed on all carbon surfaces, DA primarily adopts configurations in which its aromatic ring is parallel to the surface, as seen from the dominant peak, which is close to $\phi = 0°$ in all cases. This configuration maximizes the π–π interactions and is seen in most of the structures shown in Figure 8c. However, a second, asymmetric peak is observed in a subset of the cases at $\phi \approx 15°$ and corresponds to the tentlike configurations seen in structures *(i)* and *(ii)* in Figure 8c. The relative probability of these two tilt angles clearly depends on the surface curvature—the peak at $\phi \approx 0°$ is strongest on the most concave surface, whereas the peak at $\phi \approx 15°$ is strongest on the most convex surface.

The tilt angle distributions also display a clear dependence on charge, as can be seen on solvated flat graphene in Figure 9e, where there is substantial probability around $\phi \approx 15°$ for DA and DOQ but no such density for DAH$^+$ and DOQH$^+$. From the amine group distributions for these positively charged species in Figure 7, we know that they adopt configurations in which the amine group stretches out into the bulk water, which precludes the more tilted tentlike structures like *(i)* and *(ii)* in Figure 8c.

The tilt angle distribution also depends on solvation. As can be seen in Figure 9d, the curvature-dependence observed at the carbon:water surface is also present at the carbon:vacuum surface. However, the population of the tilted configuration increases in all cases, which corresponds well to the shift in the amine distance distribution to values that are closer to the surface for the carbon:vacuum surfaces in Figure 7. Similar results were obtained for DOQ at the carbon:vacuum interface, see Figure S6a.

Adsorbate alignment with CNT axis also depends on curvature and solvation. In Figure 10, the orientational alignment of DA with the axis of the CNT, as defined by θ in Figure 10a,b, is shown on differently curved carbon surfaces at the carbon:water interface (Figure 10c) and at the carbon:vacuum interface (Figure 10d). The θ distributions of DA, DOQ, and their protonated species are also shown for flat graphene at the aqueous interface in Figure 10e.

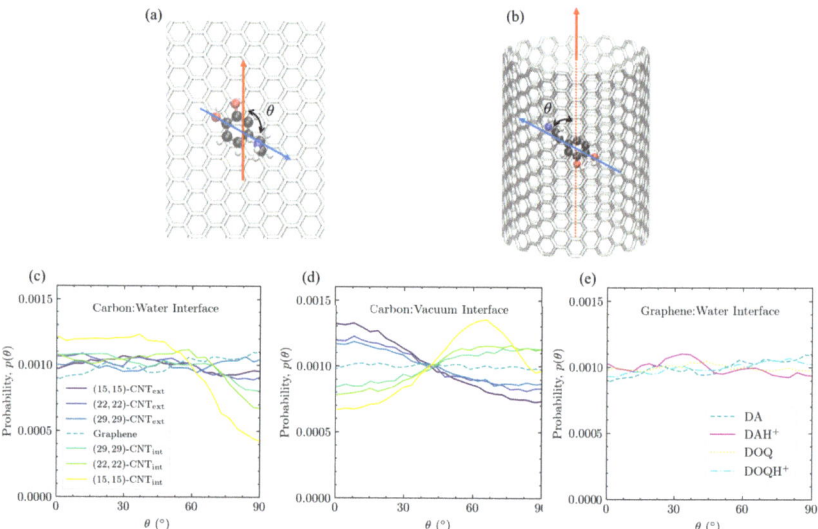

Figure 10. Orientational alignment of DA and other adsorbates with the CNT axis direction on differently curved and solvated CNT and graphene surfaces. The orientational angle, θ, is defined as the angle between the C2–C7 vector (blue arrows) and the CNT axis direction (red arrows), as shown in (**a,b**). θ distributions of DA on differently curved surfaces, plotted as histograms with a binwidth of 3.6°, are shown in (**c**) for the carbon:water interface and in (**d**) for the carbon:vacuum interface. The same results for DA, DOQ, and their protonated counterparts are shown in (**e**) on solvated flat graphene. θ has a range of $[0, 180°]$; however, the results are wrapped so that $p(\theta) = p(180° − \theta)$, for all $\theta > 90°$, due to the symmetry of the system.

At the carbon:water interface, the θ distribution of DA is uniform on flat graphene and on the exterior of the CNTs, as can be seen in Figure 10c. In addition, charge does not seem to influence this orientation for the solvated flat graphene case shown in Figure 10e. Even the flat graphene case at the carbon:vacuum interface in Figure 10d shows no change in the probability with θ. This invariance of the probability of a given θ orientation on flat graphene is to be expected, given the lack of curvature to break the symmetries present in the flat graphene case as well as the lack of significant lateral distribution patterning in Figure 4.

In contrast, on the solvated CNT interior in Figure 10c, there is a marked decrease in the orientational probability as θ approaches $90°$, and the effect becomes more dramatic as the concavity increases. These highly curved interior surfaces favor orientations where the longest axis of DA is oriented along the CNT axis ($\theta = 0 \pm 40°$). This orientational preference is linked to the rightward shift in the aromatic ring's vertical distribution as the surface changes from flat to concave, as shown in Figure 7a. In configurations where DA is not aligned with the CNT axis, its interactions with the inward-curving walls will force the center of the ring slightly away from its optimal distance above the surface. The data obtained from ten trajectories show that, on the solvated interior of the $(15, 15)$-CNT nanotube, where this orientational preference is strongest, the average vertical distance of the ring's COM for all configurations in which DA is closely aligned with the CNT axis ($|\theta| < 5°$) is 3.66 ± 0.15 Å, whereas the average vertical distance for the configurations where DA is perpendicularly aligned to the CNT axis ($85° < |\theta| < 95°$) is 3.90 ± 0.17 Å.

The θ distribution is entirely different at the carbon:vacuum interface, however. Orientations aligned with the CNT axis are disfavored on the CNT interior, and the most favorable orientation on the CNT interior shifts to $\approx 65°$. At the same time, orientations aligned with the CNT axis are favored on the CNT exterior. Both trends grow stronger with increased curvature, and the same trends were observed for DOQ at the carbon:vacuum interface (Figure S6b).

Adsorbate solvation shell depends on curvature and influences R_H. According to the Stokes–Einstein equation, the diffusion constant, $D \propto (1/R_H)$, where R_H is the effective hydrodynamic radius, which depends on the magnitude of attractions between the diffusing particle and the nearby solvent molecules. In the case of a particle adsorbed to a surface, solvation is necessarily limited by the presence and geometry of that surface. Although the Stokes–Einstein relation cannot be directly applied in that situation, it does provide a way to think about the influence of the degree of solvation on diffusion, as the magnitude of any favorable interactions between the particle and nearby solvent will influence the particle's effective hydrodynamic radius, R_H. To investigate this effect, we calculated the number of solvating water molecules within the first water shell around the DA or DOQ atoms for each surface architecture. A distance of 5 Å was chosen as the cutoff of that first water shell based on the distribution shown in Figure S5. The results are shown in Figure 11a and display a clear trend from fewest solvating waters on the smallest CNT's interior to the most solvating waters on the smallest CNT's exterior—as expected given the geometric constraints of the surface. This trend matches that seen in the diffusion constants on different surface curvatures, as seen in Figure 3c. To determine how well this solvation effect can explain the trend in diffusivities, we plotted in Figure 11b the diffusivities from Figure 3c vs. $(N_{water})^{-1/3}$, where N_{water} is the number of waters within 5 Å of a DA atom, since $D \propto (1/R_H)$, and R_H is roughly $\propto (N_{water})^{1/3}$. The correspondence is quite strong, and this effect is even able to explain the overlapping values seen in the diffusivities even as curvature steadily changes for the CNT exteriors and for the $(22, 22)$-CNT_{int} and $(29, 29)$-CNT_{int} cases. Since there is a clear geometric trend across these different diameter CNTs, the fact that the number of solvating waters is the same implies that a change in the adsorbate structures, as documented above, must compensate for that change in a way that maintains a similar degree of solvation.

Overall, we find here that the vertical placement of the adsorbate and its moieties above the carbon surface, as well as its tilt angle and alignment with the CNT axis depend in a complex manner on curvature, solvation, and charge. In addition, the degree of DA solvation varies with curvature and can explain much of the trend observed as D varies across curvatures.

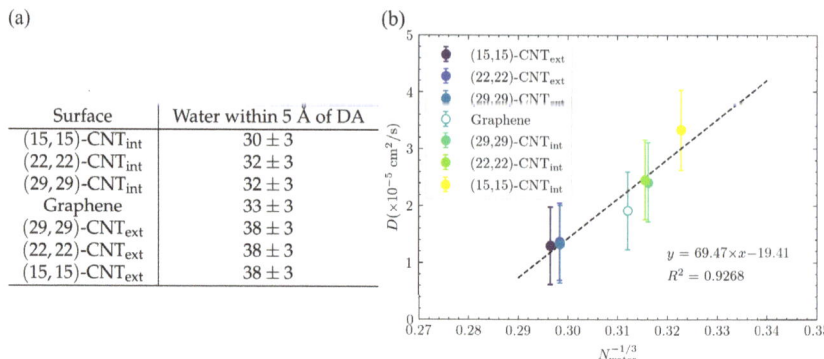

Figure 11. Correspondence between CNT surface, solvating waters, and D. (**a**) The number of waters in the first solvation shell around DA are calculated across the different surfaces. For a given water molecule, its distance to DA is the shortest distance between its oxygen atom and any the atoms of DA. Only the water molecules that are on the same side of the surface as DA are counted. N_{water} and its statistical errors were computed from 10 trajectories. (**b**) The diffusion constants, D, from Figure 3c are plotted vs. $N_{water}^{-1/3}$ for DA on a range of differently curved surfaces. A linear fit line is shown here along with the coefficient of determination, R^2.

3.4. DA Localizes and Diffuses within a CNT Groove

Since a pair of aligned CNTs is the simplest multi-CNT structure expected within CNT-based material, we also investigated how DA behaves on a groove surface, both for the solvated and vacuum cases.

In all the simulations, DA localized to the groove between the two CNTs within 2–8 ns and remained there. Given this strong structural preference, we ran each simulations for at least 5 ns after it found its way to the groove. All results presented in this section were obtained from the portions of the trajectories where DA is within the CNT groove.

A typical configuration from a groove simulation is shown in Figure 12a, the lateral distribution of DA is shown in Figure 12b, and the 3D distribution is shown in Figure 12c. There is a slight dependence on the underlying hexagonal structure in the lateral density distribution in Figure 12b, but only the axial direction, as the adsorbate's location around the circumference is determined by the optimal distance from the other CNT surface, as can be seen in Figure 12c. Note that any lateral patterning will depend on the degree to which the neighboring CNTs are in register. There is a clear separation in the 3D density plot between configurations with DA adsorbed to one CNT surface vs. the other. Jumps between the two CNT surfaces are rare in the solvated case (1.9 ± 0.4 ns^{-1}), but were more frequently for DA adsorbed at the carbon:vacuum interface (49.2 ± 7.4 ns^{-1}). Jump trajectories across both the carbon:water and carbon:vacuum CNT grooves can be seen in Figure S7.

Figure 13a compares $D_\parallel$ and $D_\perp$ for DA in the solvated groove to the same values for DA on the exterior of a single $(15, 15)$-CNT, since the groove is constructed of two aligned $(15, 15)$-CNTs. Results directly obtained from the 100 Å-length CNT groove system are shown in the top section of the table, while the extrapolation to the infinite CNT groove is shown at the bottom. Importantly, the observed trends hold for both the finite size results and the infinite size extrapolations. As expected, $D_\perp$ drops to almost zero when DA remains in the groove. In contrast, DA's diffusivity along the groove, $D_\parallel$, is significantly faster than the corresponding axial diffusivity on the exterior surface of a single CNT. We then calculated N_{water} for DA in the groove and found 26 ± 3 waters within 5 Å. This value is lower than those reported in Figure 11a for the other surface structures and explains the faster diffusion within the solvated groove.

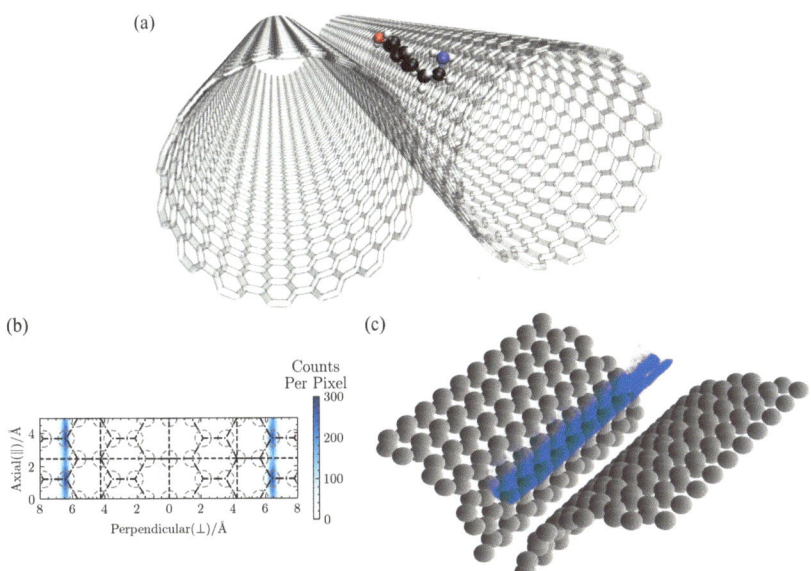

Figure 12. Spatial distributions of DA in a solvated CNT groove. The COM coordinates of DA within a solvated CNT groove formed by two parallel CNT, as seen in a typical configuration shown in (**a**), are plotted here in both (**b**) 2D and (**c**) 3D. The CNT groove is constructed of two parallel, 100 Å (15, 15)-CNTs. In the 2D distribution plot in (**b**), locations along the axial direction were wrapped into two unit cells. The gray dashed circles represent the location of the surface carbon atoms, and the black dashed line in the middle at $\perp = 0$ Å represents the location on the CNT circumference where the distance between the two CNTs is smallest. The distribution density in region to the left of that dashed line results from configurations where the adsorbate is closest to the CNT on the left, while the density to the right results from configurations where the adsorbate is closest to the CNT on the right. In the 3D distribution in (**c**), the COM coordinates along the axial direction were wrapped into ten unit cells for plotting.

Interestingly, this trend is reversed for DA's diffusivity in the groove at the carbon:vacuum interface. Figure 13b shows the comparison of the axial MSD of DA in the groove to that of DA on other CNT and graphene surfaces, all at the carbon:vacuum interface. Without solvent, displacement along the groove is reduced as compared to that on any other surface, which can be readily explained by the presence of two variegated surfaces that can impact DA's inertial motion rather than just one.

The results for the diffusion of all four adsorbate species within the 100 Å CNT groove are shown in Table 3. The previously observed trends between oxidized and reduced species (oxidized diffuses more rapidly) and between protonated and neutral species (neutral diffuses more rapidly) both hold within the groove architecture.

Table 3. Diffusion coefficients of DA, DOQ, DAH$^+$, and DOQH$^+$ in a solvated CNT groove. The CNT groove results shown here are reported directly from the finite 100 Å-long CNT simulations.

Adsorbate	$D_\parallel$ ($\times 10^{-5}$ cm^2/s)	$D_\perp$ ($\times 10^{-5}$ cm^2/s)
DA	1.82 ± 0.09	0.02 ± 0.01
DOQ	1.98 ± 0.17	0.04 ± 0.03
DAH$^+$	1.60 ± 0.10	0.02 ± 0.01
DOQH$^+$	1.63 ± 0.05	0.02 ± 0.00

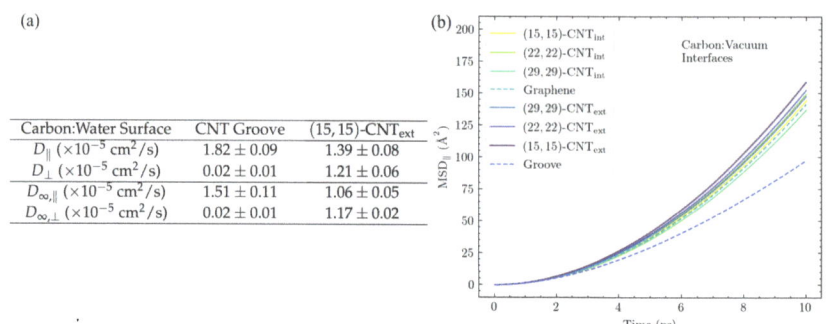

Figure 13. Diffusion coefficients of DA within a CNT groove. The CNT groove is constructed of two 100 Å long, aligned, $(15,15)$-CNTs. (a) Diffusion constants for the solvated CNT groove and a solvated $(15,15)$-CNT$_{ext}$ surface are shown here, both from the 100 Å simulation directly (top rows) and from the infinite-system size extrapolation (bottom rows). $D_\parallel$ is the 1D diffusion coefficient for motion along the CNT groove and axis, and $D_\perp$ is the 1D diffusion coefficient around the CNT circumference. (b) The axial mean squared displacement of DA is plotted for various surfaces at the carbon:vacuum interface. These MSD results are taken directly from simulations done in the vacuum on 100 Å CNTs and 100×100 Å^2 graphene.

4. Conclusions

Overall, we find that DA and DOQ rapidly diffuse on the surface of pristine CNTs, just as they do on the flat graphene surface [18]. Diffusion on a single CNT is rapid both along the CNT axis and around its circumference. This observation corresponds to results from Kim et al., who developed a continuum model on the μm scale to demonstrate the catalytic activity of the exterior sidewall of individual CNTs. The model shows evidence that the entire length of the CNT is uniformly accessible to the electrochemically active analytes, which matched their spatially resolved scanning electrochemical microscopy results [12].

At the same time, we find that the adsorbate diffusivity also depends on the CNT curvature. We observed enhanced adsorbate diffusion as the surface changes from convex to flat to concave. Although this trend is similar to that observed previously for atomic adsorbates on CNT surfaces [23,24], its origin differs. In our study, where molecular adsorbates are diffusing on a solvated surface, the curvature-dependent diffusion cannot be attributed to changes in the underlying surface energy roughness with curvature, as the lateral distributions of the molecular adsorbates do not depend on curvature. In addition, we find that the diffusion constants on the zigzag and armchair CNTs are indistinguishable. Finally, in the absence of solvent, the curvature dependence disappears.

Why, then, does adsorbate diffusivity change with curvature? First and foremost, the degree of solvation depends upon the surface geometry and will influence the adsorbate's effective hydrodynamic radius, R_H, and the Stokes–Einstein equation, although not quantitatively applicable here, tells us that the diffusion constant goes as $1/R_H$. Second, we also observe systematic shifts in the adsorbate tilt angle and axial orientation with surface curvature, which are also influenced by solvation. Last, multiple studies have shown changes in solvent dynamics within a CNT [25,27,28,30,31], which could influence adsorbate dynamics in our simulation. While most of these effects are for CNTs with diameters significantly smaller than ours, enhancements in solvent diffusion have been seen at the interior of narrow CNTs and are more dramatic close to the CNT surface [25,27]. We also note that we observe more significant finite size effects in the CNT interior systems (see Figure S4); however, the observed trend with curvature holds even when the correction is made to an infinitely long CNT system (see Table 1).

Directional diffusion of adsorbates on the surface of CNTs is of general interest for several applications [23,41,49–51]. Prior work studying adatom diffusion on the CNT surface noted substantial differences between diffusion pathways on armchair and zigzag

CNTs, with the adatom diffusing exclusively around the zigzag CNT's circumference, while on the armchair CNT, the adatom moved axially as well [23]. It may be concluded that CNT helicity could play an important role in determining mass transport on these nanoscale surfaces. However, we found no such effect on the surface of a single CNT in our system; the larger molecular structure of DA and DOQ decreased the importance of the direction of strain in the underlying CNT hexagonal surface. More importantly, solvation at room temperature removes the helicity dependence for even the adatom(DA) in our simulations, despite the fact that its lateral placement depends on the direction of curvature (see Figure 4, top row). As a result, we do not expect CNT helicity to play an important role in determining the directionality of diffusive transport for adsorbates on solvated surfaces at room temperature. At the same time, we did observe significant changes in the direction of diffusion for DA at the groove junction between two aligned CNTs. Once the adsorbate encountered the groove, it stayed there and subsequent diffusion was restricted to the axial direction. This directional effect could therefore have a significant impact on mass transport within CNT-based nanomaterials.

Although the work in this paper focuses on single-walled CNTs and graphene, we expect that our key findings can be extended to other carbon nanostructures. On multi-walled CNTs, we anticipate dopamine structures, diffusion timescales, and curvature trends that are similar to single-walled CNTs with the same interface curvature, since we found previously that dopamine diffusion on one layer of pristine graphene was indistinguishable from that on a triple layer of graphene [18]. Dopamine diffusion on the exterior of fullerenes will also be similar to that on the exterior of the highly curved CNTs. However, the slow "hopping" rate we observed from one CNT surface to another—even when both surfaces share an extended edge where they are in close proximity—makes it clear that adsorption of DA to fullerene, or other 0D nanostructures, would localize DA for long timescales. Thus, we expect that some fraction of the mass transport of adsorbed DA would be arrested on a composite surface that incorporates fullerenes. Diffusion of molecular adsorbates on extended and 3D carbon surfaces are likely to differ significantly from our observations on CNTs, as these structures may have highly confined waters, where dynamics are known to differ significantly from that of bulk water [27–29]. In addition, we have found that the degree of adsorbate solvation at the carbon:aqueous interface, coupled with the local water dynamics, is essential for determining adsorbate diffusivities across a range of molecular carbon surfaces.

CNTs have become common materials for electrochemical sensors but the diffusion of common analytes, such as dopamine, has not been understood on their surface. Here, we find that diffusion is fast on CNTs, about as fast as on flat graphene. However, CNT-based electrodes are not made of single CNTs, and many electrodes consist of aligned CNT materials, such as CNT forests or CNT yarns [3–5]. Thus, modeling a CNT groove shows that interactions between CNTs also affect dopamine dynamics. The CNT groove provides directionality for movement and localizes the dopamine on one part of the CNT. In future studies, we could introduce a voltage and examine electrochemistry. We expect that the observed shifts in tilt angle, axial orientation, and analyte–surface distance that occur upon changes to CNT curvature will be important for electron transfer. These are the first studies of dopamine diffusion on CNT electrodes and provide foundational information about the surface structure and dynamics of dopamine adsorbates on electrode surfaces.

Supplementary Materials: The following supporting information can be downloaded at: https://www.mdpi.com/article/10.3390/molecules27123768/s1. References [52–54] are cited in the supplementary materials.

Author Contributions: Conceptualization, Q.J., B.J.V., K.H.D.; methodology, Q.J., K.H.D.; formal analysis, Q.J., K.H.D.; investigation, Q.J.; resources, B.J.V., K.H.D.; data curation, Q.J., B.J.V., K.H.D.; writing—original draft preparation, Q.J., B.J.V., K.H.D.; writing—review and editing, Q.J., B.J.V., K.H.D.; visualization, Q.J.; supervision, K.H.D., B.J.V.; project administration, K.H.D.; funding acquisition, B.J.V., K.H.D. All authors have read and agreed to the published version of the manuscript.

Funding: This work was supported by an NIH grant, NIH R01EB026497, to B.J.V. Additional support was provided by funding from the University of Virginia.

Institutional Review Board Statement: Not applicable.

Informed Consent Statement: Not applicable.

Data Availability Statement: The data presented in this study, along with submission and analysis scripts, are openly available on GitHub at https://github.com/dubayresearchgroup/DopaDiff.

Acknowledgments: The authors also acknowledge Research Computing at the University of Virginia (https://rc.virginia.edu, accessed on 4 May 2022) for providing computational resources and technical support. The authors would like to thank Cheng Yang for helpful conversations on this project.

Conflicts of Interest: The authors declare no conflict of interest.

Sample Availability: Not applicable.

References

1. Cao, Q.; Hensley, D.K.; Lavrik, N.V.; Venton, B.J. Carbon nanospikes have better electrochemical properties than carbon nanotubes due to greater surface roughness and defect sites. *Carbon* **2019**, *155*, 250–257. [CrossRef] [PubMed]
2. Yang, C.; Denno, M.E.; Pyakurel, P.; Venton, B.J. Recent trends in carbon nanomaterial-based electrochemical sensors for biomolecules: A review. *Anal. Chim. Acta* **2015**, *887*, 17–37. [CrossRef] [PubMed]
3. Yang, C.; Trikantzopoulos, E.; Nguyen, M.D.; Jacobs, C.B.; Wang, Y.; Mahjouri-Samani, M.; Ivanov, I.N.; Venton, B.J. Laser Treated Carbon Nanotube Yarn Microelectrodes for Rapid and Sensitive Detection of Dopamine in Vivo. *ACS Sens.* **2016**, *1*, 508–515. [CrossRef] [PubMed]
4. Xiao, N.; Venton, B.J. Rapid, sensitive detection of neurotransmitters at microelectrodes modified with self-assembled SWCNT forests. *Anal. Chem.* **2012**, *84*, 7816–7822. [CrossRef] [PubMed]
5. Kim, H.; Kang, T.H.; Ahn, J.; Han, H.; Park, S.; Kim, S.J.; Park, M.C.; Paik, S.H.; Hwang, D.K.; Yi, H.; et al. Spirally wrapped carbon nanotube microelectrodes for fiber optoelectronic devices beyond geometrical limitations toward smart wearable E-textile applications. *ACS Nano* **2020**, *14*, 17213–17223. [CrossRef]
6. Feng, X.; Zhang, Y.; Zhou, J.; Li, Y.; Chen, S.; Zhang, L.; Ma, Y.; Wang, L.; Yan, X. Three-dimensional nitrogen-doped graphene as an ultrasensitive electrochemical sensor for the detection of dopamine. *Nanoscale* **2015**, *7*, 2427–2432. [CrossRef]
7. Salamon, J.; Sathishkumar, Y.; Ramachandran, K.; Lee, Y.S.; Yoo, D.J.; Kim, A.R.; Kumar, G.G. One-pot synthesis of magnetite nanorods/graphene composites and its catalytic activity toward electrochemical detection of dopamine. *Biosens. Bioelectron.* **2015**, *64*, 269–276. [CrossRef]
8. Taylor, I.M.; Robbins, E.M.; Catt, K.A.; Cody, P.A.; Happe, C.L.; Cui, X.T. Enhanced dopamine detection sensitivity by PEDOT/graphene oxide coating on in vivo carbon fiber electrodes. *Biosens. Bioelectron.* **2017**, *89*, 400–410. [CrossRef]
9. Rodeberg, N.T.; Sandberg, S.G.; Johnson, J.A.; Phillips, P.E.M.; Wightman, R.M. Hitchhiker's Guide to Voltammetry: Acute and Chronic Electrodes for in Vivo Fast-Scan Cyclic Voltammetry. *ACS Chem. Neurosci.* **2017**, *8*, 221–234. [CrossRef]
10. Wightman, R.M. Probing Cellular Chemistry in Biological Systems with Microelectrodes. *Science* **2006**, *311*, 1570–1574. [CrossRef]
11. Jacobs, C.B.; Ivanov, I.N.; Nguyen, M.D.; Zestos, A.G.;Venton, B.J. High Temporal Resolution Measurements of Dopamine with Carbon Nanotube Yarn Microelectrodes. *Anal. Chem.* **2014**, *86*, 5721–5727. [CrossRef] [PubMed]
12. Kim, J.; Xiong, H.; Hofmann, M.; Kong, J.; Amemiya, S. Scanning Electrochemical Microscopy of Individual Single-Walled Carbon Nanotubes. *Anal. Chem.* **2010**, *82*, 1605–1607. [CrossRef] [PubMed]
13. Güell, A.G.; Meadows, K.E.; Dudin, P.V.; Ebejer, N.; Macpherson, J.V.; Unwin, P.R. Mapping Nanoscale Electrochemistry of Individual Single-Walled Carbon Nanotubes. *Nano Lett.* **2014**, *14*, 220–224. [CrossRef] [PubMed]
14. Byers, J.C.; Güell, A.G.; Unwin, P.R. Nanoscale Electrocatalysis: Visualizing Oxygen Reduction at Pristine, Kinked, and Oxidized Sites on Individual Carbon Nanotubes. *J. Am. Chem. Soc.* **2014**, *136*, 11252–11255. [CrossRef]
15. Carbone, M.; Gorton, L.; Antiochia, R. An overview of the latest graphene-based sensors for glucose detection: The effects of graphene defects. *Electroanalysis* **2015**, *27*, 16–31. [CrossRef]
16. Chen, B.; Perry, D.; Teahan, J.; McPherson, I.J.; Edmondson, J.; Kang, M.; Valavanis, D.; Frenguelli, B.G.; Unwin, P.R. Artificial Synapse: Spatiotemporal Heterogeneities in Dopamine Electrochemistry at a Carbon Fiber Ultramicroelectrode. *ACS Meas. Sci. Au* **2021**, *1*, 6–10. [CrossRef]
17. Ma, M.; Tocci, G.; Michaelides, A.; Aeppli, G. Fast diffusion of water nanodroplets on graphene. *Nat. Mater.* **2016**, *15*, 66–71. [CrossRef]
18. Jia, Q.; Yang, C.; Venton, B.J.; DuBay, K.H. Atomistic simulations of dopamine diffusion dynamics on a pristine graphene surface. *ChemPhysChem* **2022**, *23*, e202100783. [CrossRef]
19. Venton, B.J.; Troyer, K.P.; Wightman, R.M. Response Times of Carbon Fiber Microelectrodes to Dynamic Changes in Catecholamine Concentration. *Anal. Chem.* **2002**, *74*, 539–546. [CrossRef]

20. Bath, B.D.; Martin, H.B.; Wightman, R.M.; Anderson, M.R. Dopamine Adsorption at Surface Modified Carbon-Fiber Electrodes. *Langmuir* **2001**, *17*, 7032–7039. [CrossRef]
21. Holcman, D.; Schuss, Z. Time scale of diffusion in molecular and cellular biology. *J. Phys. A Math. Theor.* **2014**, *47*, 173001. [CrossRef]
22. Oleinick, A.; Álvarez Martos, I.; Svir, I.; Ferapontova, E.E.; Amatore, C. Surface Heterogeneities Matter in Fast Scan Cyclic Voltammetry Investigations of Catecholamines in Brain with Carbon Microelectrodes of High-Aspect Ratio: Dopamine Oxidation at Conical Carbon Microelectrodes. *J. Electrochem. Soc.* **2018**, *165*, G3057–G3065. [CrossRef]
23. Shu, D.J.; Gong, X.G. Curvature effect on surface diffusion: The nanotube. *J. Chem. Phys.* **2001**, *114*, 10922–10926. [CrossRef]
24. Liu, L.; Chen, Z.; Wang, L.; Polyakova, E.; Taniguchi, T.; Watanabe, K.; Hone, J.; Flynn, G.W.; Brus, L.E. Slow gold adatom diffusion on graphene: Effect of silicon dioxide and hexagonal boron nitride substrates. *J. Phys. Chem. B* **2013**, *117*, 4305–4312. [CrossRef] [PubMed]
25. Barati Farimani, A.; Aluru, N.R. Spatial diffusion of water in carbon nanotubes: From fickian to ballistic motion. *J. Phys. Chem. B* **2011**, *115*, 12145–12149. [CrossRef]
26. Alexiadis, A.; Kassinos, S. Molecular simulation of water in carbon nanotubes. *Chem. Rev.* **2008**, *108*, 5014–5034. [CrossRef]
27. Zheng, Y.g.; Ye, H.f.; Zhang, Z.q.; Zhang, H.w. Water diffusion inside carbon nanotubes: Mutual effects of surface and confinement. *Phys. Chem. Chem. Phys.* **2012**, *14*, 964–971. [CrossRef]
28. Hirunsit, P.; Balbuena, P.B. Effects of confinement on water structure and dynamics: A molecular simulation study. *J. Phys. Chem. C* **2007**, *111*, 1709–1715. [CrossRef]
29. Limmer, D.T.; Chandler, D. Phase diagram of supercooled water confined to hydrophilic nanopores. *J. Chem. Phys.* **2012**, *137*. [CrossRef]
30. Striolo, A. The mechanism of water diffusion in narrow carbon nanotubes. *Nano Lett.* **2006**, *6*, 633–639. [CrossRef]
31. Falk, K.; Sedlmeier, F.; Joly, L.; Netz, R.R.; Bocquet, L. Molecular Origin of Fast Water Transport in Carbon Nanotube Membranes: Superlubricity versus Curvature Dependent Friction. *Nano Lett.* **2010**, *10*, 4067–4073. [CrossRef] [PubMed]
32. Plimpton, S. Fast Parallel Algorithms for Short-Range Molecular Dynamics. *J. Comput. Phys.* **1995**, *117*, 1–19. [CrossRef]
33. Jorgensen, W.L.; Maxwell, D.S.; Tirado-Rives, J. Development and Testing of the OPLS All-Atom Force Field on Conformational Energetics and Properties of Organic Liquids. *J. Am. Chem. Soc.* **1996**, *118*, 11225–11236. [CrossRef]
34. Lazar, P.; Karlický, F.; Jurečka, P.; Kocman, M.; Otyepková, E.; Šafářová, K.; Otyepka, M. Adsorption of Small Organic Molecules on Graphene. *J. Am. Chem. Soc.* **2013**, *135*, 6372–6377. [CrossRef]
35. Björk, J.; Hanke, F.; Palma, C.A.; Samori, P.; Cecchini, M.; Persson, M. Adsorption of Aromatic and Anti-Aromatic Systems on Graphene through $\pi - \pi$ Stacking. *J. Phys. Chem. Lett.* **2010**, *1*, 3407–3412. [CrossRef]
36. Li, Z. *Nanofluidics: An Introduction*; CRC Press: Boca Raton, FL, USA, 2018.
37. Yeh, I.C.; Hummer, G. System-size dependence of diffusion coefficients and viscosities from molecular dynamics simulations with periodic boundary conditions. *J. Phys. Chem. B* **2004**, *108*, 15873–15879. [CrossRef]
38. Jamali, S.H.; Wolff, L.; Becker, T.M.; Bardow, A.; Vlugt, T.J.; Moultos, O.A. Finite-size effects of binary mutual diffusion coefficients from molecular dynamics. *J. Chem. Theory Comput.* **2018**, *14*, 2667–2677. [CrossRef]
39. Fushiki, M. System size dependence of the diffusion coefficient in a simple liquid. *Phys. Rev. E* **2003**, *68*, 021203. [CrossRef]
40. Celebi, A.T.; Jamali, S.H.; Bardow, A.; Vlugt, T.J.; Moultos, O.A. Finite-size effects of diffusion coefficients computed from molecular dynamics: A review of what we have learned so far. *Mol. Simul.* **2020**, *47*, 831–845. [CrossRef]
41. Lohrasebi, A.; Neek-Amal, M.; Ejtehadi, M. Directed motion of C_{60} on a graphene sheet subjected to a temperature gradient. *Phys. Rev. E* **2011**, *83*, 042601. [CrossRef]
42. Nishihira, J.; Tachikawa, H. Theoretical Study on the Interaction Between Dopamine and its Receptor byab initioMolecular Orbital Calculation. *J. Theor. Biol.* **1997**, *185*, 157–163. [CrossRef] [PubMed]
43. Meiser, J.; Weindl, D.; Hiller, K. Complexity of dopamine metabolism. *Cell Commun. Signal.* **2013**, *11*, 34. [CrossRef] [PubMed]
44. Frenkel, D.; Smit, B. *Understanding Molecular Simulation: From Algorithm to Applications*; Academic Press: Cambridge, MA, USA, 2001.
45. Tomanek, D. *Guide through the Nanocarbon Jungle*; 2053-2571; Morgan & Claypool Publishers: Williston, VT, USA 2014.
46. Simonnin, P.; Noetinger, B.; Nieto-Draghi, C.; Marry, V.; Rotenberg, B. Diffusion under confinement: Hydrodynamic finite-size effects in simulation. *J. Chem. Theory Comput.* **2017**, *13*, 2881–2889. [CrossRef] [PubMed]
47. Gerhardt, G.; Adams, R.N. Determination of diffusion coefficients by flow injection analysis. *Anal. Chem.* **1982**, *54*, 2618–2620. [CrossRef]
48. Wu, M.C.; Li, C.L.; Hu, C.K.; Chang, Y.C.; Liaw, Y.H.; Huang, L.W.; Chang, C.S.; Tsong, T.T.; Hsu, T. Curvature effect on the surface diffusion of silver adatoms on carbon nanotubes: Deposition experiments and numerical simulations. *Phys. Rev. B* **2006**, *74*, 125424. [CrossRef]
49. Neek-Amal, M.; Abedpour, N.; Rasuli, S.; Naji, A.; Ejtehadi, M. Diffusive motion of C_{60} on a graphene sheet. *Phys. Rev. E* **2010**, *82*, 051605. [CrossRef]
50. Rurali, R.; Hernandez, E. Thermally induced directed motion of fullerene clusters encapsulated in carbon nanotubes. *Chem. Phys. Lett.* **2010**, *497*, 62–65. [CrossRef]
51. Khodabakhshi, M.; Moosavi, A. Unidirectional transport of water through an asymmetrically charged rotating carbon nanotube. *J. Phys. Chem. C* **2017**, *121*, 23649–23658. [CrossRef]

52. Arefin, M.S. Empirical equation based chirality (n, m) assignment of semiconducting single wall carbon nanotubes from resonant Raman scattering data. *Nanomaterials* **2013**, *3*, 1–21. [CrossRef]
53. Qin, L.-C. Determination of the chiral indices (n, m) of carbon nanotubes by electron diffraction. *Phys. Chem. Chem. Phys.* **2007**, *9*, 31–48. [CrossRef]
54. Castro-Villarreal, P. Brownian motion meets Riemann curvature. *J. Stat. Mech. Theory Exp.* **2010**, *2010*, P08006. [CrossRef]

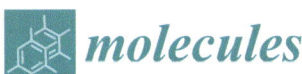

Article

Nanochannel Array on Electrochemically Polarized Screen Printed Carbon Electrode for Rapid and Sensitive Electrochemical Determination of Clozapine in Human Whole Blood

Kai Wang [1,†], Luoxing Yang [2,†], Huili Huang [3], Ning Lv [4], Jiyang Liu [2,*] and Youshi Liu [1,*]

[1] Key Laboratory of Integrated Oncology and Intelligent Medicine of Zhejiang Province, Department of Hepatobiliary and Pancreatic Surgery, Affiliated Hangzhou First People's Hospital, Zhejiang University School of Medicine, Hangzhou 310006, China; kaiw3@zju.edu.cn
[2] Key Laboratory of Surface & Interface Science of Polymer Materials of Zhejiang Province, Department of Chemistry, Zhejiang Sci-Tech University, Hangzhou 310018, China; 17858903877@163.com
[3] Department of Psychiatry, Affiliated Xiaoshan Hospital, Hangzhou Normal University, Hangzhou 310018, China; hhl1626@163.com
[4] Department of Pharmacy, The First Affiliated Hospital, School of Medicine, Zhejiang University, Hangzhou 310018, China; lvn1987@zju.edu.cn
* Correspondence: liujyxx@126.com (J.L.); liuyoushi@zju.edu.cn (Y.L.)
† These authors contributed equally to this work.

Abstract: Rapid and highly sensitive determination of clozapine (CLZ), a psychotropic drug for the treatment of refractory schizophrenia, in patients is of great significance to reduce the risk of disease recurrence. However, direct electroanalysis of CLZ in human whole blood remains a great challenge owing to the remarkable fouling that occurs in a complex matrix. In this work, a miniaturized, integrated, disposable electrochemical sensing platform based on the integration of nanochannel arrays on the surface of screen-printed carbon electrodes (SPCE) is demonstrated. The device achieves high determination sensitivity while also offering the electrode anti-fouling and anti-interference capabilities. To enhance the electrochemical performance of SPCE, simple electrochemical polarization including anodic oxidation and cathodic reduction is applied to pretreat SPCE. The electrochemically polarized SPCE (p-SPCE) exhibits an enhanced electrochemical peak signal toward CLZ compared with bare SPCE. An electrochemically assisted self-assembly method (EASA) is utilized to conveniently electrodeposit a vertically ordered mesoporous silica nanomembrane film (VMSF) on the p-SPCE, which could further enrich CLZ through electrostatic interactions. Owing to the dual signal amplification based on the p-SPCE and VMSF nanochannels, the developed VMSF/SPCE sensor enables determination of CLZ in the range from 50 nM to 20 μM with a low limit of detection (LOD) of 28 nM (S/N = 3). Combined with the excellent anti-fouling and anti-interference abilities of VMSF, direct and sensitive determination of CLZ in human blood is also achieved.

Keywords: nanochannel array; screen-printed carbon electrode; electrochemical polarization; electrochemical determination of clozapine; human blood

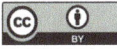

1. Introduction

Schizophrenia is a common mental illness that places a great burden on society. Some 20–30% of patients suffer from treatment-resistant schizophrenia (TRS) [1]. Research has shown that clozapine (CLZ) is the only drug with good therapeutic effect on TRS [2–4]. The intake of CLZ plays a crucial role in the recovery of patients. Excessive CLZ results in a lot of side effects including excessive salivation [5], agranulocytosis [6], seizures [7], weight gain [8], and mumps [9], which will cause secondary damage to the patient's health [10]. Therefore, real-time determination of CLZ is of great significance to reduce the risk of relapse and readmission of patients.

Until now, the determination of clozapine has mainly relied on liquid chromatography-tandem mass spectrometry (LC-MS/MS), gas chromatography-mass spectrometry (GC-MS), colorimetric analysis and fluorescence sensing, etc. [11–13]. However, these detection strategies typically require expensive instruments and a professional operator. In addition, the pretreatment process for real sample analyses is often complex and time-consuming, and requires the use of a large amount of organic solvents [14–19]. Electrochemical methods have the characteristics of fast detection, simple instrumentation, high sensitivity, and convenient operation, and have been widely used in analyses of environmental, biological, medical, clinical or food samples [20–28]. Researchers have carried out electrochemical determination of CLZ using differential pulse voltammetry (DPV), square wave voltammetry (SWV), cyclic voltammetry (CV), etc. The determination sensitivity can be improved by introducing metal nanoparticles, carbon-based materials, etc. to the electrode surface [29–31]. However, the determination of CLZ in complex samples remains a great challenge. Complex biological or clinical samples (e.g., whole blood, serum, etc.) usually have complex matrices containing a large number of co-existing components including particulate matter (e.g., red blood cells, etc.), biological macromolecules (e.g., protein, DNA, etc.) and other electroactive small molecules (e.g., ascorbic acid-AA, uric acid-UA, etc.). On the one hand, particles or biological macromolecules will contaminate the surface of the electrode through non-specific adsorption, which will significantly reduce the detection sensitivity. On the other hand, co-existing electroactive small molecules can generate interfering signals. In addition, conventional electrochemical determination uses conventional electrodes (e.g., glassy carbon, gold, platinum, etc. with a diameter of 3 mm), so detection requires a larger sample volume. Therefore, it is very important to improve the antifouling, anti-interference ability and detection selectivity of the electrode while maintaining high detection sensitivity and low sample consumption.

The introduction of nanochannel arrays on the electrode surface is an effective strategy to improve its anti-fouling and anti-interference properties. In this regard, vertically ordered mesoporous silica nanomembrane films (VMSFs) have attracted much attention. VMSFs are composed of an array of silica nanochannels with uniform pore size (commonly 2–3 nm) and high porosity (up to 12×10^{12} cm^{-2}). The high porosity ensures the mass transfer of small molecules within the film [32,33]. In addition, ultra-small nanochannels allow VMSF to achieve significant size exclusion for proteins or particles. On the other hand, the silanol groups (pK_a = 2–3) on the nanochannel surface endow VMSF with a certain charge selectivity [34–36], which can achieve selective permeation of charged species. In general, small molecules with negative charge will be repelled, making it difficult to for them enter the nanochannels and reach the electrode surface. In contrast, positively charged small molecules will be enriched, leading to signal amplification and high detection sensitivity [37–39]. Owing to the excellent anti-fouling [40] and anti-interference ability and potential enrichment effect, the VMSF modified electrode has great potential for direct and sensitive analyses of CLZ in complex samples.

Screen-printed electrodes (SPEs) are miniaturized and integrated electrodes prepared using screen-printing technology; they can disposable and entail low production costs. Since SPEs integrate the traditional three-electrode system (working electrode, counter electrode and reference electrode), the amount of sample used for detection can be very small. Among them, screen-printed carbon electrodes (SPCEs) have the advantages of a wide potential window, low background current, high biocompatibility and excellent chemical stability [41–43]. In this work, we constructed a miniaturized electrochemical sensing platform by equipping a SPCE with a nanochannel array which is able to directly and sensitively detect CLZ in human whole blood. In order to improve the electrochemical performance and achieve stable binding with VMSF, simple electrochemical polarization, including anodic oxidation at high potential and cathodic reduction at low potential, is applied to pretreat the SPCE. The electrochemically polarized SPCE (p-SPCE) exhibits a strong electrochemical peak signal in response to CLZ. An electrochemically assisted self-assembly method (EASA) is further utilized to conveniently electrodeposit VMSF on p-SPCE, which could further improve the electrochemical response to CLZ. Combined with the excellent anti-fouling and anti-interference abilities of VMSF, the constructed sensor can realize rapid and sensitive determination of CLZ in human blood. This work demonstrates a new strategy for the construction of a reliable, miniaturized, disposable and integrated electrochemical sensor with an anti-fouling layer and high detection sensitivity and selectivity.

2. Results and Discussion

2.1. Electrochemical Polarization of SPCE

As illustrated in Figure 1, SPCE was first treated by simple electrochemical polarization to enhance its electrochemical performance. Electrochemical polarization is a simple and green method to prepare highly active carbon electrodes. This method usually involves the electrochemical oxidization and reduction of electrodes in conventional electrolyte solutions. Usually, the electrode is first electrochemically oxidized at a high potential and then electrochemically reduced at a low potential. Thus, no complex chemical reagents and tedious operations are needed. During the polarization process, the sp^2-conjugated carbon on the surface of the carbon electrode is oxidatively etched at high potential, resulting in abundant edge carbon, defects and oxygen-containing functional groups. These groups serve as electrocatalytic active sites which can not only enhance the adsorption of organic electroactive molecules, but also facilitate interfacial electron transfer reactions. In addition, electrochemical polarization facilitates the formation of porous surfaces. Therefore, electrochemically polarized carbon electrodes tend to exhibit high electrochemical response and significant electrocatalytic activity.

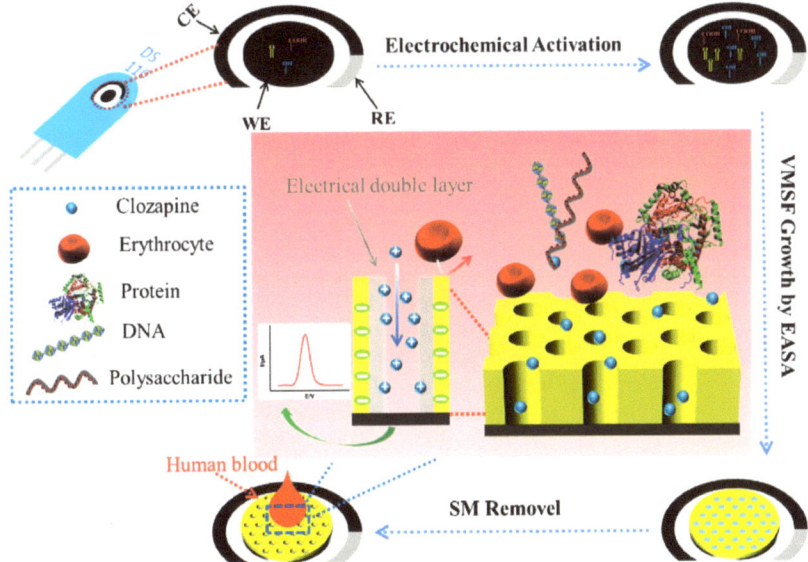

Figure 1. Schematic of the VMSF equipment on the electrochemically polarized SPCE and the direct determination of CLZ in human whole blood with high anti-fouling and anti-interference abilities.

The cyclic voltammetry curves obtained in the electrochemical electrolyte or standard electrochemical probe solution ($K_3Fe(CN)_6$) on SPCE before and after electrochemical polarization are shown in Figure 2a. Compared with SPCE, p-SPCE showed a significantly increased charging current (Inset in Figure 2a), indicating an increase in the electroactive area of the electrode through electrochemical polarization. In the case of a redox probe, p-SPCE exhibited higher peak current and lower peak-to-peak separation, showing an improved electron transfer rate after electrochemical polarization. This phenomenon was further confirmed by electrochemical impedance spectroscopy (EIS), as shown in Figure 2b. It is well known that the charge transfer resistance (R_{ct}) of an electrode is related to the diameter of the semicircular curve in the high frequency region. When the SPCE was electrochemically polarized, the p-SPCE displayed a reduced R_{ct} owing to the increased electron transfer rate.

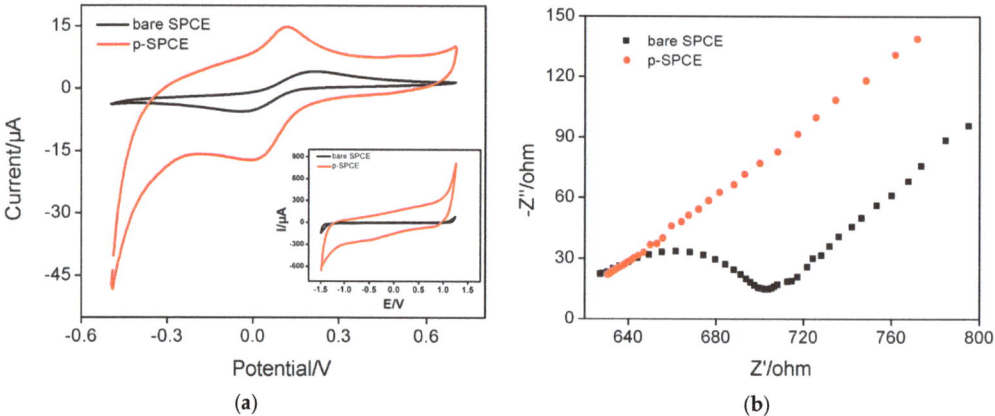

Figure 2. (a) CV curves obtained using different electrodes in 0.05 M KHP solution containing 0.5 mM $Fe(CN)_6^{3+}$. Inset: CV curves obtained with SPCE or p-SPCE in PBS (0.1 M, pH = 6). (b) Nyquist plots of different electrodes obtained in 0.1 M KCl solution containing 2.5 mM $K_3Fe(CN)_6$ and 2.5 mM $K_4Fe(CN)_6$.

2.2. VMSF Enquipment on the p-SPCE

After electrochemical polarization of the SPCE, VMSF was then electrodeposited on the electrode surface by the EASA method (Figure 1). EASA is a convenient method by which to apply VMSF to conductive substrates; it can complete the rapid growth of VMSF within 10 s. When the p-SPCE was immersed in an acidic precursor solution containing siloxane (TEOS) and cetyltrimethylammonium bromide (CTAB) micelles, a negative current was applied to the electrode and OH- was generated. This local pH increase induced the self-assembly of surfactant micelles (SM) and the polycondensation of siloxane, leading to a hexagonally packed pore structure. The stable binding of VMSF with p-SPCE was attributed to two factors. First, the negatively charged oxygen-containing functional groups on the surface of p-SPCE facilitated the electrostatic adsorption of the cationic SM. Second, the OH groups on p-SPCE formed Si-O bonds with VMSF through a co-condensation reaction, bestowing the adhesion of VMSF on p-SPCE with high mechanical stability. Finally, the SM in the nanochannels was removed with HCl-EtOH solution to obtain a VMSF/p-SPCE with open nanochannels.

Transmission electron microscopy (TEM) was used to characterize the morphology of the nanopore/channel structure of VMSF. Figure 3 demonstrates top-view and cross-sectional TEM images of the VMSF nanochannel. As shown in Figure 3a, the VMSF had a well-ordered structure with uniform pore size. The diameter of the nanopores was between 2 nm and 3 nm. The cross-sectional view in Figure 3b clearly reveals the parallel nanochannel structure.

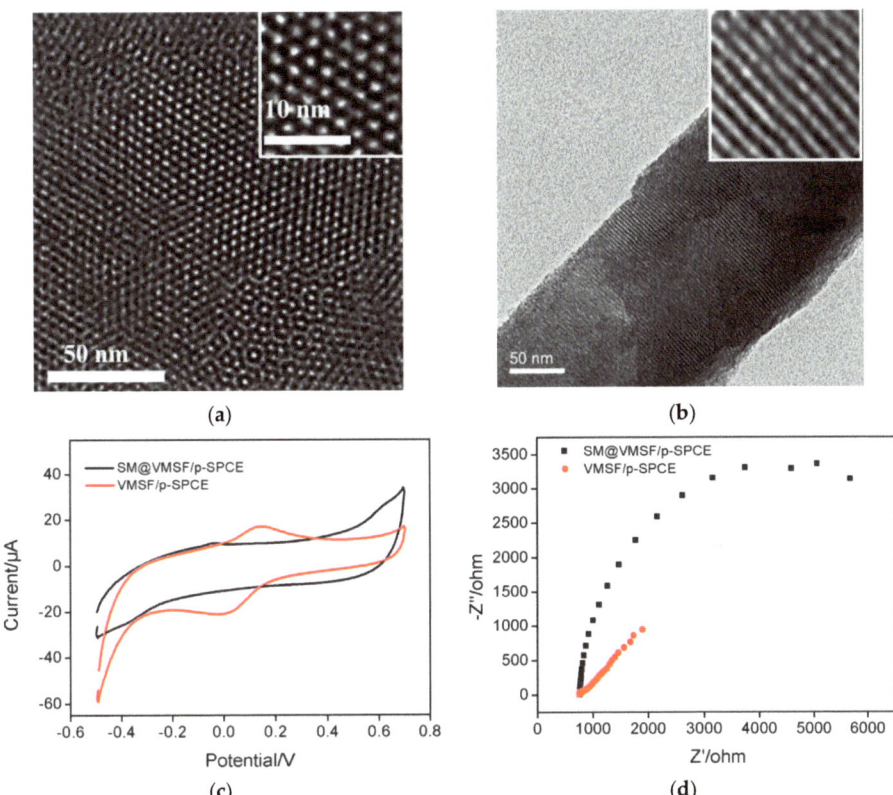

Figure 3. Top-view (**a**) and cross-sectional (**b**) TEM images of VMSF at different magnifications. (**c**) CV curves obtained at different electrodes in 0.05 M KHP solution containing 0.5 mM Fe(CN)$_6^{3+}$. (**d**) Nyquist plots of different electrodes obtained in 0.1 M KCl solution containing 2.5 mM K$_3$Fe(CN)$_6$ and 2.5 mM K$_4$Fe(CN)$_6$.

The integrity of VMSF was further proven through electrochemical characterization. The CV curves and Nyquist plots of the obtained on SM@VMSF/p-SPCE and VMSF/p-SPCE are shown in Figure 3c,d. As seen, SM@VMSF/p-SPCE exhibited almost no peak current while VMSF/p-SPCE had remarkable peaks (Figure 3c). Thus, the filling of SM inside VMSF nanochannels inhibited the mass transfer of the redox probe through the nanochannels and then prohibited the subsequent electron transfer of between the electrode. EIS experiments also demonstrated the same phenomenon (Figure 3d). An electrode containing micelles in nanochannels showed extremely high charge transfer resistance. On the other hand, the VMSF/p-SPCE with open nanochannels presented significantly lower charge transfer resistance. The above results demonstrate the successful modification of VMSF on a p-SPCE and the integrity of the nanofilm.

2.3. Dual Signal Amplification and Significantly Enhanced CLZ Response on VMSF/p-SPCE

The CV and DPV curves of CLZ on different electrodes are compared in Figure 4. It can be seen that CLZ exhibited a pair of reversible redox peaks, which were attributed to its redox reaction on the electrode surface (Figure 4a). The response of bare SPCE to CLZ had the lowest peak current (Figure 4b). In contrast, the response of p-SPCE to CLZ was significantly enhanced. This was attributed to the enhancement of electrode performance by electrochemical polarization. On the one hand, electrochemical polarization increased the electroactive area, thereby increasing the interaction with the CLZ. On the other hand, the active groups generated by electrochemical polarization enhanced the electron transfer rate of p-SPCE. Therefore, electrochemical polarization can enhance the sensitivity to CLZ. When VSMF was grown on the surface of p-SPCE, VMSF/p-SPCE showed the highest peak current, demonstrating the enrichment of CLZ by VMSF nanochannels. This was attributed to the electron sieving effect of the nanochannels. In the electrolyte solution, the silanol groups on the surface of VMSF were negatively charged (pK_a = 2–3), which allowed electrostatic adsorption of CLZ (pK_a = 7.6) to occur. Thus, the VMSF/p-SPCE had a dual signal amplification effect on the determination of CLZ, indicating its potential for as a sensitive CLZ detector.

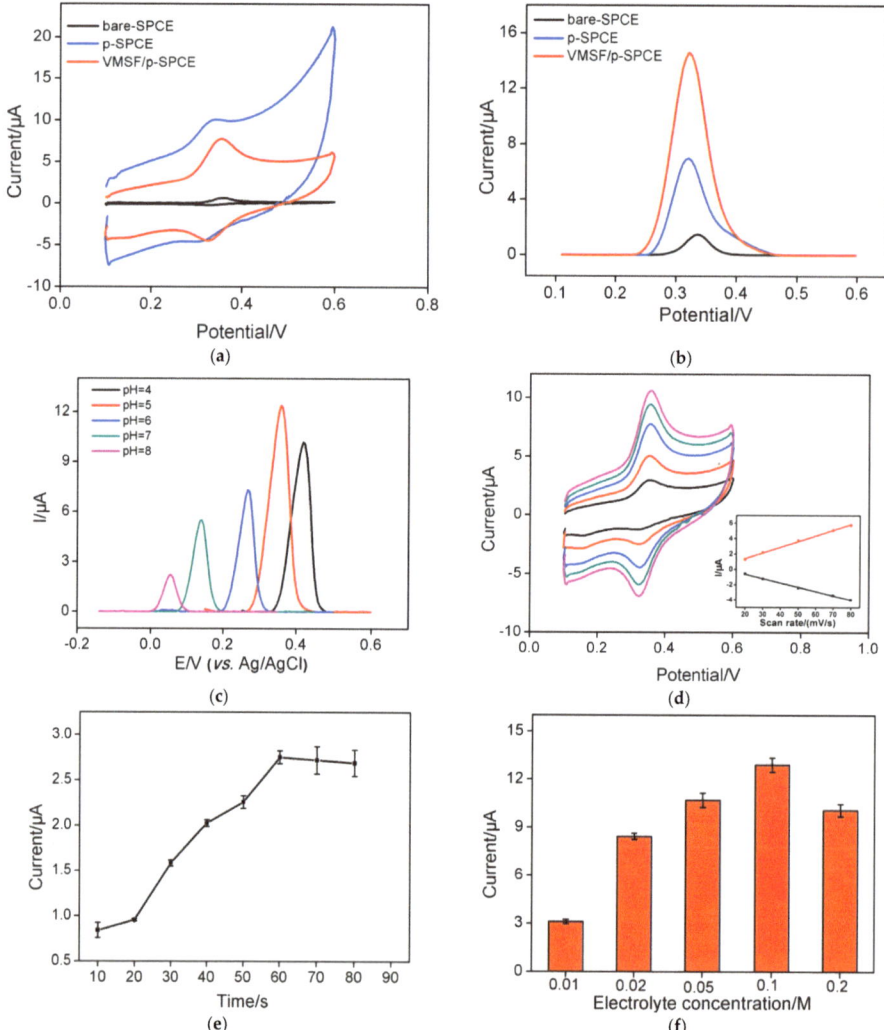

Figure 4. (a) CV or DPV (b) curves of CLZ on different electrodes. (c) DPV curves of CLZ at different pH. (d) CV curves of CLZ at different scan rates. The inset shows the linear regression curve between the peak current and the scan rate. (e) Effect of enrichment time on the peak current of CLZ. (f) Effect of the concentration of the electrolyte on the peak current of CLZ.

2.4. Optimization of Conditions for the Determination of CLZ

To improve the sensitivity to CLZ, conditions such as pH, enrichment time, and ionic strength were optimized. Figure 4c shows the DPV curves of CLZ on VMSF/p-SPCE at different pH. With the increase of pH, the oxidation peak potential of CLZ moved to the negative potential, and the peak current also changed greatly. The highest peak current was observed at pH 6. This was attributed to the effect of pH on the electrostatic interaction between the nanochannels with CLZ. An excessively low pH would reduce the negative charge on the surface of the VMSF nanochannels, which reduced the electrostatic force on CLZ. On the other hand, an overly high pH would reduce the positive charge of CLZ. Thus, pH = 6 was chosen for further investigation. Figure 4d displays the CV curves of CLZ at different scan rates. With the increase of scan rate, both the oxidation peak current and reduction peak current increased accordingly. Good linearity was observed between the peak current and the scan rate, indicating an adsorption-controlled process (inset in Figure 4d). Thus, the effect of enrichment time on the peak current of CLZ was investigate. As shown in Figure 4e, the peak current reached equilibrium after 60 s, indicating very short time for CLZ to reach mass transfer equilibrium on the electrode surface. This was attributed to the good permeability of VMSF and dual enrichment of the VMSF/p-SPCE. The ionic strength of the electrolyte solution affected the thickness of the electric double layer of the nanochannels, which changed the electrostatic interaction between the nanochannel and CLZ. Figure 4f shows the current responses of CLZ at different ionic strengths. When the ionic strength of the electrolyte solution was high, the electric double layer (EDL) did not overlap and the nanochannel exhibited electrostatic attraction to positively charged substances [44]. Thus, 0.1 M PBS was chosen as the electrolyte solution for the determination of CLZ.

2.5. Determination of CLZ Using VMSF/SPCE

The performance of the developed VMSF/p-SPCE sensor for the determination of CLZ using was investigated. Figure 5a displays the DPV curves obtained on the VMSF/p-SPCE in the presence of different concentrations of CLZ. As shown, the peak current gradually increased when the concentration of CLZ increased. A linear correlation was revealed between the oxidation peak current (I, μA) and concentration of CLZ (C, μM) in the range from 50 nM to 20 μM ($I = 2.6\ C - 0.05$, $R^2 = 0.996$) (Figure 5b). The limit of detection (LOD) was 28 nM with a signal-to-noise ratio of 3. For comparison, linear detection of CLZ ranging from 1 μM to 15 μM was obtained on a bare SPCE ($I = 0.647\ C + 0.052$, $R^2 = 0.997$). In the case of the p-SPCE, CLZ could be linearly detected from 0.5 to 20 μM ($I = 1.44\ C + 0.11$, $R^2 = 0.993$). Thus, VMSF/p-SPCE exhibited the highest sensitivity. The LOD obtained on the VMSF/p-SPCE was lower than that on GCE modified by multiwall carbon nanotubes or on WO_3 nanoparticles hydride modified by α-terpineol [45], Bi–Sn nanoparticles applied to carbon aerogel-modified SPCE (Bi–Sn NP/CAG/SPCE) [46], ruthenium (IV) oxide nanoparticle-modified SPCE (RuO_2NPs/SPE) [31] or a TiO_2 nanoparticle-modified carbon paste electrode (TiO_2NP-MCPE) [47]. The low LOD of the developed sensor may be attributed to the dual amplification effects resulting from both the p-SPCE and VMSF nanochannels.

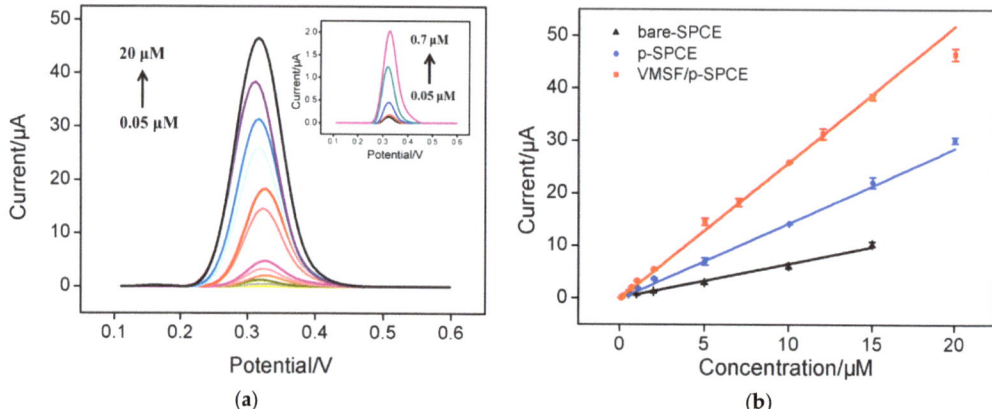

Figure 5. (a) Differential pulse voltametric curves of VMSF/p-SPCE toward various concentrations (0.05, 0.1, 0.2, 0.5, 0.7, 1, 2, 5, 7, 10, 12, 15, 20 μM) of CLZ. The inset is an enlarged image of the curves at low concentrations. (b) Corresponding calibration curves for the determination of CLZ using VMSF/p-SPCE, p-SPCE, or bare SPCE.

2.6. Anti-Interference and Anti-Fouling Properties of the VMSF/p-SPCE Sensor

Anti-interference and anti-fouling capabilities are important characteristics of electrochemical sensors, and are especially important for analyses of real samples with complex matrices. To study the anti-interference ability of the developed VMSF/p-SPCE sensor, the effects of common substances in human blood on the determination of CLZ were investigated. Briefly, electrolyte ions (K^+, Na^+, Mg^{2+}, Ca^{2+}), common redox small molecules (ascorbic acid-AA, dopamine-DA, uric acid-UA) and metabolites (urea, glucose-Glu) were tested. As shown in Figure 6a, determinations of CLZ were not affected even when the concentrations of the above substances were 25 times higher than that of CLZ, proving the good anti-interference characteristic of the sensor. It is particularly noteworthy that three electroactive small molecules, i.e., AA, DA, and UA, did not interfere with the determination of CLZ, indicating that the constructed VMSF/p-SPCE sensor has excellent potential resolution. Blood samples or tablets associated with CLZ often contain large amounts proteins, hydroxypropyl methyl cellulose (HPMC) and starch. Therefore, the effects of bovine serum albumin (BSA), HPMC and soluble starch on the determination of CLZ were investigated. As shown in Figure 6b–d, these three species did not interfere with the determination of CLZ, further revealing the good anti-fouling ability of the electrode. In contrast, the responses changed significantly in presence or absence of these species (inset in Figure 6b–d). The excellent anti-fouling performance of the VMSF/p-SPCE sensor was attributed to the size and electrostatic exclusion effect of the VMSF nanochannels.

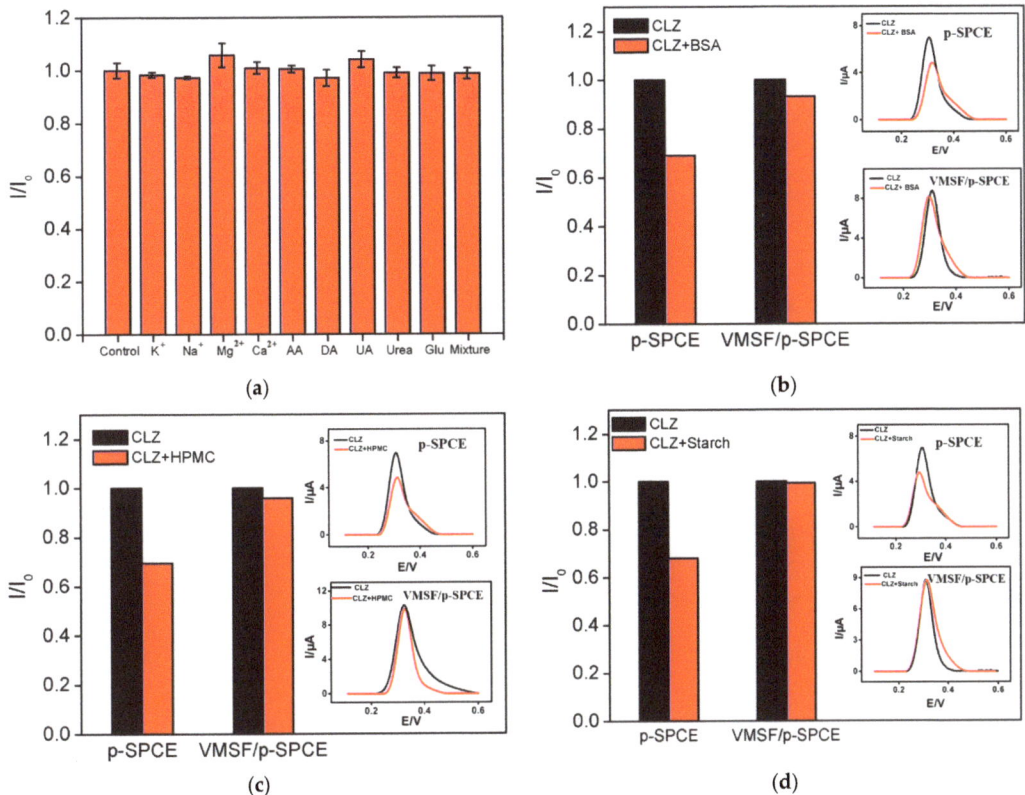

Figure 6. (a) The peak current ratio of CLZ on the VMSF/p-SPCE in the absence (I_0) or presence (I) of the indicated substance or mixtures thereof. (**b**–**d**) The peak current ratio of CLZ on the VMSF/p-SPCE or p-SPCE in the absence (I_0) or presence (I) of BSA (**b**), HPMC (**c**) and starch (**d**). Insets are the corresponding DPV curves obtained using single CLZ (black) or the binary mixture (red).

2.7. Determination of CLZ in Human Whole Blood with Low Sample Consumption

The excellent anti-fouling and anti-interference properties of the constructed VMSF/p-SPCE sensor show its great potential for use in direct electroanalyses of CLZ in complex samples. As a proof-of-concept, electrochemical determination of CLZ in human whole blood was investigated. Human whole blood was applied as the detection medium after dilution by a factor of 100. For comparison, determinations using a bare SPCE or p-SPCE were also undertaken. As shown in Figure 7a, the DPV peak current on the VMSF/p-SPCE increased with an increase in the concentration of CLZ. Although the detection sensitivity was reduced compared with that of the buffer system, the VMSF/p-SPCE sensor could still linearly detect CLZ from 0.5 µM to 12 µM ($I = 0.563 C + 0.04$, $R^2 = 0.996$) with a LOD of 110 nM (Figure 7b). In contrast, the CLZ signal on both the bare SPCE and p-SPCE showed a non-linear relationship with its concentration, indicating that the electrode was seriously contaminated. The regeneration and reusability of the constructed VMSF/p-SPCE sensor was investigated. The performance of the p-SPCE was also examined for comparison. The sensor can easily be regenerated by soaking in a hydrochloric acid–ethanol solution (0.1 M) for 2 min. As shown in Figure 7c,d, both electrodes can be easily regenerated, although the CLZ signals on the regenerated electrodes were almost undetectable in the electrolyte. In addition, the VMSF/p-SPCE sensor can be reused with no significant change in its response to CLZ (Figure 7c). However, the peak currents for CLZ obtained on the p-SPCE were significantly reduced (Figure 7d). This phenomenon once again serves as evidence of the excellent anti-fouling performance of VMSF.

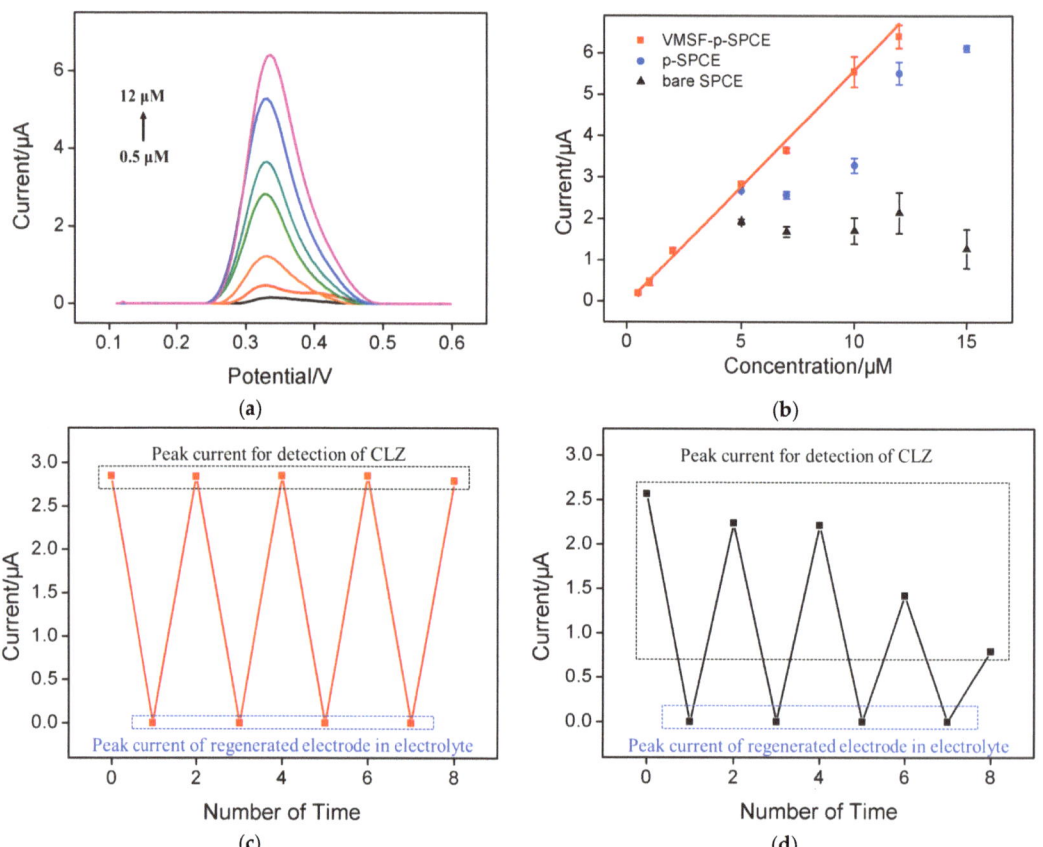

Figure 7. (**a**) DPV curves obtained on VMSF/p-SPCE in diluted human whole blood with the addition of different concentrations of CLZ (from bottom to top: 0.5, 1, 2, 5, 7, 10, 12 µM). (**b**) The corresponding calibration curve obtained on the VMSF/p-SPCE and DPV peak currents obtained on both the p-SPCE and bare SPCE. The regeneration and reuse performance of the VMSF/p-SPCE (**c**) and p-SPCE (**d**). The first peak current was obtained using the original electrode. Other peak currents were obtained in electrolyte (**bottom**) or CLZ solution (**top**) using the regenerated electrodes. The detected CLZ was 5 µM in diluted human blood (i.e., by a factor of 100).

The reliability of the device was further investigated by the standard addition method. Different concentrations of CLZ were artificially added to the human whole blood. Then, the whole blood was diluted by a factor of 10. As shown, the recovery of the concentration of CLZ ranged from 97.3% to 104%, with a relative standard deviation (RSD) of no more than 3.2% (Table 1), indicating good reliability for direct measurements of CLZ in complex samples. Since the SPCE features an integrated working electrode, a counter electrode and a reference electrode, a very small amount of sample (50 µL) can be dropped directly onto the surface of the electrode during tests. Therefore, the constructed VMSF/p-SPCE sensor can achieve rapid, direct and sensitive determinations of CLZ with very low sample consumption, indicating its great potential for use with fingertip blood.

Table 1. Determination of CLZ in human whole blood samples.

Sample [a]	Added (μM)	Found (μM)	RSD (%)	Recovery (%)
Human whole blood [a]	10.0	10.4	2.9	104
	30.0	29.2	3.2	97.3
	50.0	51.0	2.6	102

[a] Samples with added CLZ were diluted 10 times using PBS electrolyte. The concentration of CLZ is before dilution.

3. Materials and Methods

3.1. Chemicals and Materials

Tetraethyl orthosilicate (TEOS), hexadecyl trimethyl ammonium bromide (CTAB), potassium ferricyanide ($K_3[Fe(CN)_6]$), tetrapotassium hexacyanoferrate trihydrate ($K_4[Fe(CN)_6]$), sodium phosphate dibasic dodecahydrate ($Na_2HPO_4 \bullet 12H_2O$), potassium hydrogen phthalate (KHP), glucose (Glu), ascorbic acid (AA), uric acid (UA), dopamine hydrochloride (DA), bovine serum albumin (BSA), hydroxypropyl methylcellulose (HPMC), soluble starch (Starch), sodium dodecyl sulfate (SDS) and clozapine (CLZ) were purchased from Aladdin Biochemical Technology Co., Ltd. (Shanghai, China). Potassium chloride (KCl), anhydrous calcium chloride ($CaCl_2$) and anhydrous ethanol (EtOH) were purchased from Hangzhou Gaojing Fine Chemical Co., Ltd. (Hangzhou, China). Magnesium chloride ($MgCl_2$) and sodium dihydrogen phosphate dihydrate ($Na_2H_2PO_4 \bullet 2H_2O$) were purchased from Shanghai Macklin Biochemical Technology Co., Ltd. (Shanghai, China). Sodium chloride (NaCl) and urea (Urea) were purchased from Tianjin Yongda Chemical Reagent Co., Ltd. (Tianjing, China). Screen-printed carbon electrodes (SPCEs) were purchased from Metrohm (Bern, Switzerland). Briefly, SPCEs contain three integrated electrodes, i.e., working and counter electrodes made up of conductive graphite paste and an Ag reference electrode comprising conductive silver paste. Human whole blood (healthy male) was provided by the Hangzhou Occupational Disease Prevention and Control Institute (Hangzhou, China). All reagents used in the experiment were of analytical grade and did not require further processing. The ultrawater (18 MΩ·cm) used in the experiments was prepared by the Mill-Q system (Millipore Corporation, Burlington, MA, USA).

3.2. Experiments and Instrumentations

The pore structure and vertically ordered nanochannels of the VMSF were characterized by transmission electron microscopy (TEM). Images were obtained on a transmission electron microscope (HT7700, Hitachi, Japan). The accelerating voltage was 100 kV. VMSF was gently scraped from p-SPCE, then dispersed in ethanol. Before characterization, the VMSF dispersion was dropped onto a copper grid. All electrochemical experiments, including cyclic voltammetry (CV), differential pulse voltammetry (DPV) and electrochemical impedance spectroscopy (EIS), were performed using an Autolab electrochemical workstation (PGSTAT302N, Metrohm, Herisau, Switzerland). The CV scan rate was 50 mV/s. During the DPV test, the step potential was 0.005 V, the pulse amplitude was 0.05 V, the pulse time was 0.05 s and the interval time was 0.2 s. EIS measurement was performed in $K_3Fe(CN)_6/K_4Fe(CN)_6$ (2.5 mM) solution containing KCl (0.1 M) with a frequency range of 10^4 to 10^{-1} Hz.

3.3. Electrochemical Polarization of SPCE

Electrochemical polishing was performed to remove impurities such as organics and polymers from the surface of SPCE electrodes. Briefly, H_2SO_4 (0.05 M) was used as the medium and CV scans were then performed for 10 cycles between 0.4 and 1.0 V. After the electrode was rinsed with ultrapure water and dried with N_2, it was placed in a phosphate buffer solution (PBS, 0.1 M, pH = 5). The subsequent electrochemical polarization included anodic oxidation and cathodic reduction. Firstly, the electrode was anodized by applying a constant potential of 1.8 V for 300 s. The oxidized SPCE was then cathodically reduced by CV scanning for three cycles (initial potential: 0 V; minimum potential: −1.3 V; maximum potential: 1.25 V; and scan rate: 100 mV/s). The obtained electrochemically polarized SPCE, that is, p-SPCE, was washed with ultrapure water and then dried with N_2.

3.4. Preparation of VMSF-Modified p-SPCE

VMSF was electrodeposited on the surface of p-SPCE by the EASA method. To prepare the precursor solution for VMSF deposition, ethanol (20 mL) was mixed with an equal volume of $NaNO_3$ (0.1 M, pH = 2.6). Then, CTAB (1.585 g) was added under magnetic stirring until the solution became clear. After TEOS (3050 µL) was added, the obtained solution was stirred at room temperature for 2.5 h. To grow VMSF, a p-SPCE electrode was placed in the precursor solution and a galvanostatic current (−52.2 µA) was applied for 10 s. As surfactant micelles (SM) were present within VMSF nanochannels, the obtained electrode was denoted as SM@VMSF/p-SPCE. After thorough rinsing with ultrapure water, the SM@VMSF/p-SPCE was aged at 80 °C for 10 h. Then, SM was removed by immersing the SM@VMSF/p-SPCE in 0.1 M HCl-EtOH solution ($v:v$ = 1:1) for 5 min with stirring. An electrode with open nanochannels was finally obtained and named VMSF/p-SPCE.

3.5. Electrochemical Determination of CLZ

PBS (0.1 M, pH = 6) was used as the detection electrolyte. To investigate the effect of a complex medium on detection, human whole blood was also applied as the detection medium after diluting by a factor of 100 using PBS electrolyte. Electrochemical determination of clozapine was carried out by DPV. After adding different concentrations of CLZ, a DPV curve was recorded. For the real sample analysis, different concentrations of CLZ were added to the human whole blood to simulate changes in CLZ levels in patient blood after taking the drug. Then, human whole blood with added CLZ was diluted by a factor of 10 using PBS electrolyte. Next, 50 µL of the obtained solution was dropped on the surface of VMSF/p-SPCE electrode. After static enrichment for 1 min, a DPV curve was recorded.

4. Conclusions

In summary, using simple equipment, a miniaturized, integrated and disposable electrochemical sensing platform was constructed comprising a vertically ordered mesoporous silica nanomembrane film (VMSF) on electrochemically polarized SPCE (p-SPCE). The p-SPCE was characterized by increased active area and improved electron transfer rate, thereby improving the determination sensitivity of CLZ. The nanochannels of the VMSF also achieved electrostatic enrichment toward CLZ. Due to the excellent size/charge exclusion effect of the nanochannels and the high potential resolution ability of p-SPCE, the constructed VMSF/p-SPCE sensor had excellent anti-interference and anti-fouling properties, allowing it to realize rapid, direct and sensitive determinations of CLZ in human whole blood. In addition, the developed VMSF/p-SPCE sensor has the advantage of very low sample consumption (50 µL), indicating great potential for use with fingertip blood. The nanochannel array on SPCE established here also provides a new strategy for rapid, direct and sensitive electroanalyses of complex samples.

Author Contributions: Investigation, K.W.; data curation, L.Y.; writing—original draft preparation, H.H.; writing—review and editing, N.L.; conceptualization and supervision, J.L.; writing—review and editing, Y.L. All authors have read and agreed to the published version of the manuscript.

Funding: This research was funded by the National Natural Science Foundation of China (21904117), the Construction Fund of Key Medical Disciplines of Hangzhou (OO20200093), and the Zhejiang Provincial Natural Science Foundation of China (LY20B050007).

Institutional Review Board Statement: Not applicable.

Informed Consent Statement: Not applicable.

Data Availability Statement: The data presented in this study are available on request from the corresponding author.

Conflicts of Interest: The authors declare no conflict of interest.

Sample Availability: Samples of the compounds are available from the authors.

References

1. Verdoux, H.; Quiles, C.; Bachmann, C.J.; Siskind, D. Prescriber and institutional barriers and facilitators of clozapine use: A systematic review. *Schizophr. Res.* **2018**, *201*, 10–19. [CrossRef]
2. Rowntree, R.; Murray, S.; Fanning, F.; Keating, D.; Szigeti, A.; Doyle, R.; McWilliams, S.; Clarke, M. Clozapine use–has practice changed? *J. Psychopharmacol. Oxford* **2020**, *34*, 567–573. [CrossRef] [PubMed]
3. Kane, J.; Honigfeld, G.; Singer, J.; Meltzer, H. Clozapine for the treatment-resistant schizophrenic: A double-blind comparison with chlorpromazine. *Arch. Gerontol. Geriatr.* **1988**, *45*, 789–796. [CrossRef] [PubMed]
4. Ereshefsky, L.; Watanabe, M.D.; Tran-Johnson, T.K. Clozapine: An atypical antipsychotic agent. *Clin. Pharm.* **1989**, *8*, 691–709. [PubMed]
5. Schoretsanitis, G.; Kuzin, M.; Kane, J.M.; Hiemke, C.; Paulzen, M.; Haen, E. Elevated clozapine concentrations in clozapine-treated patients with hypersalivation. *Clin. Pharmacokinet.* **2021**, *60*, 329–335. [CrossRef] [PubMed]
6. Alvir, J.M.J.; Lieberman, J.A.; Safferman, A.Z.; Schwimmer, J.L.; Schaaf, J.A. Clozapine-induced agranulocytosis—Incidence and risk factors in the United States. *N. Engl. J. Med.* **1993**, *329*, 162–167. [CrossRef] [PubMed]
7. Hiemke, C.; Baumann, P.; Bergemann, N.; Conca, A.; Dietmaier, O.; Egberts, K.; Fric, M.; Gerlach, M.; Greiner, C.; Grunder, G.; et al. AGNP consensus guidelines for therapeutic drug monitoring in psychiatry: Update 2011. *Pharmacopsychiatry* **2011**, *44*, 195–235. [CrossRef] [PubMed]
8. Jessurun, N.T.; Derijks, H.J.; van Marum, R.J.; Jongkind, A.; Giraud, E.L.; van Puijenbroek, E.P.; Grootens, K.P. Body weight gain in clozapine-treated patients: Is norclozapine the culprit? *Br. J. Clin. Pharmacol.* **2021**, *88*, 853–857. [CrossRef] [PubMed]
9. Jerónimo, J.; Santos, J.; Bastos, L. Uncommon effects of clozapine. *Eur. Psychiatry* **2016**, *33*, S614. [CrossRef]
10. Jann, M.W.; Grimsley, S.R.; Gray, E.C.; Chang, W.-H. Pharmacokinetics and pharmacodynamics of clozapine. *Clin. Pharm.* **1993**, *24*, 161–176. [CrossRef]
11. Saint-Marcoux, F.; Sauvage, F.L.; Marquet, P. Current role of LC-MS in therapeutic drug monitoring. *Anal. Bioanal. Chem.* **2007**, *388*, 1327–1349. [CrossRef] [PubMed]
12. Chen, X.; Zheng, S.; Le, J.; Qian, Z.Y.; Zhang, R.S.; Hong, Z.Y.; Chai, Y.F. Ultrasound-assisted low-density solvent dispersive liquid–liquid microextraction for the simultaneous determination of 12 new antidepressants and 2 antipsychotics in whole blood by gas chromatography–mass spectrometry. *J. Pharm. Biomed. Anal.* **2017**, *142*, 19–27. [CrossRef] [PubMed]
13. Schulte, P.F.J.; Bogers, J.; Bond-Veerman, S.R.T.; Cohen, D. Moving forward with clozapine. *Acta Psychiatr. Scand.* **2020**, *142*, 75–77. [CrossRef] [PubMed]
14. Li, Z.; Zhu, M. Detection of pollutants in water bodies: Electrochemical detection or photo-electrochemical detection? *Chem. Commun.* **2020**, *56*, 14541–14552. [CrossRef] [PubMed]
15. Cui, Y.; Duan, W.; Jin, Y.; Wo, F.J.; Xi, F.N.; Wu, J.M. Graphene quantum dot-decorated luminescent porous silicon dressing for theranostics of diabetic wounds. *Acta Biomater.* **2021**, *131*, 544–554. [CrossRef] [PubMed]
16. Duan, W.; Jin, Y.; Cui, Y.; Xi, F.N.; Liu, X.Y.; Wo, F.J.; Wu, J.M. A co-delivery platform for synergistic promotion of angiogenesis based on biodegradable, therapeutic and self-reporting luminescent porous silicon microparticles. *Biomaterials* **2021**, *272*, 120772. [CrossRef]
17. Wan, Y.J.; Zhao, J.W.; Deng, X.C.; Chen, J.; Xi, F.N.; Wang, X.B. Colorimetric and fluorescent dual-modality sensing platform based on fluorescent nanozyme. *Front. Chem.* **2021**, *9*, 774486. [CrossRef]
18. Deng, X.C.; Zhao, J.W.; Ding, Y.; Tang, H.L.; Xi, F.N. Iron and nitrogen co-doped graphene quantum dots as highly active peroxidases for the sensitive detection of l-cysteine. *New J. Chem.* **2021**, *45*, 19056–19064. [CrossRef]
19. Cui, Y.X.; Jin, Y.; Wo, F.J.; Xi, F.N.; Wu, J.M. Ratiometric fluorescent nanohybrid for noninvasive and visual monitoring of sweat glucose. *ACS Sens.* **2020**, *5*, 2096–2105. [CrossRef]
20. Zhang, Y.N.; Niu, Q.; Gu, X.; Yang, N.; Zhao, G. Recent progress on carbon nanomaterials for the electrochemical detection and removal of environmental pollutants. *Nanoscale* **2019**, *11*, 11992–12014. [CrossRef] [PubMed]
21. Liu, G.; Xiong, Z.; Yang, L.; Shi, H.; Fang, D.; Wang, M.; Shao, P.; Luo, X. Electrochemical approach toward reduced graphene oxide-based electrodes for environmental applications: A review. *Sci. Total Environ.* **2021**, *778*, 146301. [CrossRef] [PubMed]
22. Zhu, M.; Zhao, Z.; Liu, X.; Chen, P.; Fan, F.; Wu, X.; Hua, R.; Wang, Y. A novel near-infrared fluorometric method for point-of-care monitoring of Fe^{2+} and its application in bioimaging. *J. Hazard. Mater.* **2021**, *406*, 124767. [CrossRef] [PubMed]
23. Vinoth, S.; Shalini Devi, K.S.; Pandikumar, A. A comprehensive review on graphitic carbon nitride based electrochemical and biosensors for environmental and healthcare applications. *Trends. Analyt. Chem.* **2021**, *140*, 116274. [CrossRef]
24. Guo, J. Smartphone-Powered Electrochemical Dongle for point-of-care monitoring of blood beta-ketone. *Anal. Chem.* **2017**, *89*, 8609–8613. [CrossRef]
25. Xuan, L.L.; Liao, W.Y.; Wang, M.F.; Zhou, H.X.; Ding, Y.; Yan, F.; Liu, J.Y.; Tang, H.L.; Xi, F.N. Integration of vertically-ordered mesoporous silica-nanochannel film with electro-activated glassy carbon electrode for improved electroanalysis in complex samples. *Talanta* **2021**, *225*, 122066. [CrossRef] [PubMed]
26. Zhang, Y.; Lei, Y.; Lu, H.; Shi, L.; Wang, P.; Ali, Z.; Li, J. Electrochemical detection of bisphenols in food: A review. *Food Chem.* **2021**, *346*, 128895. [CrossRef]
27. Xing, X.; Yao, L.; Yan, C.; Xu, Z.L.; Xu, J.G.; Liu, G.D.; Yao, B.B.; Chen, W. Recent progress of personal glucose meters integrated methods in food safety hazards detection. *Crit. Rev. Food Sci. Nutr.* **2021**. [CrossRef]

28. Liu, Q.S.; Zhong, H.G.; Chen, M.; Zhao, C.; Liu, Y.; Xi, F.N.; Luo, T. Functional nanostructure-loaded three-dimensional graphene foam as a non-enzymatic electrochemical sensor for reagentless glucose detection. *RSC Adv.* **2020**, *10*, 33739–33746. [CrossRef]
29. Farhadi, K.; Karimpour, A. Electrochemical behavior and determination of clozapine on a glassy carbon electrode modified by electrochemical oxidation. *Anal. Sci.* **2007**, *23*, 479–483. [CrossRef]
30. Tammari, E.; Nezhadali, A.; Lotfi, S.; Veisi, H. Fabrication of an electrochemical sensor based on magnetic nanocomposite Fe_3O_4/β-alanine/Pd modified glassy carbon electrode for determination of nanomolar level of clozapine in biological model and pharmaceutical samples. *Sens. Actuators B Chem.* **2017**, *241*, 879–886. [CrossRef]
31. Aflatoonian, M.R.; Tajik, S.; Mohtat, B.; Aflatoonian, B.; Shoaie, I.S.; Beitollahi, H.; Zhang, K.Q.; Jang, H.W.; Shokouhimehr, M. Direct electrochemical detection of clozapine by RuO_2 nanoparticles-modified screen-printed electrode. *RSC Adv.* **2020**, *10*, 13021–13028. [CrossRef]
32. Walcarius, A.; Sibottier, E.; Etienne, M.; Ghanbaja, J. Electrochemically assisted self-assembly of mesoporous silica thin films. *Nat. Mater.* **2007**, *6*, 602–608. [CrossRef] [PubMed]
33. Teng, Z.; Zheng, G.; Dou, Y.; Li, W.; Mou, C.Y.; Zhang, X.; Asiri, A.M.; Zhao, D. Highly ordered mesoporous silica films with perpendicular mesochannels by a simple Stober-solution growth approach. *Angew. Chem. Int. Ed.* **2012**, *51*, 2173–2177. [CrossRef]
34. Yang, Q.; Lin, X.; Su, B. Molecular filtration by ultrathin and highly porous silica nanochannel membranes: Permeability and selectivity. *Anal. Chem.* **2016**, *88*, 10252–10258. [CrossRef] [PubMed]
35. Calvo, A.; Yameen, B.; Williams, F.J.; Soler-Illia, G.J.; Azzaroni, O. Mesoporous films and polymer brushes helping each other to modulate ionic transport in nanoconfined environments. An interesting example of synergism in functional hybrid assemblies. *JACS* **2009**, *131*, 10866–10868. [CrossRef] [PubMed]
36. Ma, K.; Yang, L.X.; Liu, J.; Liu, J.Y. Electrochemical sensor nanoarchitectonics for sensitive detection of uric acid in human whole blood based on screen-printed carbon electrode equipped with vertically-ordered mesoporous silica-nanochannel film. *Nanomaterials* **2022**, *12*, 1157. [CrossRef] [PubMed]
37. Sun, Q.; Yan, F.; Yao, L.; Su, B. Anti-biofouling isoporous silica-micelle membrane enabling drug detection in human whole blood. *Anal. Chem.* **2016**, *88*, 8364–8368. [CrossRef] [PubMed]
38. Yan, F.; Wang, M.; Jin, Q.; Zhou, H.X.; Xie, L.H.; Tang, H.L.; Liu, J.Y. Vertically-ordered mesoporous silica films on graphene for anti-fouling electrochemical detection of tert-butylhydroquinone in cosmetics and edible oils. *J. ElectroAnal. Chem.* **2021**, *881*, 114969. [CrossRef]
39. Ma, K.; Zheng, Y.Y.; Liu, J.; Liu, J.Y. Ultrasensitive immunosensor for prostate-specific antigen based on enhanced electrochemiluminescence by vertically ordered mesoporous silica-nanochannel film. *Front. Chem.* **2022**, *10*, 851178. [CrossRef]
40. Zhou, H.X.; Ma, X.Y.; Sailjoi, A.; Zou, Y.Q.; Lin, X.Y.; Yan, F.; Su, B.; Liu, J.Y. Vertical silica nanochannels supported by nanocarbon composite for simultaneous detection of serotonin and melatonin in biological fluids. *Sens. Actuators B Chem.* **2022**, *353*, 131101. [CrossRef]
41. Razzino, C.A.; Serafín, V.; Gamella, M.; Pedrero, M.; Montero-Calle, A.; Barderas, R.; Calero, M.; Lobo, A.O.; Yáñnez-Sedeño, P.; Campuzano, S.; et al. An electrochemical immunosensor using gold nanoparticles-PAMAM-nanostructured screen-printed carbon electrodes for tau protein determination in plasma and brain tissues from Alzheimer patients. *Biosens. Bioelectron.* **2020**, *163*, 112238. [CrossRef] [PubMed]
42. Castrovilli, M.C.; Bolognesi, P.; Chiarinelli, J.; Avaldi, L.; Cartoni, A.; Calandra, P.; Tempesta EGiardi, M.T.; Antonacci, A.; Arduini, F.; Scognamiglio, V. Electrospray deposition as a smart technique for laccase immobilisation on carbon black-nanomodified screen-printed electrodes. *Biosens. Bioelectron.* **2020**, *163*, 112299. [CrossRef] [PubMed]
43. Fabiani, L.; Saroglia, M.; Galatà, G.; De Santis, R.; Fillo, S.; Luca, V.; Faggioni, G.; D'Amore, N.; Regalbuto, E.; Salvatori, P.; et al. Magnetic beads combined with carbon black-based screen-printed electrodes for COVID-19: A reliable and miniaturized electrochemical immunosensor for SARS-CoV-2 detection in saliva. *Biosens. Bioelectron.* **2021**, *171*, 112686. [CrossRef] [PubMed]
44. Nasir, T.; Herzog, G.; Hebrant, M.; Despas, C.; Liu, L.; Walcarius, A. Mesoporous Silica Thin Films for Improved Electrochemical Detection of Paraquat. *ACS Sens.* **2018**, *3*, 484–493. [CrossRef]
45. Fathi, M.R.; Almasifar, D. Electrochemical sensor for square wave voltammetric determination of clozapine by glassy carbon electrode modified by WO_3 nanoparticles. *IEEE Sens. J.* **2017**, *17*, 6069–6076. [CrossRef]
46. Veerakumar, P.; Manavalan, S.; Chen, S.M.; Pandikumar, A.; Lin, K.C. Ultrafine Bi–Sn nanoparticles decorated on carbon aerogels for electrochemical simultaneous determination of dopamine (neurotransmitter) and clozapine (antipsychotic drug). *Nanoscale* **2020**, *12*, 22217–22233. [CrossRef]
47. Mashhadizadeh, M.H.; Afshar, E. Electrochemical investigation of clozapine at TiO_2 nanoparticles modified carbon paste electrode and simultaneous adsorptive voltammetric determination of two antipsychotic drugs. *Electrochim. Acta* **2013**, *87*, 816–823. [CrossRef]

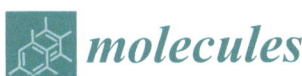

Article

The Facile Preparation of PBA-GO-CuO-Modified Electrochemical Biosensor Used for the Measurement of α-Amylase Inhibitors' Activit

Min Li [1], Xiaoying Yin [1,2,*], Hongli Shan [1,2], Chenting Meng [1], Shengxue Chen [1] and Yinan Yan [1,3,*]

[1] College of Chemistry and Chemical Engineering, Shanghai University of Engineering Science, Shanghai 201620, China; 18516629660@163.com (M.L.); mli19960904@163.com (H.S.); kamiyahc@163.com (C.M.); sxchen1009@163.com (S.C.)
[2] School of Chemistry and Chemical Engineering, Institute for Frontier Medical Technology, Shanghai 201620, China
[3] National Engineering Research Center for Nanotechnology, 28 East Jiang Chuan Road, Shanghai 200241, China
* Correspondence: ncyxoy@163.com (X.Y.); melyan@163.com (Y.Y.)

Citation: Li, M.; Yin, X.; Shan, H.; Meng, C.; Chen, S.; Yan, Y. The Facile Preparation of PBA-GO-CuO-Modified Electrochemical Biosensor Used for the Measurement of α-Amylase Inhibitors' Activity. *Molecules* 2022, *27*, 2395. https://doi.org/10.3390/molecules27082395

Academic Editors: Luca Tortora and Gianlorenzo Bussetti

Received: 26 March 2022
Accepted: 6 April 2022
Published: 7 April 2022

Publisher's Note: MDPI stays neutral with regard to jurisdictional claims in published maps and institutional affiliations.

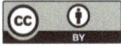

Copyright: © 2022 by the authors. Licensee MDPI, Basel, Switzerland. This article is an open access article distributed under the terms and conditions of the Creative Commons Attribution (CC BY) license (https://creativecommons.org/licenses/by/4.0/).

Abstract: Element doping and nanoparticle decoration of graphene is an effective strategy to fabricate biosensor electrodes for specific biomedical signal detections. In this study, a novel nonenzymatic glucose sensor electrode was developed with copper oxide (CuO) and boron-doped graphene oxide (B-GO), which was firstly used to reveal rhubarb extraction's inhibitive activity toward α-amylase. The 1-pyreneboronic acid (PBA)-GO-CuO nanocomposite was prepared by a hydrothermal method, and its successful boron doping was confirmed by transmission electron microscopy (TEM) and X-ray photoelectron spectroscopy (XPS), in which the boron doping rate is unprecedentedly up to 9.6%. The CuO load reaches ~12.5 wt.%. Further electrochemical results showed that in the enlarged cyclic voltammograms diagram, the electron-deficient boron doping sites made it easier for the electron transfer in graphene, promoting the valence transition from CuO to the electrode surface. Moreover, the sensor platform was ultrasensitive to glucose with a detection limit of 0.7 μM and high sensitivity of 906 μA mM^{-1} cm^{-2}, ensuring the sensitive monitoring of enzyme activity. The inhibition rate of acarbose, a model inhibitor, is proportional to the logarithm of concentration in the range of 10^{-9}–10^{-3} M with the correlation coefficient of R^2 = 0.996, and an ultralow limit of detection of ~1×10^{-9} M by the developed method using the PBA-GO-CuO electrode. The inhibiting ability of Rhein-8-b-D-glucopyranoside, which is isolated from natural medicines, was also evaluated. The constructed sensor platform was proven to be sensitive and selective as well as cost-effective, facile, and reliable, making it promising as a candidate for α-amylase inhibitor screening.

Keywords: graphene; nonenzymatic glucose sensor; boron-doped; copper oxide

1. Introduction

The inhibitors of α-amylase can prevent some late complications by suppressing the postprandial rise of blood glucose. The analysis methods applied for α-amylase inhibitor measurement are studied by many researchers [1,2].

Electrochemical sensor strategies are prevailing and deserve more attention due to intrinsic advantages such as high sensitivity and selectivity [3–6] and direct monitoring of the target enzymes without complicated pretreatment [7–10]. In the construction of an electrochemical sensor, chemically modified electrodes improve electron transport rate at a low potential, resulting in a decrease in the interference of impurities and an increase in the sensitivity of the current response [11,12]. The performance of the sensors improved due to development of nanotechnology such as the detection limit and a wide range of detection of target molecules. These advantages allow electroanalytical methods to be widely used in the determination of biological and environmental analysis.

Recently, considerable attention has been focused on developing nonenzymatic glucose sensors since it overcomes such drawbacks of traditional enzyme glucose sensors as instability, high cost of enzymes, complicated immobilization procedure, critical operating situations, etc., [13–16]. This also provided a new idea for identifying and detecting α-amylase inhibitors. Metals alloys, metal nanoparticles, and noble metals have been extended to develop nonenzymatic glucose sensors [17–20]. However, these electrodes have such disadvantages as high cost, low selectivity, or poisoning of chloride ions, which greatly limit their applications [21–25]. Thus, developing a highly selective, fast, reliable, and cheap nonenzymatic glucose sensor is still imperatively demanded.

Graphene is a well-known conductive material composed of two-dimensional honeycomb lattice-structured carbon atoms connected by an sp^2 monolayer [26–29]. Studies have shown that doping heterogeneous elements, such as nitrogen, boron, oxygen, sulfur, and halogens can effectively improve electrochemical performance [30–32]. First, boron doping can enhance the contact area between graphene, CuO nanoparticle, and electrolyte [33]. Furthermore, the electron deficiency of the boron element doped on the graphene acts as a superior electron receiver [34]. The materials mentioned above acting as a substrate to support CuO nanoparticles can vastly improve conductivity and sensing ability [35]. On the other hand, as a p-type semiconductor with a narrow bandgap of 1.2 eV, CuO has been widely studied because of its numerous applications in semiconductors, catalysis, biosensors, field transistors, and gas sensors. The CuO nanowires are an important nanoparticle in modifying electrodes with high sensitivity. However, the synthesis of CuO nanowires is tedious and time-consuming [34].

In this study, a novel PBA-GO-CuO nanoparticle was prepared through the hydrothermal method, and the synergistic effect of PBA and GO dramatically improved the electrocatalytic properties of glucose oxidation and detection. The developed detection platform using PBA-GO-CuO nanoparticles provided an acceptable detection limit of 0.95 nM to acarbose at a signal-to-noise ratio of 3, indicating ultra-sensitivity to α-amylase inhibitors. Rhein-8-b-D-glucopyranoside isolated from natural products was screened by the proposed sensing platform, demonstrating the excellent applicability [36]. The correctness was also verified using the iodine assay colorimetric method [37]. The constructed sensor platform was proven to be facile and cost-effective as well as highly sensitive, selective, and reliable, making it promising as a candidate for trace inhibitor screening of natural products.

2. Results and Discussion

2.1. Characterization of PBA-GO-CuO Nanocomposite

SEM images of various aggregates are shown in Figure 1, displaying distinct morphologies during the synthesis of PBA-GO-CuO nanomaterials. Figure 1a presents typical ellipsoidal CuO particles with a size of ~23 nm. In Figure 1b, graphene oxide aggregates appeared as ruffled wrinkles abound on surface areas. As shown in Figure 1c, the macroscopic stacked structure becomes predominant after boron doping. Moreover, Figure 1d displays the SEM images of CuO-GO hybrid material. The pronounced aggregates are observed due to the CuO load on graphene oxide [38–40]. Figure 1e portrays the PBA-GO-CuO nanomaterials' rich pore structure and high specific surface area. From the enlarged picture in Figure 1f, we can see with more detailed information that the size of CuO is smaller than that in Figure 1a.

The TEM and energy dispersive X-ray spectra (EDS) are exhibited in Figure 2. In Figure 2a,b, massive amounts of CuO particles are decorated on the graphene oxide surface, affirming the SEM observation. From the EDS mapping surface scan (Figure 2c), we can see that the elements of carbon (green), boron (red), and oxygen (yellow) are uniformly overlapped, proving once again that CuO particles are homogeneously braced on graphene oxide. The FTIR images in Figure 2d confirm the boron doping with the characteristic absorption bands of B–O at 1350 cm^{-1} and B–C at 1180 cm^{-1} [35].

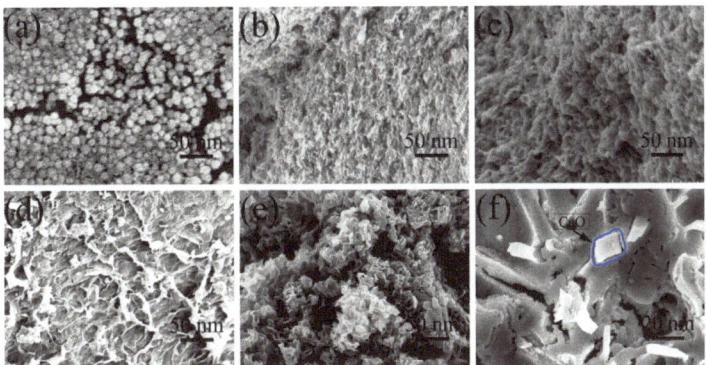

Figure 1. SEM image of (**a**) CuO, (**b**) GO, (**c**) PBA-GO, (**d**) GO-CuO, (**e**) PBA-GO-CuO, (**f**) PBA-GO-CuO.

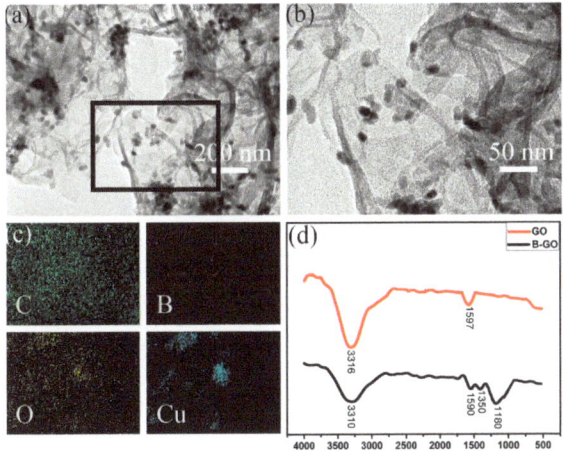

Figure 2. (**a**) TEM image of PBA-GO-CuO, (**b**,**c**) EDS mappings of PBA-GO-CuO for C (green), B (red), O (yellow), and Cu (blue), (**d**) FTIR image.

We performed XPS tests to understand the diverse valence states of boron doping and the variation in the element composition of PBA-GO-CuO nanomaterials, as shown in Figure 3. The curve fitting and analysis of C_{1s} and B_{1s} signals are presented in Table 1. The C_{1s} peak at 290.2 eV, O_{1s} peak at 530.9 eV, and the peak at 195.2 eV is related to the B_{1s} peak in Figure 3a. The high-resolution C_{1s} spectrum of PBA-GO-CuO consists of five characteristic peaks in Figure 3b, corresponding to C–B (288.3 eV), C–C (289 eV), C–O (291.2 eV), C=O (292.5 eV), and O–C=O (287.5 eV) structures. The high-resolution B_{1s} peak was synthesized into four peaks (Figure 3c), representing the structures of B_4C (187.8 eV, attributed to the graphene lattice defects), BC_3 (189.9 eV, may indicate that boron atoms replace carbon atoms in the graphene skeleton), BC_2O (191.2 eV, may suggest that boron atoms replace carbon atoms in the edge or defect position of the graphene skeleton), and BCO_2 (192.3 eV, same as BC_2O) [39–42]. Figure 3d is a high-resolution spectrum of Cu, where the peaks observed at 933.2 and 953.8 eV are due to $Cu_{2p3/2}$ and $Cu_{2p1/2}$, which are attributed to oxidized Cu (II) [41].

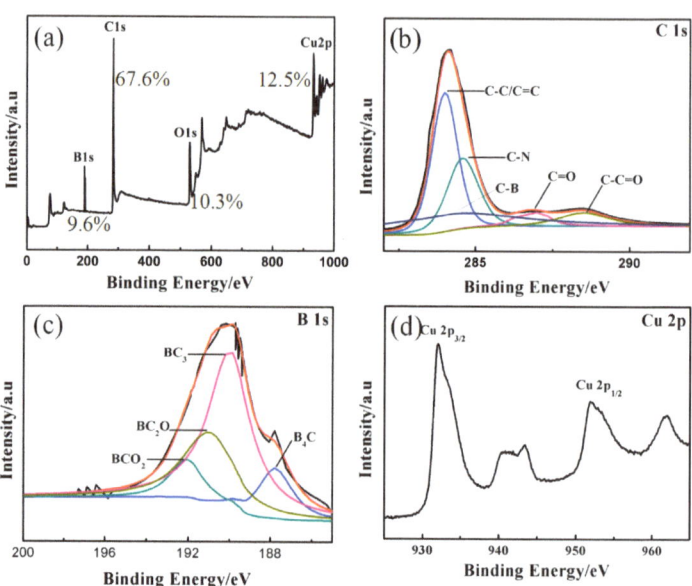

Figure 3. XPS curves: (**a**) whole spectra of PBA-GO-CuO, (**b**) C1s of PBA-GO-CuO, (**c**) B1s of PBA-GO-CuO, (**d**) Cu2p of PBA-GO-CuO.

Table 1. XPS elemental analysis of PBA-GO-CuO.

Element	Species	Binding Energy(eV)	Relative Intensity (%)
	C-C/C=C	284.01	71.26
	C-N	284.62	18.30
C 1s	C-C=O	288.50	5.29
	C=O	287.07	3.08
	C-B	284.81	2.07
	BC3	189.92	67.21
B 1s	BC2O	191.04	18.26
	BCO2	192.13	8.25
	B4C	187.81	6.34

2.2. Electrochemical Characteristics of Modified Electrodes

Electrochemical impedance spectroscopy is a valuable method to reflect the interfacial changes in the sensor in which the semicircle portion at a higher frequency expresses the electron-transfer-limited process, and the line at a lower frequency characterizes the diffusion process. The semicircle diameter order in Figure 4 is equal to that of the electron-transfer resistance: bare Glassy Carbon electrode (GCE) > CuO-GCE > PBA-GO-CuO-GCE. PBA-GO-CuO-GCE's diffusion uniformity (more parallel to the X-axis) is more excellent than other modified materials. In summary, the PBA-GO-CuO-GCE has the best response to glucose.

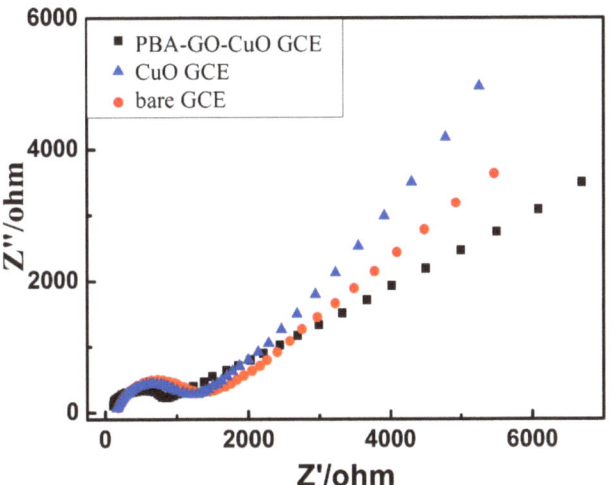

Figure 4. Impedance diagram of bare GCE, CuO-GCE, and PBA-GO-CuO-GCE in 0.1 KCl electrolyte solution containing 5 mM Fe(CN)$_6^{3-/4-}$.

2.3. Electrochemical Response of Modified Electrode to Glucose

Cu (II)/Cu (III) redox peaks are essential in nonenzymatic electrochemical glucose signal enlargement. As shown in the blue curve in Figure 5, CuO was oxidized to Cu (III) species, including CuO(OH) or another compound at an oxidation peak of about +0.4 V, and the generated Cu (III) species catalyzed the oxidation of glucose to glycoside at a scanning rate of 0.4 V/s. The PBA-GO-CuO-GCE displays poor redox peaks in 0.1 M NaOH without glucose (Figure 5). At the same time, Cu (III) was reduced to Cu (II) at the reduction peak of about +0.6 V. It is evident in Figure 5 that the bare GCE displays an inconspicuous redox peak at 0–0.8 V, which also confirms the signal amplification effect of the copper pair. After added glucose, electrons were quickly transferred from the glucose to the electrode. Cu (III) ions received electrons and functioned as electron-transfer carriers [43]. The black and red curves represent the redox peaks of PBA-GO-CuO-GCE and GO-CuO-GCE, respectively. Additionally, the approximate ratio of the closed-loop area of the four cyclic voltammetry curves in Figure 5 is 2.2: 1.57: 1.04: 0.07. The synergic signal enhancement is due to two reasons. Firstly, the electronic defects of the B element can cause the positively charged PBA-GO to be more likely to function as an electron receiver, absorbing electrons on the electrode; secondly, the CuO deposited on the PBA-GO is uniformly distributed, providing highly catalytically active sites and a high-efficiency glucose oxidation platform.

Prior to nonenzymatic glucose detection, the alkaline medium may be favorable to improve the electrocatalytic activity of the transition metal-based catalysts. Hence, the impact of NaOH concentrations was investigated in amperometry measurements of 0.1 M glucose. As shown in Figure 6, the amperometry currents increase correspondingly when the electrolyte concentration increases from 0.01 to 0.10 M because glucose is more easily oxidized, and the electrocatalytic activity of NN-CuO is greatly enhanced at high OH-. However, the peak current is decreased by further increasing the electrolyte concentration from 0.10 to 0.20 M. A possible reason may be that too much OH- can block the further electro-adsorption of glucose anion and result in a decrease in the current signal.

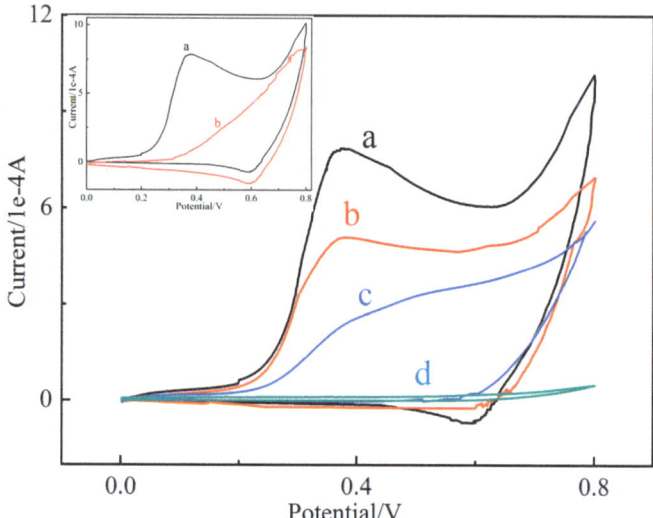

Figure 5. The cyclic voltammograms of bare GCE (**d**), CuO GCE (**c**), GO-CuO-GCE (**b**), and PBA-GO-CuO-GCE (**a**) in 0.1 M NaOH solution with 10 mM glucose (scan rate: 0.4 V/s); inset: PBA-GO-CuO-GCE in 0.2 M NaOH with (**a**) and without (**b**) the injection of 10 mM glucose.

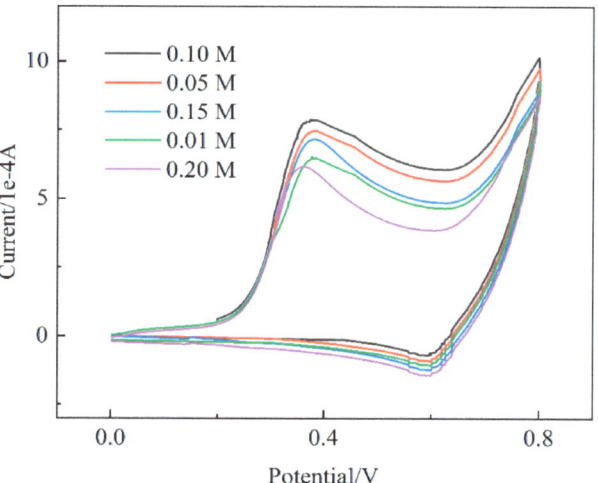

Figure 6. CVs of PBA-GO-CuO-GCE toward 10 mM glucose at 0.4 V under different NaOH concentrations (0.01, 0.05, 0.10, 0.15, 0.20); scan rate: 0.4 mV/s.

2.4. Chronoamperometry Studies

The chronoamperometry and a calibration curve of the PBA-GO-CuO-GCE glucose sensor are shown in Figure 7. A stable and fast stair-shape current-time signal responsive diagram can be observed in Figure 7a. In the first portion of the stair diagram, a 0.10 mM glucose solution was repeatedly added into a 0.10 M NaOH electrolyte after every 50 s, resulting in a current increase by 7.1×10^{-6} after each operation; in the second part of the stair diagram, a 1 mM glucose solution was repetitively added over 10 times, and the enlarged stair-shape signal occurred. The second part of the current is three times faster than the first. However, the current-time signal noise fluctuates after repeated glucose addition because the intermediate products are overlapped on the electrode due to signal interference [44]. With the continuous increase in glucose concentration of 1.5 mM and 2 mM, the current tends are stable, so the current-time relationship between 0.1 and 10 mM was selected for further study.

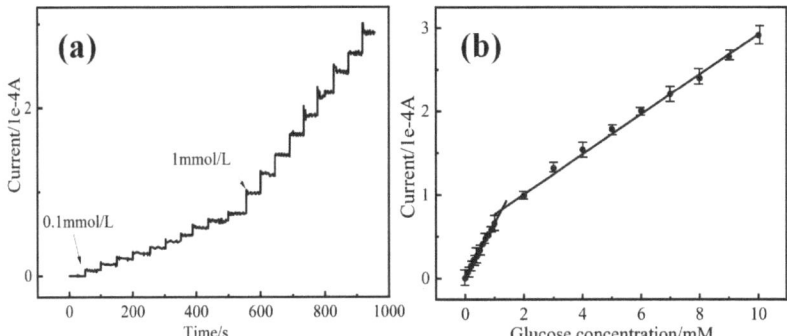

Figure 7. (a) I-t response of the PBA-GO-CuO electrode recorded at 0.4 V with the successive addition of an amount of glucose, (b) linear relationship between I vs. c of glucose.

As shown in Figure 7b, the calibrated diagram consisted of two linear current–concentration curves as follows: Y_1 (10^{-4} A) = 0.6432 X_1 (mM) + 0.0136 (R^2 = 0.99794) (low concentration range of 0.1–1 mM); Y_2 (10^{-4} A) = 0.2305 X_2 (mM) + 0.5951 (R^2 = 0.99657) (high concentration range of 1–10 mM). The detection limit is 0.7 μM (S/N = 3), and the calculated sensitivity is ~906 μA mM^{-1} cm^{-2} and 325 μA mM^{-1} cm^{-2} (the geometrical area and diameter of GCE are 7.068 and 3 mm, respectively). The sensitivity at a high concentration range is less than at a low concentration range, possibly due to the intermediate product generated by the electrocatalytic oxidation of glucose that was absorbed [45]. In contrast, the adsorption kinetics of glucose is slower at high concentrations. The detection performance of the fabricated modified electrode is compared with GO-CuO-GCE, CuO-GCE, and some other GCE-based nonenzymatic sensors. As can be seen in Table 2, the PBA-GO-CuO-GCE-modified electrode has a lower detection limit and a wider linear range [45–56].

Table 2. Comparison of detecting performance of the B-GO-CuO with other nonenzymatic glucose sensors.

Electrode Material	Electrode	Doping Element (and Its Source)	Sensitivity (μA mM^{-1} cm^{-2})	Linear Range	Detection Limit (μM)	Reference
PBA-GO-CuO	GCE	B (1-Pyrene boric acid)	906	0.1 mM–2.0 mM	0.7 μM	This work
GO-CuO	GCE	-	723	0.1 mM–2.0 mM	1.5 μM	This work
CuO	GCE	-	206	0.1 mM–2.0 mM	9.5 μM	This work
Faceted CuO nanoribbons	GCE	-	412	0.05 mM–3.5 mM	58 μM	Sahoo et al. [46]
LSC/rGO	GCE	-	330	2 μM–3.35 mM	63 μM	He et al. [47]
GO/CuO	GCE	-	37.63	0.005 mM–14 mM	5.04 μM	Foroughi et al. [48]
MWCNT/Au	GCE/CSPE	-	2.77 ± 0.14	0.1 mM–20 mM	4.1 μM	Branagan et al. [49]
Au/Cu$_2$O/GCE	GCE	-	715	0.05 mM–2.0 mM	18 μM	Su et al. [50]

Table 2. Cont.

Electrode Material	Electrode	Doping Element (and Its Source)	Sensitivity (μA mM^{-1} cm^{-2})	Linear Range	Detection Limit (μM)	Reference
Co-MOF Nanosheets	GCE	-	219.67	0.5 μM–8.065 mM	0.25 μM	Li et al. [51]
Co/MoS$_2$/CNTs	GCE	-	131.69	0–5.2 mM	80 nM	Branagan et al. [49]
Ni(II)-CP/C$_{60}$	GCE	-	614.29	0.01 mM–3.00 mM	4.3 μM	Shahhoseini et al. [52]
3D flower-like Ni$_7$S$_6$	GCE	-	271.8	5 μM–3.7 mM	0.15 μM	Wu et al. [53]
N-GR-CNTs/AuNPs	GCE	N(HNO$_3$)	0.9824	2 μM–19.6 mM	0.5 μM	Jeong et al. [55]
Microwave N-GO/CuO	GCE	N(urea)	122.336	0.01 mM–10 mM	14.52 μM	Rahsepar et al. [31]
S-rGO/CuS	GCE/RDE	S(Na$_2$S)	429.4	3.88 mM–20.17 mM	0.032 μM	Karikalan et al. [56]

2.5. Ultrasensitive Screening of Inhibitors from Natural Products

The established glucose sensor was applied to study the inhibitor of α-amylase, and the inhibiting ability can be sensitivity reported by the current responsive intensity. As described in Figure 8, the process of α-amylase inhibition limits glucose production and ultimately affects the strength of the current response. As one of the commonly used clinical α-amylase inhibitors, acarbose was tested as a positive drug. As shown in Figure 9a, the levels of current responsive intensity relative to the doses of the inhibitors after the inhibitors were added into the α-amylase reaction mixture. Serials of acarbose concentrations (1.0×10^{-9} M, 5.0×10^{-8} M, 1.0×10^{-8} M, 5.0×10^{-7} M, 1.0×10^{-7} M, 1.0×10^{-6} M, 1.0×10^{-5} M) were tested with a linear equation of I (%) = 919.426 C_{glu} + 11.602 and a good correlation coefficient of 0.997. The developed platform provided a detection of 0.95 nM at a signal-to-noise ratio of 3, indicating ultra-sensitivity. By calculating the regression equation, the IC$_{50}$ values are 48.6 μM. In order to further prove the applicability of the developed method, five compounds belonging to flavonoids (which was accomplished through our protein hybrid nanoflower technology) were screened [36]. The results of the Rhein-8-b-D-glucopyranoside are shown in Figure 10a. It can be seen that our method can efficiently detect the inhibition ability driven by Rhein-8-b-D-glucopyranoside. The good linear correlations of I (%) = 1014.056 C_{Rhe} + 216.239(R^2 = 0.997) were obtained for Rhein-8-b-D-glucopyranoside, and its limit of detection (LOD) was 1.39 nM. By calculating the regression equation, the IC$_{50}$ value of Rhein-8-b-D-glucopyranoside is 39.1 μM. The IC$_{50}$ values of acarbose (48.6 μM), Rhein-8-b-D-glucopyranoside (39.1 μM), indicated that Rhein-8-b-D-glucopyranoside possessed the most powerful inhibiting activity followed by acarbose. Moreover, the inhibiting ability of acarbose and Rhein-8-b-D-glucopyranoside were also investigated by the Iodine assay colorimetric method, and results are shown in Figures 9b and 10b [37]. The above results of the iodine assay colorimetric method powerfully demonstrate that the new sensing platform is capable of screening α-amylase. Because α-amylase is an important target in diabetes, these results further verified that the natural medicines containing Rhein-8-b-D-glucopyranoside often possess anti-diabetes activity.

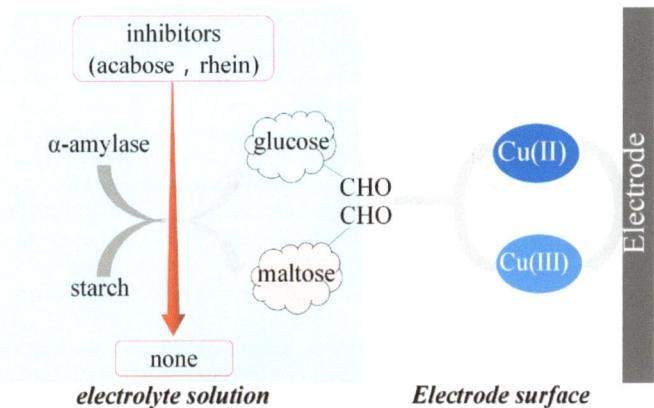

Figure 8. Schematic diagram of the mechanism of the method.

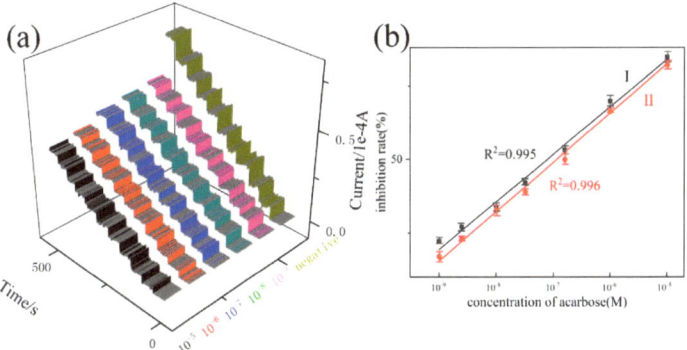

Figure 9. (**a**) The current-time curve with acarbose concentration of 1.0×10^{-9} M, 5.0×10^{-8} M, 1.0×10^{-8} M, 5.0×10^{-7} M, 1.0×10^{-7} M, 1.0×10^{-6} M, 1.0×10^{-5} M, (**b**) I: electrochemical standard curve; II: iodine assay colorimetric method standard curve.

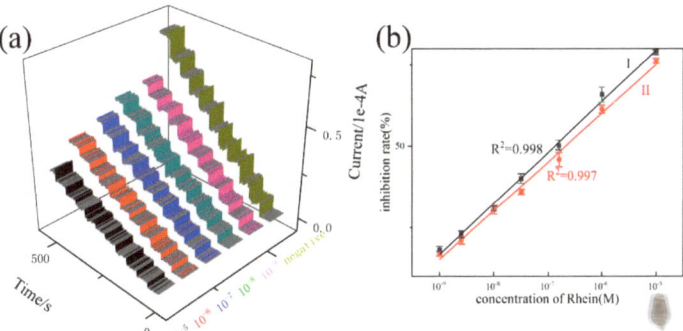

Figure 10. (**a**) The current-time curves with Rhein concentrations of 1.0×10^{-9} M, 5.0×10^{-8} M, 1.0×10^{-8} M, 5.0×10^{-7} M, 1.0×10^{-7} M, 1.0×10^{-6} M, 1.0×10^{-5} M, (**b**) I: electrochemical standard curve; II: iodine assay colorimetric standard curve.

2.6. Sensor Repeatability, Selectivity, and Stability

Superior repeatability and stability are critical factors in measuring electrode preparation success. We examine the stability of the electrode from the following two aspects. First, five freshly prepared PBA-GO-CuO electrodes were used to measure a 0.2 M NaOH solution (adding 10.0 mM glucose). The relative standard deviation of the electrode is 2.8% ($n = 5$), indicating that the designed and prepared PBA-GO-CuO electrode has excellent repeatability. Then, one of the electrodes was tested five consecutive times and washed with distilled water after each test. The relative standard deviation of the measured oxidation peak was 2.6%. In conclusion, the PBA-GO-CuO electrode prepared using this design method has good repeatability.

Moreover, the prepared PBA-GO-CuO electrode was stored in the dark for 2 months. After 2 months, it was used to measure a 0.2 M NaOH solution (10.0 mM glucose added). The oxidation current peak remained at 96%, signifying that the PBA-GO-CuO electrode prepared using this design method has excellent stability.

Additionally, some interfering ions, starch, inhibitor, and components in herbal medicine which may be present in the electrolyte solution were used to influence the determination results. It was observed that the tested substances had no practical influence on our detection platform. The high selectivity of the developed method is due to the specific response of the detection platform.

3. Materials and Methods

3.1. Materials and Apparatus

Graphene oxide aqueous solution (GOs-325, 2 mg/mL, $\geq$99.9%), 1-pyreneboronic acid (PBA), copper (II) acetate monohydrate, acarbose (98%), α-amylase (from porcine pancreas, type VI-B, $\geq$10 units/mg), soluble starch, potassium hexacyanoferrate (II) trihydrate, potassium hexacyanoferrate (III), D-(+)-glucose, and Nafion dispersion solution were purchased from Sigma-Aldrich (Sigma-Aldrich, Shanghai Titan Technology Co., Ltd., Shanghai, China). Rhubarb was purchased from Jiangxi Zhihetang Chinese Medicine Decoction Pieces Co., Ltd. (Jiangxi, China, batch numbers 160501 and 160801).

Electrochemical measurements were tested by a CHI800D electrochemical workstation (Shanghai Chenhua Instrument Co., Ltd., Shanghai, China). All electrochemical experiments were carried out on a three-electrode system, including a bare or modified GCE as the working electrode (WE)) (prior to surface coating, the GCE was polished carefully with 1.0, 0.3, and 0.05 μm alumina powder, respectively. Then, the polished GCE was cleaned sequentially with 1:1 HNO_3, ethanol, and water by continuous sonication, respectively. The electrode was allowed to dry at ambient temperature for further use). A Pt piece electrode was used as the counter electrode (CE), and an Ag/AgCl (3 M KCl) as the reference electrode (RE). All electrodes were purchased from Sigma-Aldrich (Sigma-Aldrich Company, Shanghai, China). Transmission electron microscopy (TEM) images were obtained by a Hitachi HT7700 (Shanghai, China), scanning electron microscopy (TEM) images were recorded by a JEOL JSM-6700 (Shanghai, China), X-ray photoelectron spectroscopy (XPS) images were recorded by a PHI5000V VersaProbe (Shanghai, China), and Fourier transform infrared (FTIR) images were recorded by a Nicolet Avatar 370 spectrometer (Jiangsu Skyray instruments Co., Ltd., Shanghai, China).

3.2. Preparation of PBA-GO-CuO Nanocomposite

CuO, GO-CuO, and PBA-GO-CuO were synthesized according to the reported studies with minor revisions to boron doping [40]. Then, 175 mg of a 5 mg/mL PBA was added into 35 mL of a 1.5 mg/mL GO suspension by intense agitation for 60 min. Then, the amount of Cu $(CH_3COO)_2$ H_2O was added dropwise to allow the copper source to adsorb on the graphene oxide; subsequently, the as-obtained turbid suspension was transferred into a high-temperature high-pressure autoclave and subjected to the hydrothermal reduction at 180 °C for 12 h. For comparison experiments, both CuO (without adding PBA and GO, the other steps remained the same) and GO-CuO (replaced PBA and GO with GO, the other steps remained the same) were synthesized according to a similar procedure. Afterward, the resulting dark precipitates were collected by centrifugation and washed with deionized water. Finally, the purified precipitate was freeze-dried overnight, and the CuO, GO-CuO, and PBA-GO-CuO were obtained for further characterization and preparation of the sensor.

3.3. Preparation and Measurement of the Glucose Sensor

The modified glassy carbon electrode (GCE) was formed through a conventional technique. In simple terms, the above-collected PBA-GO-CuO was hand-ground and dispersed with alcohol to obtain a uniform 5 mg/mL solution. A total of 10 µL of dispersion was dropped on the surface of a clean GCE and dried at room temperature. Subsequently, 5 µL of 0.1% Nafion solution was dropped on the surface of a GCE and dried at room temperature to obtain a PBA-GO-CuO-modified electrode, which we labeled PBA-GO-CuO-GCE. CuO, GO, and GO-CuO were prepared using a similar procedure for comparison.

3.4. Trace α-Amylase Inhibitor Screening from Natural Product

As a typical α-amylase inhibitor, acarbose was employed to verify the feasibility of the α-amylase inhibitor screening platform. Five natural compounds (i.e., aloe-emodin-8-O-b-D-glucopyranoside, 6-O-cinnamamoyglucose, L-epicatechin, 2-O-cinnamoyl-1-O-galloy-b-D-glucose, and Rhein-8-b-D-glucopyranoside) were also screened. Different concentrations of the tested compounds were prepared by ethanol-water solution (70:30, v/v). The assay for α-amylase inhibitors was as follows: (1) 0.5 mL of α-amylase (0.1 U/mL) was incubated in Phosphate Buffer (PBS, pH = 6.8) with different doses of inhibitors, then, 5 mL 30 g/L soluble starch was added dropwise at 37 °C for 20 min, and dried with a flow of N_2. The blank group, negative control group, and positive control group were prepared using a similar procedure; the glucose content of each reaction system was detected by a glucose sensor. (2) According to the following calculation formula (Equation (1)) for inhibition rate, the inhibition rate of each inhibitor and the positive drug acarbose on α-amylase can be calculated.

$$I/\% = \frac{C_B - C_D}{C_B - C_A} \quad (1)$$

where I is the enzyme inhibition rate (%), C_A is the glucose concentration (M) measured in the blank group, C_B is the glucose concentration (M) measured in the negative control group, and C_D is the glucose concentration (M) measured in the sample group. The IC_{50} was calculated from the inhibition rate-concentration curve.

4. Conclusions

In summary, we successfully synthesized a glucose sensor consisting of a PBA-GO-CuO nanocomposite where the boron doping rate remarkably reaches up to 9.6%, and the CuO load is ~12.5 wt.%, leading to rich pore structure and high specific surface area. This sensor acquires an enhanced signal amplification effect, a more comprehensive linear range (0.1–10 mM), lower detection limit (0.7 µM), higher sensitivity (906 µA mM^{-1} cm^{-2}), and lower detection potential (+0.4 V). The prepared sensor application in acarbose and Rhein's inhibitory activity measurer has the advantages of easy preparation, charting, and convenience, providing a reference value and feasible basis for electrochemistry in the additional calculation and activity verification of traditional Chinese medicine.

Author Contributions: Conceptualization of the compounds, M.L. and X.Y.; synthesis, methodology, M.L. and Y.Y.; supervision over the project, S.C. and C.M.; data curation, M.L. and H.S.; writing—original draft preparation, M.L.; writing—review and editing, M.L. and Y.Y.; funding acquisition, X.Y. All authors have read and agreed to the published version of the manuscript.

Funding: This research was funded by the Construction Project of Shanghai Engineering Research Center of Pharmaceutical Intelligent Equipment (20DZ2255900).

Institutional Review Board Statement: Not applicable.

Informed Consent Statement: Not applicable.

Data Availability Statement: Not applicable.

Acknowledgments: This work was financially supported by the Construction Project of Shanghai Engineering Research Center of Pharmaceutical Intelligent Equipment (20DZ2255900) and Shanghai Frontiers Science Research Center for Druggability of Cardiovascular noncoding RNA.

Conflicts of Interest: The authors declare no conflict of interest.

Sample Availability: Samples of the compounds are not available from the authors.

References

1. Liu, L.L.; Cen, Y.; Liu, F.; Yu, J.G.; Jiang, X.Y.; Chen, X.Q. Analysis of α-amylase inhibitor from corni fructus by coupling magnetic cross-linked enzyme aggregates of α-amylase with HPLC-MS. *J. Chromatogr. B* **2015**, *15*, 30008. [CrossRef] [PubMed]
2. Malene, J.P.; Rita, D.C.; Louise, K.; Dan, S. Immobilized α-amylase magnetic beads for ligand fishing: Proof of concept and identification of α-amylase inhibitors in Ginkgo biloba. *Phytochemistry* **2019**, *164*, 94.
3. Lima, H.R.; Silva, J.; Farias, E. Electrochemical sensors and biosensors for the analysis of antineoplastic drugs. *Biosens. Bioelectron.* **2018**, *108*, 15. [CrossRef] [PubMed]
4. Mourzina, Y.G.; Ermolenko, Y.E.; Offenhäusser, A. Synthesizing Electrodes into Electrochemical Sensor Systems. *Front. Chem.* **2021**, *9*, 641. [CrossRef] [PubMed]
5. Ye, Y.L.; Ji, J.; Sun, Z.Y. Recent advances in electrochemical biosensors for antioxidant analysis in foodstuff. *TrAC Trends Anal. Chem.* **2019**, *122*, 155718. [CrossRef]
6. Cortina, M.E.; Melli, L.J.; Roberti, M. Electrochemical magnetic microbeads-based biosensor for point-of-care serodiagnosis of infectious diseases. *Biosens. Bioelectron.* **2016**, *80*, 15. [CrossRef]
7. Lv, M.; Liu, Y.; Geng, J.H. Engineering nanomaterials-based biosensors for food safety detection. *Biosens. Bioelectron.* **2018**, *106*, 30. [CrossRef]
8. Zhang, X.L.; Wu, D.; Zhou, X.X. Recent progress on the construction of nanozymes-based biosensors and their applications to food safety assay. *TrAC Trends Anal. Chem.* **2019**, *121*, 115668. [CrossRef]
9. Silva, N.F.; Magalhães, J.M.; Freire, C. Electrochemical biosensors for Salmonella: State of the art and challenges in food safety assessment. *Biosens. Bioelectron.* **2018**, *99*, 15. [CrossRef]
10. Hovancová, J.; Šišoláková, I.; Oriňaková, R. Nanomaterial-based electrochemical sensors for detection of glucose and insulin. *J. Solid-State Electrochem.* **2017**, *21*, 2147. [CrossRef]
11. Tajik, S.; Beitollahi, H.; Ahmadi, S.A. Screen-printed electrode surface modification with NiCo2O4/RGO nanocomposite for hydroxylamine detection. *Nanomaterials* **2021**, *11*, 3208. [CrossRef] [PubMed]
12. Beitollahi, H.; Shahsavari, M.; Sheikhshoaie, I. Amplified electrochemical sensor employing screen-printed electrode modified with Ni-ZIF-67 nanocomposite for high sensitive analysis of Sudan I in present bisphenol A. *Food Chem. Toxicol.* **2022**, *161*, 112824. [CrossRef]
13. Adeel, M.; Rahman, M.M.; Caligiuri, I. Recent advances of electrochemical and optical enzyme-free glucose sensors operating at physiological conditions. *Biosens. Bioelectron.* **2020**, *165*, 112. [CrossRef] [PubMed]
14. Han, T.; Noda, S.; Haneda, K. Development of a glucose sensor using palladium electrode. *Diabetes* **2018**, *67* (Suppl. 1), 2265-PUB. [CrossRef]
15. Zhu, H.; Li, L.; Zhou, W. Advances in non-enzymatic glucose sensors based on metal oxides. *J. Mater. Chem. B* **2016**, *4*, 7333. [CrossRef]
16. Qian, J.C.; Wang, Y.P.; Pan, J. Non-enzymatic glucose sensor based on ZnO–CeO$_2$ whiskers. *MCP* **2020**, *239*, 122051. [CrossRef]
17. Sode, K.J.; Loew, N.Y.; Ohnishi, Y.S. Novel fungal FAD glucose dehydrogenase derived from Aspergillus niger for glucose enzyme sensor strips. *Biosens. Bioelectron.* **2017**, *87*, 305. [CrossRef]
18. Lee, H.; Hong, Y.J.; Baik, S. Enzyme-based glucose sensor: From invasive to wearable device. *Adv. Healthc. Mater.* **2018**, *7*, 1701150. [CrossRef]
19. Chen, D.; Wang, X.H.; Zhang, K.X. Glucose photoelectrochemical enzyme sensor based on competitive reaction of ascorbic acid. *Biosens. Bioelectron.* **2020**, *166*, 112466. [CrossRef]
20. Salazar, P.; Rico, V.; Rodríguez-Amaro, R. New Copper wide range nanosensor electrode prepared by physical vapor deposition at oblique angles for the non-enzimatic determination of glucose. *Electrochim. Acta* **2015**, *169*, 195. [CrossRef]
21. Liu, L.; Wang, M.; Wang, C.Y. In-situ synthesis of graphitic carbon nitride/iron oxide−copper composites and their application in the electrochemical detection of glucose. *Electrochim. Acta* **2018**, *265*, 275. [CrossRef]
22. Duan, X.X.; Liu, K.L.; Xu, Y. Nonenzymatic electrochemical glucose biosensor constructed by NiCo$_2$O$_4$@Ppy nanowires on nickel foam substrate. *Sens. Actuators B Chem.* **2019**, *292*, 121. [CrossRef]
23. Wei, M.; Qiao, Y.X.; Zhao, H.T. Electrochemical non-enzymatic glucose sensors: Recent progress and perspectives. *ChemComm* **2020**, *56*, 14553. [CrossRef] [PubMed]
24. Sun, C.; Miao, J.J.; Yan, J. Applications of antibiofouling PEG-coating in electrochemical biosensors for determination of glucose in whole blood. *Electrochim. Acta* **2013**, *89*, 549. [CrossRef]

25. Wang, J.; Zhang, W.D. Fabrication of CuO nanoplatelets for highly sensitive enzyme-free determination of glucose. *Electrochim. Acta* **2011**, *56*, 7510. [CrossRef]
26. Fleischmann, M.; Korinek, K.; Pletcher, D. The kinetics and mechanism of the oxidation of amines and alcohols at oxide-covered nickel, silver, copper, and cobalt electrodes. *J. Chem. Soc. Perkin Trans.* **1972**, *2*, 1396. [CrossRef]
27. Seunghee, H.C.; Sun, S.K.; Jaeseok, Y. Chemical and biological sensors based on defect-engineered graphene mesh field-effect transistors. *Nano Converg.* **2016**, *14*, 2056.
28. Zhang, Y.P.; Liu, X.T.; Qiu, S. A Flexible Acetylcholinesterase-Modified Graphene for Chiral Pesticide Sensor. *J. Am. Chem. Soc.* **2019**, *141*, 14643. [CrossRef]
29. Sehit, E.; Altintas, Z. Significance of nanomaterials in electrochemical glucose sensors: An updated review (2016–2020). *Biosens. Bioelectron.* **2020**, *159*, 112. [CrossRef]
30. Wei, S.J.; Hao, Y.B.; Ying, Z. Transfer-free CVD graphene for highly sensitive glucose sensors. *J. Mater. Sci. Technol.* **2020**, *37*, 71. [CrossRef]
31. Rahsepar, M.; Foroughi, F.; Kim, H. A new enzyme-free biosensor based on nitrogen-doped graphene with high sensing performance for electrochemical detection of glucose at biological pH value. *Sens. Actuators B Chem.* **2019**, *282*, 322. [CrossRef]
32. Paraknowitsch, J.P.; Thomas, A. Doping carbons beyond nitrogen: An overview of advanced heteroatom doped carbons with boron, sulphur and phosphorus for energy applications. *Energy Environ. Sci.* **2013**, *6*, 2839. [CrossRef]
33. Li, Y.F.; Zhang, W.W.; Guo, B. Interlayer shear of nanomaterials: Graphene-graphene, boron nitride-boron nitride and graphene-boron nitride. *Acta Mech. Solida Sin.* **2017**, *30*, 234. [CrossRef]
34. Yu, X.M.; Han, P.; Wei, Z.X. Boron-Doped Graphene for Electrocatalytic N2 Reduction. *Joule* **2018**, *2*, 1610. [CrossRef]
35. Justino, C.; Gomes, A.R.; Freitas, A.C. Graphene based sensors and biosensors. *Trac-Trend Anal. Chem.* **2017**, *91*, 53. [CrossRef]
36. Qian, K.; Wang, H.; Liu, J.M. Synthesis of α-glycosidase hybrid nano-flowers and their application for enriching and screening α-glycosidase inhibitors. *New J. Chem.* **2017**, *42*, 429. [CrossRef]
37. Xie, Y.S.; Li, D.W.; Li, Y.F. The activity of α-amylase inhibitor was determined by colorimetric method of iodine test solution. *Jiangsu Agric. Sci.* **2015**, *43*, 301.
38. Rotte, N.K.; Naresh, V.; Muduli, S. Microwave aided scalable synthesis of sulfur, nitrogen co-doped few-layered graphene material for high-performance supercapacitors. *Electrochim. Acta* **2020**, *363*, 137209. [CrossRef]
39. Jiang, B.; Liang, K.M.; Yang, Z.J. FeCoNiB@Boron-doped vertically aligned graphene arrays: A self-supported electrocatalyst for overall water splitting in a wide pH range. *Electrochim. Acta* **2021**, *386*, 138459. [CrossRef]
40. Zhou, X.Y.; Zhang, J.; Su, Q.M. Nanoleaf-on-sheet CuO/graphene composites: Microwave-assisted assemble and excellent electrochemical performances for lithium-ion batteries. *Electrochim. Acta* **2014**, *125*, 615. [CrossRef]
41. Gao, J.P.; Qiu, G.J.; Li, H.J. Boron-doped graphene/TiO2 nanotube-based aqueous lithium-ion capacitors with high energy density. *Electrochim. Acta* **2020**, *329*, 135175. [CrossRef]
42. Shumba, M.; Nyokong, T. Electrode modification using nanocomposites of boron or nitrogen doped graphene oxide and cobalt (II) tetra aminophenoxy phthalocyanine nanoparticles. *Electrochim. Acta* **2016**, *196*, 457. [CrossRef]
43. Yang, S.L.; Li, G.; Wang, D. Synthesis of nanoneedle-like copper oxide on N-doped reduced graphene oxide: A three-dimensional hybrid for nonenzymatic glucose sensor. *Sens. Actuators B Chem.* **2017**, *238*, 588. [CrossRef]
44. Li, Y.R.; Wang, X.; Yang, Q. Ultra-fine CuO Nanoparticles Embedded in Three-dimensional Graphene Network Nanostructure for High-performance Flexible Supercapacitors. *Electrochim. Acta* **2017**, *234*, 63. [CrossRef]
45. Yadav, H.M.; Lee, J.J. One-pot synthesis of copper nanoparticles on glass: Applications for non-enzymatic glucose detection and catalytic reduction of 4-nitrophenol. *J. Solid State Electrochem.* **2019**, *23*, 503. [CrossRef]
46. Sahoo, R.K.; Das, A.; Samantaray, K. Electrochemical glucose Sensing characteristics of two-dimensional faceted and non-faceted CuO nanoribbons. *Crystengcomm* **2019**, *244*, 1607. [CrossRef]
47. He, J.; Sunarso, J.; Zhu, Y.L. High-performance non-enzymatic perovskite sensor for hydrogen peroxide and glucose electrochemical detection. *Sens. Actuators B Chem.* **2017**, *21*, 482. [CrossRef]
48. Foroughi, F.; Rahsepar, M.; Hadianfard, M.J.; Kim, H. Microwave-assisted synthesis of graphene modified CuO nanoparticles for voltammetric enzyme-free sensing of glucose at biological pH values. *Microchim. Acta* **2017**, *185*, 57. [CrossRef]
49. Branagan, D.; Breslin, C.B. Electrochemical detection of glucose at physiological pH using gold nanoparticles deposited on carbon nanotubes. *Sens. Actuators B Chem.* **2019**, *282*, 490. [CrossRef]
50. Su, Y.; Guo, H.; Wang, Z.S. Au@Cu2O core-shell structure for high sensitive non-enzymatic glucose sensor. *Sens. Actuators B Chem.* **2018**, *255*, 2510. [CrossRef]
51. Li, Q.; Shao, Z.F.; Han, T. A High-Efficiency Electrocatalyst for Oxidizing Glucose: Ultrathin Nanosheet Co-Based Organic Framework Assemblies. *ACS Sustain. Chem. Eng.* **2019**, *7*, 8986. [CrossRef]
52. Shahhoseini, L.; Mohammadi, R.; Ghanbari, B. Ni (II) 1D-coordination polymer/C60-modified glassy carbon electrode as a highly sensitive non-enzymatic glucose electrochemical sensor. *Appl. Surf. Sci.* **2019**, *478*, 361. [CrossRef]
53. Wu, W.Q.; Li, Y.B.; Jin, J.Y. A novel nonenzymatic electrochemical sensor based on 3D flower-like Ni7S6 for hydrogen peroxide and glucose. *Sens. Actuators B Chem.* **2016**, *232*, 633. [CrossRef]
54. Zhang, Y.; Wang, L.; Yu, J. Three-dimensional macroporous carbon supported hierarchical ZnO-NiO nanosheets for electrochemical glucose sensing. *J. Alloys Compd.* **2016**, *698*, 800. [CrossRef]

55. Jeong, H.; Nguyen, D.M.; Lee, M.S. N-doped graphene-carbon nanotube hybrid networks attaching with gold nanoparticles for glucose non-enzymatic sensor. *Sci. Eng. Compos. Mater.* **2018**, *90*, 38. [CrossRef]
56. Karikalan, N.; Karthik, R.; Chen, S.M. Sonochemical Synthesis of Sulfur Doped Reduced Graphene Oxide Supported CuS Nanoparticles for the Non-Enzymatic Glucose Sensor Applications. *Sci. Rep.* **2017**, *7*, 2494. [CrossRef]

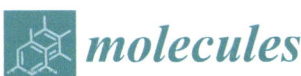

Article

Analytical Performance of Clay Paste Electrode and Graphene Paste Electrode-Comparative Study

Ewelina Skowron [1], Kaja Spilarewicz-Stanek [2], Dariusz Guziejewski [3], Kamila Koszelska [3,*], Radovan Metelka [4] and Sylwia Smarzewska [3,*]

1. Polfarmex S.A., Jozefow 9, 99-300 Kutno, Poland; ewelina.skowron96@onet.pl
2. Faculty of Chemistry, Jagiellonian University, Gronostajowa 2, 30-387 Krakow, Poland; kaja.spilarewicz-stanek@uj.edu.pl
3. Department of Inorganic and Analytical Chemistry, Faculty of Chemistry, University of Lodz, Tamka 12, 91-403 Lodz, Poland; dariusz.guziejewski@chemia.uni.lodz.pl
4. Department of Analytical Chemistry, Faculty of Chemical Technology, University of Pardubice, Studentska 573, 53210 Pardubice, Czech Republic; radovan.metelka@upce.cz
* Correspondence: kamila.koszelska@chemia.uni.lodz.pl (K.K.); sylwia.smarzewska@chemia.uni.lodz.pl (S.S.); Tel.: +48-(42)-635-58-10 (K.K.); +48-(42)-635-58-08 (S.S.)

Abstract: The analytical performance of the clay paste electrode and graphene paste electrode was compared using square wave voltammetry (SWV) and cyclic voltammetry (CV). The comparison was made on the basis of a paracetamol (PA) determination on both working electrodes. The influence of pH and SWV parameters was investigated. The linear concentration ranges were found to be 6.0×10^{-7}–3.0×10^{-5} and 2.0×10^{-6}–8.0×10^{-5} mol L^{-1} for clay paste electrode (ClPE) and graphene paste electrode (GrPE), respectively. The detection and quantification limits were calculated as 1.4×10^{-7} and 4.7×10^{-7} mol L^{-1} for ClPE and 3.7×10^{-7} and 1.2×10^{-6} mol L^{-1} for GrPE, respectively. Developed methods were successfully applied to pharmaceutical formulations analyses. Scanning electron microscopy and energy-dispersive X-ray spectroscopy were used to characterize ClPE and GrPE surfaces. Clay composition was examined with wavelength dispersive X-ray (WDXRF).

Keywords: square wave voltammetry; paracetamol; graphene; clay; carbon paste electrodes; sensors

1. Introduction

It is well known that chemical sensors are devices that transform chemical information into an analytically useful signal. Among all the chemical sensors reported in the literature, electrochemical sensors are the most attractive because of their remarkable sensitivity, experimental simplicity and low cost. Carbon paste electrodes (CPE) are widely used as working electrodes for the determination of electrochemically active compounds. Paste electrodes have received much attention due to their advantages, such as easily renewable surfaces, inexpensiveness, biocompatibility, and relatively wide potential windows [1–5]. Moreover, the incorporation of modifiers into carbon paste material makes it even more attractive in electroanalytical applications [6–12]. The performance of chemically modified carbon paste electrodes depends on the properties of the modifier, which affect the selectivity of the electrodes, kinetics of an electrochemical reaction, and sometimes even the electrode reaction product [13,14]. Nowadays, graphene and its derivatives are one of the most popular working electrodes modifiers used in electrochemical studies [15–19]. Graphene is a two-dimensional, sp^2 hybridized carbon sheet, where atoms are arranged in a honeycomb-shaped lattice [20,21]. Graphene exhibits high thermal conductivity, flexibility, transparency, lightness, and has an extremely high surface area [22–25]. Because of its interesting properties, graphene has shown great promise in many applications, such as electronics, energy storage and conversion, and electroanalysis or electrocatalysis [24].

Graphene paste electrodes are commonly applied in electrochemistry [26–28]. Clays are minerals dominantly made from a colloid fraction of soils, sediments, rocks and water [29]. Grim et al. described clays as an aggregate of minerals and colloidal substances, which are made from a stacking of tetrahedral and octahedral sheets interspersed with a space called the interlayer space. Clay minerals are classified into three families according to the thickness of the sheets, corresponding to a number of tetrahedral and octahedral layers. The gap between sheets can contain water and ions. The tetrahedral sheets are arranged in hexagonal meshes and consist of oxygen tetrahedral surrounding a silicon or aluminum atom. The octahedral sheets are formed by two planes of oxygens-hydroxyl framing broader atoms, such as Al, Fe, Mg and Li [30]. Clay, as an electrode modifier, is a less popular material than, e.g., graphene, although results obtained at such modified electrodes are exceptional [31–34]. The reason for highly attractive characteristics for electroanalytical purposes are mainly found in the stability of such easily disposable modifiers, both chemical and mechanical, but are also reasoned due to their strong sorptive properties [35]. Therefore, clay and its excellent properties may be revealed in high cation and anion exchange capacity, porosity that imparts changes into the electrical conductivity but also catalytic activity towards electrochemical processes [36–38]. The not to be missed advantage of the clay paste electrodes is its extremely low cost, especially when compared to graphene paste electrodes. The aim of this research is to collate differences and similarities in the analytical performance of clay paste and graphene paste electrodes.

2. Results and Discussion

2.1. Preliminary Studies

Initially, the surfaces of the prepared working electrodes were examined with a scanning electron microscope. In Figure 1, representative SEM images at low magnification of the graphene paste and clay paste coatings are presented. The surface texturing of both coatings is similar. Consecutive SEM images at high magnification are presented in Figure 2, demonstrating the surfaces in detail. Graphene paste exhibits a layered structure, mainly based on graphite plates. However, clay paste has a more heterogeneous structure, showing grains of clay deposited between the graphite plates. The even distribution of grains in the whole film is observed. The investigation of the chemical composition of each type of coatings was also performed with the use of the EDX method (presented in detail in the Supplementary Material). EDX results are in good agreement with data obtained from the WDXRF analysis.

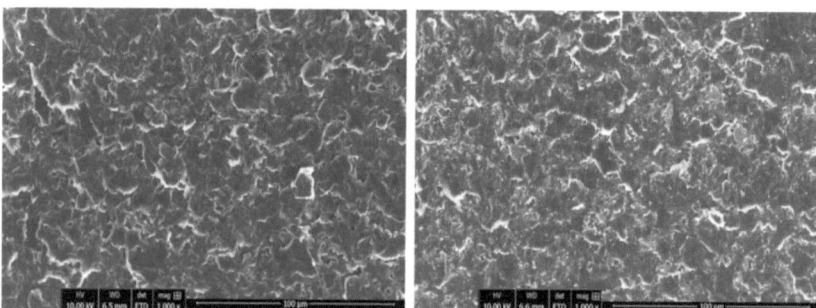

Figure 1. SEM images of graphene paste electrode (**left**) and clay paste electrode (**right**), 1000×.

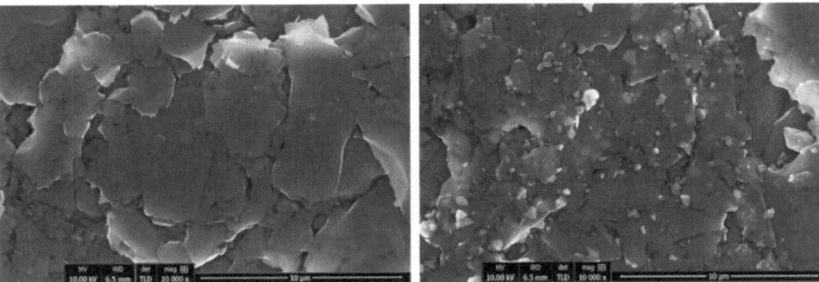

Figure 2. SEM images of graphene paste electrode (**left**) and clay paste electrode (**right**), 10,000×.

The electroactive surface of ClPE and GrPE was examined with cyclic voltammetry and a 1.0 mM hexacyanoferrate redox system. The relation between redox peak currents and the square root of the scan rate was found to be linear and the electroactive surface area was calculated with the Randles–Sevcik equation: $I_p = 2.69 \times 10^5 \times n^{3/2} \times A \times C^* \times D^{1/2} \times v^{1/2}$, where I_p refers to the peak current, n is the number of electrons transferred, A is the electroactive surface, D is the diffusion coefficient, v is the scan rate and C^* is the concentration. A values were found to be 1.07 and 1.03 mm^2 for ClPE and GrPE, respectively.

2.2. Voltammetric Studies of Paracetamol

To compare the electroanalytical performance of ClPE and GrPE, paracetamol was chosen, as its electrochemical behavior was thoroughly investigated by many researchers in various pH using many kinds of working electrodes [14,39–41]. This makes it possible to draw up reliable conclusions about observed phenomena. According to the available literature, two possible paths of the oxidation mechanism of paracetamol are known: the one-proton mechanism or the two-proton mechanism, depending on the experimental conditions [39,40,42–44]. First, the one-proton mechanism was proposed by Kang et al. (2010) [40]. The latter one, the most commonly observed, involves two electrons and two protons, in which a relatively stable product—N-acetyl-p-benzoquinone-imine (NAPQI) is generated [39,41–43]. The occurrence of the follow-up chemical reactions of NAPQI is pH-dependent [39,43]. The electrochemical behavior of paracetamol, on both working electrodes, was first analyzed with cyclic voltammetry. The dependence of scan rate on the PA peak currents was investigated. Figure 3 presents cyclic voltammograms of PA recorded on GrPE and ClPE. As can be seen at both working electrodes, the single anodic peak is visible. The corresponding cathodic signal is much smaller, which is consistent with previous reports discussing paracetamol electrochemical behavior [41].

For the clay paste electrode, it was observed that the logarithm of the peak current is linearly proportional to the logarithm of the scan rate (slope = 0.97), indicating an adsorption-controlled electrode reaction (Figure 3A, right inset). This was confirmed by a linear correlation between the PA peak current and the scan rate (Figure 3A, left inset). For graphene paste, electrode adsorption was not observed as the PA peak current was linearly dependent on the square root of the scan rate (Figure 3B, left inset), and the dependence between the logarithm of the peak current and logarithm of the scan rate gave a slope of 0.44 (Figure 3B, right inset), which is close to a theoretical value of 0.5—characteristic for electrode reactions controlled by depolarizer diffusion. Observed differences are in good agreement with previous reports, where it was proven that the paracetamol electrode reaction is dependent on the working electrode surface and material [14,44]. Next, as supporting electrolyte composition may significantly affect the electrochemical behavior of electroactive compounds, the effect of supporting electrolyte pH on PA peak currents was investigated. For this purpose, BR buffers pH 2.0–10.0 were chosen. Similar behavior of paracetamol was observed for both working electrodes. The PA peak current increased with pH to reach the maximum at pH 3.0 on both electrodes and then decreased. At higher pH values (pH ≥ 7), neither the peak currents nor the peak potentials were stable, thus results obtained in pH 7 and higher were not taken into account in further data analyses. Dependences between the PA peak currents and pH of Britton–Robinson buffer obtained on both working electrodes are shown in Figure 4. Based on these dependencies, in order to obtain the highest PA response, BR buffer pH 3.0 was chosen as the optimum supporting electrolyte and used in further studies with both working electrodes. Together, with the peak current, the paracetamol peak potential was also checked, as it frequently is pH-dependent. The PA peak potentials shifted toward less positive values with an increase in the pH for both electrodes. Dependences between the paracetamol peak potentials and pH of the BR buffer were linear for ClPE and GrPE, and could be described using the following equations: $E_p = -0.046\,\text{pH} + 0.817$, and $E_p = -0.048\,\text{pH} + 0.833$, respectively (as can be seen in the inset of Figure 4).

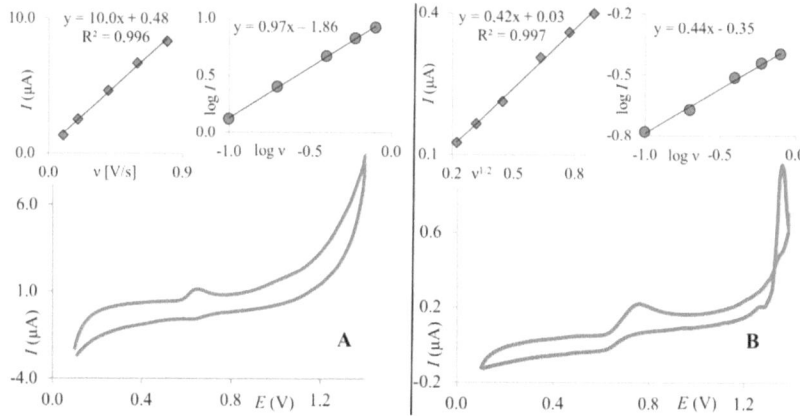

Figure 3. Cyclic voltammograms (scan rate 50 mV × s^{-1}) of 1.0×10^{-5} mol L^{-1} PA were recorded on ClPE (**A**) and GrPE (**B**). Insets: the relationship between PA peak current and scan rate (**A**-left) or the square root of scan rate (**B**-left); the relationship between the logarithm of PA peak current and logarithm of scan rate (**A**-right, **B**-right).

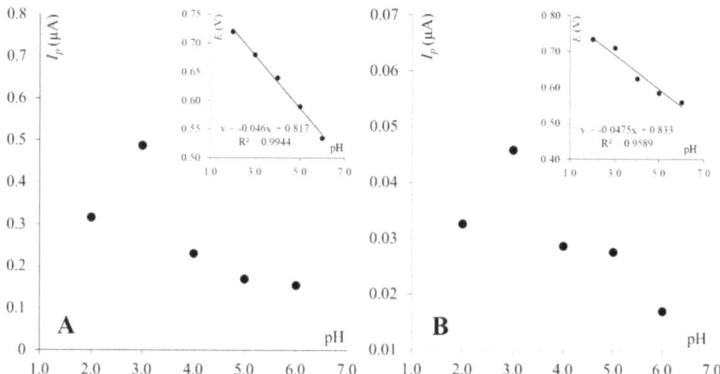

Figure 4. Dependence between PA peak currents and pH of BR buffer for ClPE (**A**) and GrPE (**B**). Insets: dependence between PA peak potentials and pH of BR buffer.

As SWV parameters are interrelated and exert a combined effect on the registered peak currents, in the next experimental step, the influence of SW amplitude, step potential, and frequency on PA signals was studied for ClPE and GrPE. Amplitude (ΔE), step potential

(ΔE_s), and frequency (f) were evaluated in the range of 10–100 mV, 3–21 mV, and 10–100 Hz, respectively. In the case of ClPE, the parabolic dependence of the amplitude on PA signals was observed, the peak current increased from 10 mV to 40 mV, and then decreased. The best results were obtained at 40 mV, and thus this value of amplitude was adopted in subsequent studies. Similarly, a parabolic dependence was observed for frequency analysis, the best-shaped peaks were obtained at 70 Hz. Consequently, 70 Hz was selected for further investigations. Finally, the step potential was evaluated at a whole examined range of step potentials. The PA signals increased with the increase of the ΔE_s value, but obtained voltammograms were angularly shaped above 7 mV, thus in further studies, a step potential of 7 mV was applied. In the case of GrPE, the effect of amplitude was as follows: the PA peak currents increased from 10 mV to 70 mV, and then a non-linear growth of the peak (plateau) was observed. Therefore, an ΔE value of 70 mV was adopted in further studies. The observed PA signals increased with the increasing of f and ΔE_s values at a whole range of frequency and step potential variations. However, a significant deterioration of the peak shape was observed above 30 Hz and 7 mV, thus those values were chosen for subsequent investigations. To summarize, the optimized SW parameters, which were selected with respect to the height and shape of PA signals, were as follows: $\Delta E = 40$ mV, $f = 70$ Hz, $\Delta E_s = 7$ mV and $\Delta E = 70$ mV, $f = 30$ Hz, $\Delta E_s = 7$ mV, for ClPE and GrPE, respectively.

Next, the calibration curve was constructed under optimized SWV parameters. The peak current of PA was found to increase linearly with concentration from 6.0×10^{-7} to 3.0×10^{-5} mol L^{-1} for ClPE (Figure 5A) and from 2.0×10^{-6} to 8.0×10^{-5} mol L^{-1} for GrPE (Figure 5B).

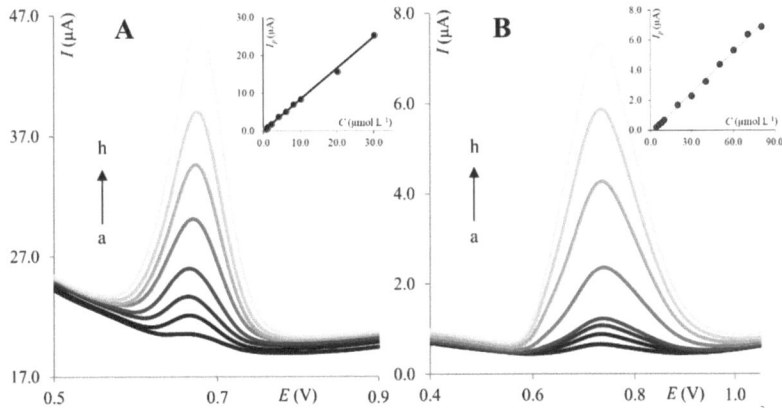

Figure 5. Voltammograms of PA recorded on the ClPE (**A**) and GrPE (**B**). (**A**): (a) 6.0×10^{-7} mol L^{-1}, (b) 1.0×10^{-6} mol L^{-1}, (c) 2.0×10^{-6} mol L^{-1}, (d) 4.0×10^{-6} mol L^{-1}, (e) 8.0×10^{-6} mol L^{-1}, (f) 1.0×10^{-5} mol L^{-1}, (g) 2.0×10^{-5} mol L^{-1}, (h) 3.0×10^{-5} mol L^{-1}; (**B**): (a) 4.0×10^{-6} mol L^{-1}, (b) 6.0×10^{-6} mol L^{-1}, (c) 8.0×10^{-6} mol L^{-1}, (d) 1.0×10^{-5} mol L^{-1}, (e) 2.0×10^{-5} mol L^{-1}, (f) 4.0×10^{-5} mol L^{-1}, (g) 6.0×10^{-5} mol L^{-1}, (h) 8.0×10^{-5} mol L^{-1}. Insets: Corresponding calibration curves.

The linear regression equations can be expressed as:

$$\text{for ClPE: } I_p\ (\mu A) = 0.83 \times C_{PA} + 1.56 \times 10^{-7}, \qquad (1)$$

$$\text{for GrPE: } I_p\ (\mu A) = 0.092 \times C_{PA} + 2.18 \times 10^{-7}. \qquad (2)$$

The limit of detection (LOD) and limit of quantification (LOQ) were calculated from the calibration curves as $k \cdot SD/b$, where: $k = 3$ for LOD, $k = 10$ for LOQ, SD is the standard deviation of the intercept, b is the slope of the calibration curve. The regression parameters for the calibration curves are listed in Table 1. To characterize the reproducibility and stability of the procedure, inter- and intra-day measurements were performed in a solution containing 5.0×10^{-6} mol L^{-1} of paracetamol on both working electrodes. The relative standard deviation (RSD) of the voltammetric responses for five repeated detections on the ClPE electrode was 3.0%, whereas, on the GrPE, it was 4.9%. The intra-day reproducibility of the ClPE and GrPE toward PA detection was investigated at the same molar concentration as paracetamol. The relative standard deviation in the peak current for 10 successive assays was 7.8% and 5.2%, respectively.

Table 1. Regression parameters for determination of PA on ClPE and GrPE, $n = 3$.

Electrode	Clay Paste Electrode	Graphene Paste Electrode
Linear range (mol L^{-1})	6.0×10^{-7}–3.0×10^{-5}	2.0×10^{-6}–8.0×10^{-5}
Correlation coefficient R^2	0.998	0.997
LOD (mol L^{-1})	1.4×10^{-7}	3.7×10^{-7}
LOQ (mol L^{-1})	4.7×10^{-7}	1.2×10^{-6}

Although the linear range length is comparable for both electrodes, the linearity observed for ClPE is shifted towards lower concentrations. Therefore, ClPE is a more sensitive sensor towards PA determination. Developed methods were successfully applied for the determination of PA in pharmaceutical formulations. Pharmaceutical formulations containing paracetamol (Paracetamol LG and Paracetamol Polfa) were purchased in a local pharmacy. The PA determination was performed by square wave voltammetry using the standard addition method. As presented in Table 2, no significant differences were observed between the values found by the SWV method and those declared by the producer. However, it is worth noting that results obtained on clay paste electrodes are characterized by a much smaller scatter.

Table 2. Determination of PA in commercial formulations, $n = 3$.

	Clay Paste Electrode	
	Paracetamol LG	Paracetamol Polfa
Content given (mg)	500.0	500.0
Content found (mg)	480.8 ± 18.0	476.1 ± 23.8
Recovery (%)	96.2	95.2
	Graphene Paste Electrode	
	Paracetamol LG	Paracetamol Polfa
Content given (mg)	500.0	500.0
Content found (mg)	481.0 ± 47.5	524.6 ± 42.2
Recovery (%)	96.2	104.9

3. Materials and Methods

3.1. Apparatus

The voltammetric experiments were performed using an EmStat3 potentiostat (PalmSens, Houten, The Netherlands) with an M164 electrode stand (mtm-Anko, Krakow, Poland). All measurements were carried out with a classical three-electrode system and a glass cell of 10 mL volume. A platinum wire and Ag/AgCl (3 mol L^{-1} KCl) were used as the auxiliary and reference electrodes, respectively. Clay paste and graphene paste electrodes were used as the working electrodes. The pH measurements were done using a CP-315 M pH-meter (Elmetron, Zabrze, Poland) with a combined glass electrode. Water was demineralized by means of PURALAB UHQ (made by Elga LabWater, High Wycombe, UK). For microscopic characterization, clay paste and graphene paste were spread onto SEM stubs covered with carbon conductive adhesive tape. SEM images were recorded by a field emission scanning microscope FEI NovaNano SEM 450 using a conventional Everhar–Thornley SE detector (ETD) for 1000× magnification and a thorough lens detector (TLD) in immersion mode for 10,000× magnification. An energy-dispersive X-ray spectroscopy (EDX) was carried out with EDAX TEAM equipped with an EDS Octane Pro detector. Spectrophotometric measurements were made using a Cary 100 Bio UV-Vis spectrophotometer (Agilent). The elemental composition of graphene was analyzed with a Vario MICRO cube: elemental analyzer. The elemental composition of clay powder was examined with the WDXRF spectrometer Panalytical AxiosmAX (lamp Rh-SST–mAX, 4 kW).

3.2. Solutions and Materials

All chemicals used in the experiments were of analytical grade and used without further purification. Paracetamol, ferricyanide and all chemicals used for buffers preparation were from Sigma Aldrich (Darmstadt, Germany). Materials used for paste preparation were purchased from Graphene Supermarket (graphite and graphene nanopowder) and Green Club Pharmacy (raw Australian red clay). All water solutions were prepared using distilled and deionized water. Graphene nanopowder was analyzed by combustion analysis (carbon content >99.7%) and UV-VIS spectrometry where one single absorption band at 270 nm was observed (this peak is characteristic for graphene materials and corresponds to the $\pi \rightarrow \pi^*$ transition of the C–C bond of the hexagonal carbon ring). The clay elemental composition was tested with a WDXRF spectrometer (page 6 in Supplementary Material).

3.3. Preparation of Working Electrodes

The body of the carbon paste electrode consisted of a Teflon rod (outer diameter of 12 mm) with a horizontal channel (diameter of 4 mm) for the carbon paste filling and metal contact. The paste was prepared by thoroughly (t = 20 min.) hand-mixing 500.0 mg of clay or graphene with 500.0 mg of carbon powder and 0.3 mL of paraffin oil. Before each experiment, the surface of the electrode was refreshed by squeezing out a small portion of paste and polishing it with wet filter paper until a smooth surface was obtained.

3.4. Voltammetric Procedure

All voltammetric measurements were carried out at ambient temperature. The general procedure used to obtain square wave (SW) or cyclic (CV) voltammograms was as follows: 10 mL of a supporting electrolyte was transferred to the electrochemical cell. After recording an initial blank, the required volumes of the analyte were added using a micropipette. Then, a sample voltammogram was recorded. For SWV, optimized parameters (amplitude (ΔE), frequency (f), and step potential (ΔE_s)) were used.

3.5. Analysis of Pharmaceutical Formulations

Commercial tablets of PA (Paracetamol Laboratorium Galenowe and Paracetamol Polfa) were obtained from a local pharmacy (Lodz, Poland). Each tablet contained 500 mg of paracetamol. The pharmaceuticals were prepared by the following procedure. The tablets were accurately weighed and carefully grounded in a mortar. Then, the appropriate amount of the powder was placed in a volumetric flask and filled to volume with distilled and deionized water.

4. Conclusions

This paper presents an electroanalytical comparison between the clay paste electrode and the graphene paste electrode. This comparison was made on the basis of a paracetamol determination. For both working electrodes, the supporting electrolyte composition and SW parameters were optimized. In optimal conditions, calibration curves were estimated. Based on the obtained results, it can be concluded that, in general, ClPE and GrPE exhibit similar analytical performance, but clay paste electrodes exhibit a higher sensitivity towards the PA determination, expressed in LOD and LOQ values. Using developed methods, the determination of paracetamol in pharmaceutical formulations was possible with very good recovery on ClPE, as well as on GrPE, however a much smaller data scatter was observed on clay paste electrode. Answering the question "do we really need expensive nanomaterials?" it has to be stated that in comparison to graphene paste electrodes, clay paste electrodes exhibited similar electroactive area and surface morphology, and as mentioned above, improved analytical performance toward paracetamol detection. Moreover, clay paste is a hundred times cheaper than graphene paste. In conclusion, in the authors' opinion, graphene is undoubtedly an excellent and very promising material but we scientists should always remain open-minded. As shown in this paper, the most expensive and popular materials do not guarantee the best results. Sometimes, ordinary materials serve with a comparable or even higher performance.

Supplementary Materials: The following supporting information can be downloaded at: https://www.mdpi.com/article/10.3390/molecules27072037/s1, EDX analysis of clay paste—Analysis no.1; EDX analysis of clay paste—Analysis no.2; EDX analysis of graphene paste; XRF analysis of clay powder.

Author Contributions: Conceptualization, S.S.; data curation, D.G., R.M. and S.S.; formal analysis, E.S., K.K., R.M. and S.S.; funding acquisition, S.S.; investigation, E.S., K.S-S., D.G., K.K. and S.S.; methodology, S.S.; project administration, S.S.; resources, D.G. and S.S.; supervision, S.S.; validation, E.S., K.K. and S.S.; visualization, K.K. and S.S.; writing—original draft, E.S., D.G. and S.S.; writing—review and editing, K.K. and S.S. All authors have read and agreed to the published version of the manuscript.

Funding: This research received funding from the University of Lodz (project number B2211100000047.01). For the purpose of Open Access, the author has applied a CC-BY public copyright license to any Author Accepted Manuscript (AAM) version arising from this submission.

Data Availability Statement: The data presented in this study are available on request from the corresponding author.

Conflicts of Interest: The authors declare no conflict of interest.

Sample Availability: Not available.

References

1. Urbaniczky, C.; Lundström, K. Voltammetric studies on carbon paste electrodes. The influence of paste composition on electrode capacity and kinetics. *J. Electroanal. Chem.* **1984**, *176*, 169–182. [CrossRef]
2. Kalcher, K. Chemically modified carbon paste electrodes in voltammetric analysis. *Electroanalysis* **1990**, *2*, 419–433. [CrossRef]
3. Pauliukaite, R.; Metelka, R.; Švancara, I.; Królicka, A.; Bobrowski, A.; Vytřas, K.; Norkus, E.; Kalcher, K. Carbon paste electrodes modified with Bi_2O_3 as sensors for the determination of Cd and Pb. *Anal. Bioanal. Chem.* **2002**, *374*, 1155–1158. [CrossRef]
4. Švancara, I.; Walcarius, A.; Kalcher, K.; Vytřas, K. Carbon paste electrodes in the new millennium. *Cent. Eur. J. Chem.* **2009**, *7*, 598–656. [CrossRef]
5. Vytřas, K.; Švancara, I.; Metelka, R. Carbon paste electrodes in electroanalytical chemistry. *J. Serb. Chem. Soc.* **2009**, *74*, 1021–1033. [CrossRef]
6. Adraoui, I.; El Rhaz, M.; Amine, A.; Idrissi, L.; Curulli, A.; Palleschi, G. Lead determination by anodic stripping voltammetry using a p-phenylenediamine modified carbon paste electrode. *Electroanalysis* **2005**, *17*, 685–693. [CrossRef]
7. Smarzewska, S.; Pokora, J.; Leniart, A.; Festinger, N.; Ciesielski, W. Carbon Paste Electrodes Modified with Graphene Oxides—Comparative Electrochemical Studies of Thioguanine. *Electroanalysis* **2016**, *28*, 1562–1569. [CrossRef]
8. Smarzewska, S.; Ciesielski, W. Application of a Graphene Oxide–Carbon Paste Electrode for the Determination of Lead in Rainbow Trout from Central Europe. *Food Anal. Methods* **2015**, *8*, 635–642. [CrossRef]
9. Chetankumar, K.; Kumara Swamy, B.E.; Sharma, S.C. Safranin amplified carbon paste electrode sensor for analysis of paracetamol and epinephrine in presence of folic acid and ascorbic acid. *Microchem. J.* **2021**, *160*, 105729. [CrossRef]
10. Winiarski, J.P.; Tavares, B.F.; de Fátima Ulbrich, K.; de Campos, C.E.M.; Souza, A.A.U.; Souza, S.M.A.G.U.; Jost, C.L. Development of a multianalyte electrochemical sensor for depression biomarkers based on a waste of the steel industry for a sustainable and one-step electrode modification. *Microchem. J.* **2022**, *175*, 107141. [CrossRef]
11. Islam, M.M.; Arifuzzaman, M.; Rushd, S.; Islam, M.K.; Rahman, M.M. Electrochemical sensor based on poly (aspartic acid) modified carbon paste electrode for paracetamol determination. *Int. J. Electrochem. Sci.* **2022**, *17*. [CrossRef]
12. De Fatima Ulbrich, K.; Winiarski, J.P.; Jost, C.L.; de Campos, C.E.M. Green and facile solvent-free synthesis of $NiTe_2$ nanocrystalline material applied to voltammetric determination of antioxidant morin. *Mater. Today Commun.* **2020**, *25*, 101251. [CrossRef]

13. Hassanein, A.; Salahuddin, N.; Matsuda, A.; Kawamura, G.; Elfiky, M. Fabrication of biosensor based on Chitosan-ZnO/Polypyrrole nanocomposite modified carbon paste electrode for electroanalytical application. *Mater. Sci. Eng. C* **2017**, *80*, 494–501. [CrossRef]
14. Tanuja, S.B.; Kumara Swamy, B.E.; Pai, K.V. Electrochemical determination of paracetamol in presence of folic acid at nevirapine modified carbon paste electrode: A cyclic voltammetric study. *J. Electroanal. Chem.* **2017**, *798*, 17–23. [CrossRef]
15. Özcan, A.; Topçuoğulları, D. Voltammetric determination of 17-B-estradiol by cysteamine self-assembled gold nanoparticle modified fumed silica decorated graphene nanoribbon nanocomposite. *Sens. Actuators B Chem.* **2017**, *250*, 85–90. [CrossRef]
16. Priya, T.; Dhanalakshmi, N.; Thinakaran, N. Electrochemical behavior of Pb (II) on a heparin modified chitosan/graphene nanocomposite film coated glassy carbon electrode and its sensitive detection. *Int. J. Biol. Macromol.* **2017**, *104*, 672–680. [CrossRef]
17. Smarzewska, S.; Metelka, R.; Festinger, N.; Guziejewski, D.; Ciesielski, W. Comparative Study on Electroanalysis of Fenthion Using Silver Amalgam Film Electrode and Glassy Carbon Electrode Modified with Reduced Graphene Oxide. *Electroanalysis* **2017**, *29*, 1154–1160. [CrossRef]
18. Smarzewska, S.; Guziejewski, D.; Leniart, A.; Ciesielski, W. Nanomaterials vs Amalgam in Electroanalysis: Comparative Electrochemical Studies of Lamotrigine. *J. Electrochem. Soc.* **2017**, *164*, B321–B329. [CrossRef]
19. Zarei, K.; Khodadadi, A. Very sensitive electrochemical determination of diuron on glassy carbon electrode modified with reduced graphene oxide–gold nanoparticle–Nafion composite film. *Ecotoxicol. Environ. Saf.* **2017**, *144*, 171–177. [CrossRef]
20. Novoselov, K.S.; Geim, A.K.; Morozov, S.V.; Jiang, D.; Zhang, Y.; Dubonos, S.V.; Grigorieva, I.V.; Firsov, A.A. Electric Field Effect in Atomically Thin Carbon Films. *Science* **2004**, *306*, 666–669. [CrossRef]
21. Katsnelson, M.I. Graphene: Carbon in two dimensions. *Mater. Today* **2007**, *10*, 20–27. [CrossRef]
22. Bolotin, K.I.; Sikes, K.J.; Jiang, Z.; Klima, M.; Fudenberg, G.; Hone, J.; Kim, P.; Stormer, H.L. Ultrahigh electron mobility in suspended graphene. *Solid State Commun.* **2008**, *146*, 351–355. [CrossRef]
23. Allen, M.J.; Tung, V.C.; Kaner, R.B. Honeycomb carbon: A review of graphene. *Chem. Rev.* **2010**, *110*, 132–145. [CrossRef] [PubMed]
24. Shao, Y.; Wang, J.; Wu, H.; Liu, J.; Aksay, I.A.; Lin, Y. Graphene based electrochemical sensors and biosensors: A review. *Electroanalysis* **2010**, *22*, 1027–1036. [CrossRef]
25. Novoselov, K.S.; Fal'Ko, V.I.; Colombo, L.; Gellert, P.R.; Schwab, M.G.; Kim, K. A roadmap for graphene. *Nature* **2012**, *490*, 192–200. [CrossRef]
26. Parvin, M.H. Graphene paste electrode for detection of chlorpromazine. *Electrochem. Commun.* **2011**, *13*, 366–369. [CrossRef]
27. Shakibaian, V.; Parvin, M.H. Determination of acetazolamide by graphene paste electrode. *J. Electroanal. Chem.* **2012**, *683*, 119–124. [CrossRef]
28. Gasnier, A.; Pedano, M.L.; Rubianes, M.D.; Rivas, G.A. Graphene paste electrode: Electrochemical behavior and analytical applications for the quantification of NADH. *Sens. Actuators B Chem.* **2013**, *176*, 921–926. [CrossRef]
29. Pinnavaia, T.J. Intercalated clay catalysts. *Science* **1983**, *220*, 365–371. [CrossRef]
30. El Kasmi, S.; Lahrich, S.; Farahi, A.; Zriouil, M.; Ahmamou, M.; Bakasse, M.; El Mhammedi, M.A. Electrochemical determination of paraquat in potato, lemon, orange and natural water samples using sensitive-rich clay carbon electrode. *J. Taiwan Inst. Chem. Eng.* **2016**, *58*, 165–172. [CrossRef]
31. Manisankar, P.; Selvanathan, G.; Vedhi, C. Utilization of sodium montmorillonite clay-modified electrode for the determination of isoproturon and carbendazim in soil and water samples. *Appl. Clay Sci.* **2005**, *29*, 249–257. [CrossRef]
32. El Mhammedi, M.A.; Bakasse, M.; Najih, R.; Chtaini, A. A carbon paste electrode modified with kaolin for the detection of diquat. *Appl. Clay Sci.* **2009**, *43*, 130–134. [CrossRef]
33. Abbaci, A.; Azzouz, N.; Bouznit, Y. A new copper doped montmorillonite modified carbon paste electrode for propineb detection. *Appl. Clay Sci.* **2014**, *90*, 130–134. [CrossRef]
34. Loudiki, A.; Hammani, H.; Boumya, W.; Lahrich, S.; Farahi, A.; Achak, M.; Bakasse, M.; El Mhammedi, M.A. Electrocatalytical effect of montmorillonite to oxidizing ibuprofen: Analytical application in river water and commercial tablets. *Appl. Clay Sci.* **2016**, *123*, 99–108. [CrossRef]
35. El-Desoky, H.S.; Ismail, I.M.; Ghoneim, M.M. Stripping voltammetry method for determination of manganese as complex with oxine at the carbon paste electrode with and without modification with montmorillonite clay. *J. Solid State Electrochem.* **2013**, *17*, 3153–3167. [CrossRef]
36. Falaras, P.; Lezou, F. Electrochemical behavior of acid activated montmorillonite modified electrodes. *J. Electroanal. Chem.* **1998**, *455*, 169–179. [CrossRef]
37. Navrátilová, Z.; Kula, P. Cation and anion exchange on clay modified electrodes. *J. Solid State Electrochem.* **2000**, *4*, 342–347. [CrossRef]
38. Navrátilová, Z.; Mucha, M. Organo-montmorillonites as carbon paste electrode modifiers. *J. Solid State Electrochem.* **2015**, *19*, 2013–2022. [CrossRef]
39. Niedziałkowski, P.; Cebula, Z.; Malinowska, N.; Białobrzeska, W.; Sobaszek, M.; Ficek, M.; Bogdanowicz, R.; Anand, J.S.; Ossowski, T. Comparison of the paracetamol electrochemical determination using boron-doped diamond electrode and boron-doped carbon nanowalls. *Biosens. Bioelectron.* **2019**, *126*, 308–314. [CrossRef]
40. Kang, X.; Wang, J.; Wu, H.; Liu, J.; Aksay, I.A.; Lin, Y. A graphene-based electrochemical sensor for sensitive detection of paracetamol. *Talanta* **2010**, *81*, 754–759. [CrossRef]

41. Silva, T.A.; Zanin, H.; Corat, E.J.; Fatibello-Filho, O. Simultaneous Voltammetric Determination of Paracetamol, Codeine and Caffeine on Diamond-like Carbon Porous Electrodes. *Electroanalysis* **2017**, *29*, 907–916. [CrossRef]
42. Nematollahi, D.; Shayani-Jam, H.; Alimoradi, M.; Niroomand, S. Electrochemical oxidation of acetaminophen in aqueous solutions: Kinetic evaluation of hydrolysis, hydroxylation and dimerization processes. *Electrochim. Acta* **2009**, *54*, 7407–7415. [CrossRef]
43. Tyszczuk-Rotko, K.; Bęczkowska, I.; Wójciak-Kosior, M.; Sowa, I. Simultaneous voltammetric determination of paracetamol and ascorbic acid using a boron-doped diamond electrode modified with Nafion and lead films. *Talanta* **2014**, *129*, 384–391. [CrossRef]
44. Karikalan, N.; Karthik, R.; Chen, S.M.; Velmurugan, M.; Karuppiah, C. Electrochemical properties of the acetaminophen on the screen printed carbon electrode towards the high performance practical sensor applications. *J. Colloid Interface Sci.* **2016**, *483*, 109–117. [CrossRef]

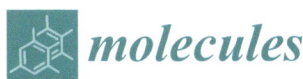

Article

Compared EC-AFM Analysis of Laser-Induced Graphene and Graphite Electrodes in Sulfuric Acid Electrolyte

Claudia Filoni [1,*], Bahram Shirzadi [1], Marco Menegazzo [1], Eugenio Martinelli [2], Corrado Di Natale [2], Andrea Li Bassi [3], Luca Magagnin [4], Lamberto Duò [1] and Gianlorenzo Bussetti [1]

[1] Department of Physics, Politecnico di Milano, p.za Leonardo da Vinci 32, I-20133 Milan, Italy; bahram.shirzadi@mail.polimi.it (B.S.); marco.menegazzo@mail.polimi.it (M.M.); lamberto.duo@polimi.it (L.D.); gianlorenzo.bussetti@polimi.it (G.B.)
[2] Department of Electronic Engineering, University of Rome Tor Vergata, v. del Politecnico, I-00133 Rome, Italy; martinelli@ing.uniroma2.it (E.M.); dinatale@eln.uniroma2.it (C.D.N.)
[3] Department of Energy, Politecnico di Milano, v. Ponzio 34/3, I-20133 Milan, Italy; andrea.libassi@polimi.it
[4] Department of Chemistry, Materials and Chemical Engineering "Giulio Natta", Politecnico di Milano, v. Mancinelli 7, I-20131 Milan, Italy; luca.magagnin@polimi.it
* Correspondence: claudia.filoni@polimi.it; Tel.: +39-0223-996-181

Abstract: Flexible and economic sensor devices are the focus of increasing interest for their potential and wide applications in medicine, food analysis, pollution, water quality, etc. In these areas, the possibility of using stable, reproducible, and pocket devices can simplify the acquisition of data. Among recent prototypes, sensors based on laser-induced graphene (LIGE) on Kapton represent a feasible choice. In particular, LIGE devices are also exploited as electrodes for sensing in liquids. Despite a characterization with electrochemical (EC) methods in the literature, a closer comparison with traditional graphite electrodes is still missing. In this study, we combine atomic force microscopy with an EC cell (EC-AFM) to study, in situ, electrode oxidation reactions when LIGE or other graphite samples are used as anodes inside an acid electrolyte. This investigation shows the quality and performance of the LIGE electrode with respect to other samples. Finally, an ex situ Raman spectroscopy analysis allows a detailed chemical analysis of the employed electrodes.

Keywords: laser-induced graphene; Kapton; graphite foils; graphite; EC-AFM; Raman spectroscopy

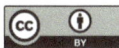

1. Introduction

The development of portable, low-cost, and effective devices has been increasing over the past few decades [1,2]. Among the different applications, electrochemical biosensors, e.g., neurotransmitters or non-enzymatic glucose sensors, have received large interest due to their high sensitivity and selectivity, easy miniaturization, efficiency, and ease of use [3–11]. The commercial versions of combined electrode systems are typically based on carbon or carbon-based materials (e.g., glassy carbon, carbon nanosheet electrodes, etc.) that have good electrical properties and are very handy materials [12–14]. These systems are usually modified with metal nanoparticles, carbon nanotubes, or graphene in order to reach the best parameters, such as faster electron transfer kinetics, low residual current, and excellent thermal conductivity [15,16]. Supercapacitors have a long history that has seen the employment of various carbon-electrode-based solid-state devices up to the development of their miniaturized form, known as micro-supercapacitors [17]. The rapid growth of portable electronics, remote control systems, radio-frequency detectors, and micro-electro-mechanical systems has significantly increased the need for device miniaturization [18–20]. Currently, their potential is becoming more evident with respect to a fast charging–discharging rate, a long cycling life, flexibility, and shape diversity, together with their functional convenient size and their lightweight [21,22]. In addition, global climate change calls for the urgent development of carbon-neutral and renewable-energy rechargeable devices, such as batteries, and hybrid technologies, including electric vehicles [23–26].

One of the current trends foresees the exposure of carbonaceous substrates to intense laser beams, which both reduces substrate thickness (down to a multi-layered graphene system) and increases the porous density of the original structure (three-dimensional (3D) porous graphene). In fact, the intense laser beam burns the pristine substrate and removes part of its mass. At the same time, the surface graphitization increases the number of defects, holes, and pores or, generally speaking, the surface's roughness [27–29]. This process acts as one-step, scalable printing to produce carbon-based electrodes patterning on a stretchable and flexible platform [30]. It is widely known how the electric properties of graphene change depending on the stacking of layers [31,32]. Graphene is a one-atom-thick, bi-dimensional (2D) carbon sheet with carbon atoms arranged in a honeycomb lattice. The hexagonally sp^2-bonded carbon atoms arrange to reach very high thermal conductivity ($\approx$5000 Wm^{-1}K^{-1}), mobility ($\approx$10,000 cm^{2}V^{-1}s^{-1}), and surface area (2630 m^{2}g^{-1}). With the aim of forming sensing prototypes, some of the other primary advantages of graphene include a high Young's modulus and high optical transparency in the visible wavelength range [33,34]. Three-dimensional, or multilayered, graphene is a sort of compromise between thick graphite and a single graphene layer that, however, can be exploited for producing portable and flexible energy storage devices. In particular, 3D porous graphene presents better mechanical stability and higher catalytic activity [35]. It is well known from the literature that graphene can be fabricated by a large variety of methods, such as chemical exfoliation of graphite and chemical vapor deposition (CVD). Nevertheless, these production techniques can be quite expensive or can have some disadvantages: CVD needs a high amount of energy, and the mechanical exfoliation process yields a low-quality graphene product with some forms of defects, e.g., microscopic corrugation [36]. Moreover, the carbon-based electrochemical devices available in the market are normally fabricated by lithography, e.g., photolithography, dry etching, or film transfer; all these techniques have a high production cost and require consistent time-consuming procedures [37,38]. To make the best laser-pattern process, it is usually necessary to combine a conductive matrix, e.g., graphene, with suitable flexible material as the substrate, such as polyurethane or polyimide, to form a novel composite [39].

In this regard, in 2014, laser-induced porous 3D graphene was synthesized on polymers by Lin et al. [40]. In this novel one-step process, the porous graphene film was patterned by pointing a CO$_2$ laser onto a commercial polyimide foil in an ambient environment. No baking step nor need of materials, other than polyimide foil, were required [41,42]. Among the different carbon-containing materials, the first material used as a precursor was Kapton, a classic polyimide developed in the 1960s by DuPont. Polyimides ($C_{22}H_{10}O_5N_2$) have been massively produced since 1955; they are lightweight, flexible, resistant to heat and chemicals, and they show natural structural anisotropy due to the preferential orientation of the polymer chains obtained during the manufacturing process. Kapton exhibits excellent physical properties and is exploited as an electrical and thermal insulator in harsh environments [43]. In the photothermal conversion process, lasing causes the propagation of a high degree of lattice vibrations through the precursor material, resulting in localized heating; meanwhile, sp^3 carbon atoms are converted into a sp^2 hybridization and C–N, C–O, C–H, and C=O bonds dissociate [44]. Laser-induced graphene's (LIGE) foam-like morphology has a direct influence on electron transfer kinetics enhancement (increased surface-to-volume ratio): The 3D porosity formed during the laser scribing process contributes to faster electron transfer rates [45,46]. The resulting product (LIGE) shows similar properties as commercial graphene but a higher porosity with respect to pristine graphene, which eases the adsorption of ions, influencing the sensitivity and selectivity of the systems [47].

The aim of this study is to compare the behavior of traditional electrodes, such as graphite electrodes (namely, Highly Oriented Pyrolytic Graphite (HOPG), graphite foil, and glassy carbon) and the innovative LIGE electrode. The electrode behavior was studied when specimens were immersed in a 1 M sulfuric (H_2SO_4) electrolyte in which the main electrochemical characteristics in graphite electrodes are known. In order to achieve this goal, by combining an electrochemical Atomic Force Microscope (EC-AFM) and ex situ Raman spectroscopy measures, we performed a detailed analysis of the employed electrodes in a liquid environment to study the electrode oxidation reaction and compared the obtained results.

2. Results and Discussion

2.1. EC Characterization

In Figure 1, we report the EC analysis of our electrodes when immersed in 1 M H_2SO_4 electrolytes. The panel shows the acquired cyclic-voltammetry (CV), i.e., a voltammogram of the flowing faradaic current (y-axis) when a potential (x-axis) is applied to the sample (working electrode, WE).

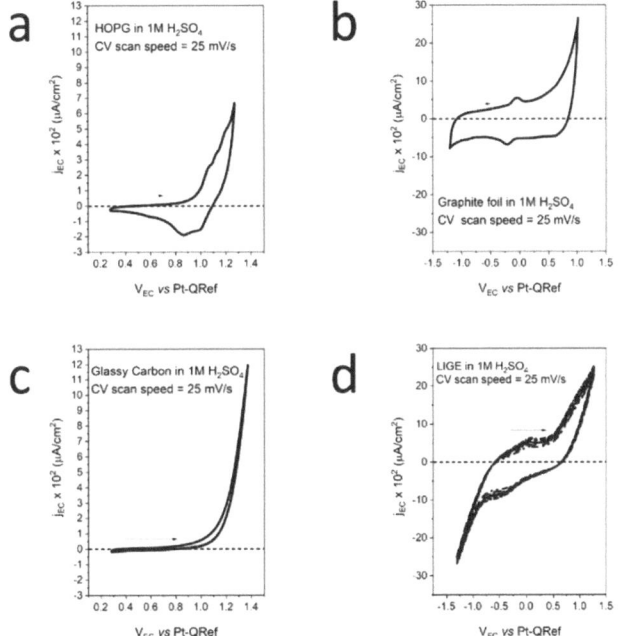

Figure 1. Cyclic-voltammetry acquired on the four exploited electrodes: (**a**) HOPG; (**b**) graphite foil; (**c**) glassy carbon; and (**d**) LIGE.

Figure 1a refers to the well-studied HOPG CV, where shoulders appear as soon as a higher EC potential with respect to the oxygen evolution reaction (OER) is applied to the WE [48]. These features are related to the solvated anion intercalation inside the graphite basal plane. The anodic exchange charge is about 20 μC. During the cathodic potential sweep, a negative current is measured. The latter is traditionally referred to as a partial de-intercalation process that is probably coupled with other processes still under discussion [49]. Anion intercalation changes graphite crystal structures because solvated anions are tidily interposed between the graphite layers (graphite intercalated compound, GIC) [50]. The overall interpretative model was developed by Goss and coworkers at the beginning of the 1990s [51]. According to this model, solvate anions can diffuse inside HOPG-stratified crystal structures through surface defects, such as steps and holes. However, following recent results obtained in our research, acid electrolytes are able to dissolve the graphite basal plane, thus increasing the defects and allowing solvated anions to easily enter the HOPG bulk [48]. When the OER is reached, gases (namely, CO, CO_2, and O_2) also evolve inside the HOPG's bulk. Here, they can produce intense pressures that are able to swell the basal plane and create blisters on the surface. As a consequence of the detailed knowledge of these processes in HOPG electrodes, we propose this electrode dynamic as a model to interpret results collected on other carbonaceous samples [52].

When graphite foil (GF) was employed, the faradaic current intensity was higher, which is reasonably due to the presence of many defects on the GF surface (see Figure 1b). These defects are preferential sites for electrolyte intercalation. In addition, the effective electrode roughness was higher with respect to the HOPG's basal plane and, consequently, the electrode surface was exposed to the electrolyte. We observed that two peaks (oxidation and reduction) were placed between −0.25 V and 0.0 V (vs. PtQRef). The exchanged anodic (cathodic) charge was approximately 180 µC (240 µC), almost an order of magnitude higher with respect to the anodic charge exchanged in the HOPG intercalation process. These voltammetric features, which can be attributed to the presence of oxygen compounds, intruded the GF sample through possible pores [53]. The intense faradaic current during the anodic evolution suggests possible anion intercalation inside the foil. However, the cathodic sweep was significantly different with respect to the HOPG voltammogram. In contrast to the HOPG electrode, gases produced at the OER can be eliminated through the pores and defects present in the GF.

Glassy carbon (GC) was produced from pyrolysis of furfuryl alcohol, phenolic resins, and similar polymers under heating up to 3000 °C. The obtained system was not graphitizable, i.e., it was not possible to convert the GC into crystalline graphite. The sample combined mechanical properties close to those of ceramics and glass. The local structure was made up almost completely of sp^2-bonded carbon atoms. As a consequence of the GC vitreous behavior, the EC performance of this electrode demonstrated faradaic current intensity enhancement due to the OER without any other feature or the presence of a negative (cathodic) current (see Figure 1c). In these conditions, anion intercalation was precluded, and the voltammogram showed an almost superimposable anodic and cathodic sweep. No de-intercalation features were detected at negative faradaic currents, confirming the picture of a very inert electrode.

The LIGE electrode CV is shown in Figure 1d. Interestingly, we observed a partial similarity with the GF CV. In fact, two features, placed between −0.5 V and 0.0 V, appeared in the CV. The anodic (cathodic)-exchanged charge was approximately 390 µC (264 µC), about a factor of 2 higher with respect to the GF. Considering both these similarities and the high surface roughness (a consequence of the Kapton burning process), we speculate that the GF CV interpretation, in terms of a significant presence of oxygen compounds, is also reasonable for the LIGE electrode. The similarity of the LIGE voltammogram with that reported for the GF suggests that, as in the previous case, anion intercalation enhances the faradaic current during the anodic sweep, but the high porosity and defect density allow gases to move out from the buried LIGE layers, without any particular signature in the voltammogram. Finally, we observed that, in Figure 1d, four CVs were reported. Their perfect superposition directly shows the stability of the LIGE electrode during subsequent EC treatments.

2.2. EC-AFM Characterization

In Figure 2, we report the topographic images acquired for HOPG (panels Figure 2a,b), GF (Figure 2c,d), and GC (Figure 2e,f) electrodes. Panels a, c, and e refer to pristine electrodes while the other panels refer to the sample after one CV in sulfuric acid electrolyte (see Figure 1).

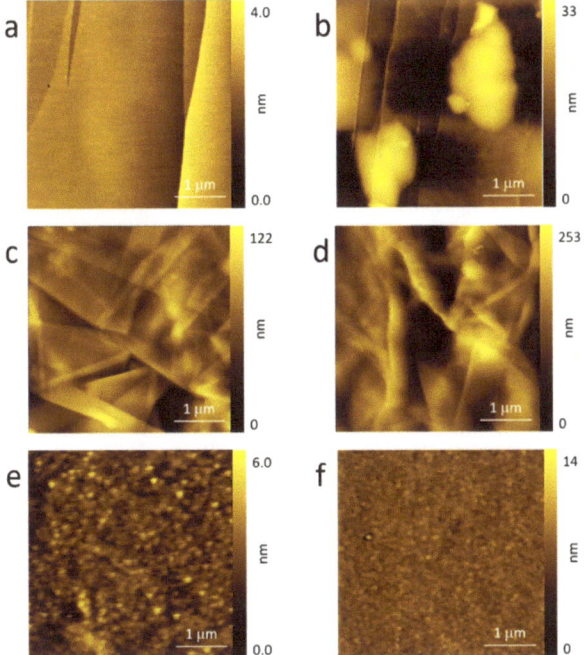

Figure 2. AFM images of the used electrodes before (HOPG (**a**); GF (**c**); GC (**e**)) and after (HOPG (**b**); GF (**d**); GC (**f**)) the EC treatment.

HOPG (see Figure 2a) was characterized by flat terraces and sharp step edges. The situation significantly changed after the intercalation process [50]: Clear blisters (Figure 2b), a consequence of the entrapped gas deformation of the basal plane, were visible close to or on the step edges. The latter were preferential regions of solvated ion intercalation [50,51].

GF is shown in Figure 2c. The surface morphology appeared as the superposition of different thin graphite layers. Many steps, defects, and pores were observed in the image. Consequently, the expected gas evolution during the anodic sweep in acid electrolytes could find more paths for its outflow, as discussed above. This hypothesis is well supported by the AFM image acquired after the CV treatment (see Figure 2d). The roughness undoubtedly increased, probably due to swelling of some GF regions, but blisters (at least, as defined for HOPG) were not clearly visible in the acquired topography. The general behavior recalls a carbonaceous surface after a partial dissolution. This process is indeed observed on HOPG and reported by the authors [48].

The GC electrode was very stable. The surface topography did not show significant changes between the pristine and used electrode (see Figure 2e,f). The former was characterized by relatively small particles and valleys that were randomly distributed as a consequence of the GC industrial production. The electrode's surface, after the EC treatment, appeared more uniform in which particles did not have a clear contrast. This effect was obviously due to the sulfuric acid electrolytes but, when working as an electrode, the GC surface did not show blisters, swelled areas, or holes as a consequence of the carbon dissolution, as already reported by the authors [48,52]. This result is reasonable when considering the mechanical properties of the GC as reported above.

LIGE required a different morphological analysis. In fact, while Kapton can be characterized by AFM, the LIGE electrode presented many difficulties due to the high surface roughness. For this reason and in view of completeness, we decided to compare Kapton morphology (see Figure 3a) with its topography after laser burning (b). In order to avoid very high rough regions, the reported AFM image (Figure 3b) refers to an area where the original Kapton was still partially visible.

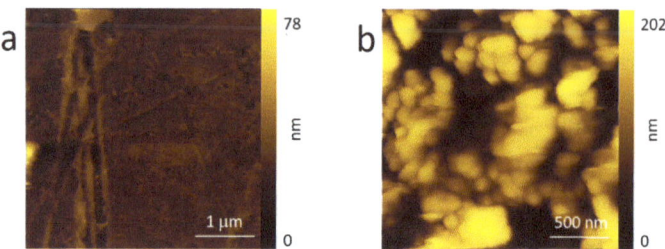

Figure 3. AFM images of the pristine Kapton (**a**) and after laser burning (**b**) acquired in air. See the text for more details.

Kapton morphology (Figure 3a) was basically flat, even if it were possible to observe scratches or bumps that are possible after industrial production. The topography of the partially burnt sample significantly changed: the roughness immediately increased, and AFM images were possible only at reduced areas (2 × 2 µm^2). Here, many roundish objects characterized the surface. The morphology was compatible with processes of polymer laser melting, which can sometimes produce periodic structures [54]. From this result, it is clear that an AFM acquisition of the total burnt Kapton sample was not possible. However, this analysis suggests that the expected increased number of defects and pores precludes any gas encapsulation (blister evolution) during the anodic sweep, which is in close agreement with the GF behavior.

2.3. Raman Spectroscopy Characterization

In Figure 4, we show the Raman spectra of the electrodes before (Figure 4a) and after (Figure 4b) the electrochemical process in 1M H_2SO_4. According to the literature [49,55], the pristine HOPG spectrum, the main reference for Raman spectroscopy evolution as a function of the EC treatment, highlights only one peak (G-peak) at approximately 1581 cm^{-1} (Figure 4a). The presence of only the G-peak is a consequence of a carbon crystal possessing sp^2 C–C bonds.

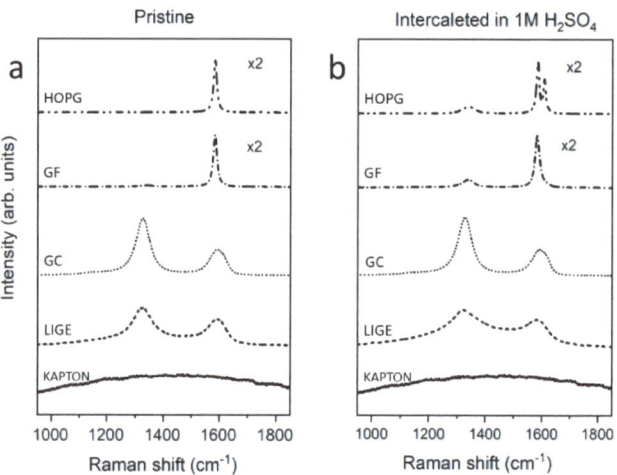

Figure 4. Raman spectra of electrodes in pristine condition (**a**) and after the EC treatment (**b**).

Surprisingly, the pristine GF Raman spectrum is mainly characterized by only the G-peak. Only a smaller feature, placed at approximately 1330 cm^{-1}, appears in the data. The latter, when investigated in other carbon compounds (see below), is labeled as the D-peak, and it is generally related to the presence of structural alterations in the graphitic structure. As a consequence, despite having more steps and defects that can enhance the faradaic current in CV (see above), the GF is characterized by a local structural behavior superimposable to the HOPG structure. Considering that the GF production foresees the mechanical compression of HOPG grains, the GF Raman spectrum reported in Figure 4a is expected.

Conversely, the GC sample is prepared by following a high-temperature process (see above) that significantly enhances the crystal structure. The Raman spectrum is, thus, characterized by a significant D-peak for which its intensity is higher than the G-peak. In addition, the latter feature is also broader with respect to the crystalline HOPG spectrum, in agreement with the GC structural properties.

The Kapton Raman spectrum did not show any signal in the region of interest while, when burned by the laser beam (LIGE), two features appeared in the same spectrum positions of the G-peaks and D-peaks. The close agreement between the GC and LIGE Raman spectra suggests that the burned Kapton is characterized by a disordered graphitic structure for which its D-peak has a higher intensity with respect to the G-peak and the latter has a wider line shape with respect to the crystalline HOPG sample.

The HOPG electrode was analyzed by Raman spectroscopy after EC treatment (see Figure 4b). Following the results reported by the authors in reference [49], the evolution of blisters and the general detriment of graphite basal plane allow the evolution of a D-peak (smaller with respect to the G-peak) and a second feature (G_i) at higher Raman shift (about 1610 cm^{-1}) strictly related to the chemical action of the intercalated acid. The G_i peak is a specific characteristic of the intercalated HOPG electrode and was not observed in any other sample.

The effect of the EC treatment was also clearly visible on the GF sample. While the G-peak seemed to be almost unaltered, the D-peak was more pronounced in the spectrum, suggesting that part of the GF surface underwent a detriment that was also visible in the AFM image (see Figure 2d).

The non-reactive behavior of the GC electrode was proved by the Raman analysis. A fast comparison between Figure 4a,b revealed that the spectra were superimposable. The stability of the GC sample was also confirmed by previous topographic analyses and justifies the acquired CV in Figure 1.

The LIGE electrode showed modified features after the EC treatment. In contrast to the GC electrode, the D-peak of the LIGE sample became broader with respect to the pristine sample, suggesting some changes (chemical and/or physical, as a disorder enhancement) in the burned Kapton region. The signal-to-noise ratio decreased substantially probably due to the fact that the uppermost part of the LIGE was mechanically removed after immersion inside the EC cell.

3. Materials and Methods

Different samples [(25 × 25 × 1) mm^3] have been exploited in this work. Their active surface, when used as electrodes, is 0.2 cm^2 in order to avoid high faradaic current intensities:

(i) The Z-grade highly oriented pyrolytic graphite (HOPG) was acquired from Optigraph and was mechanically exfoliated before each experiment by means of an adhesive tape.

(ii) Graphite foil and glassy carbon samples were provided by Goodfellow. The samples were cleaned in ethanol and deionized water before their employment.

(iii) A Trotec Speedy 100 laser cutter (Trotec Laser Inc., Marchtrenk, Austria) was used for producing porous graphene films using Kapton, a commercial polymer film [40]. Graphene production was a result of the conversion of the sp^3 carbon atoms in the

Kapton into sp^2 carbon atoms by pulsed laser irradiation. Laser cutter parameters are found in reference [56].

The electrolyte was prepared by diluting a H_2SO_4 solution (95–97% w/w, Merck Darmstadt, Germany) to obtain a 1 M concentration. Before filling the EC cell, the electrolyte was de-aerated by bubbling pure Ar in a Squibb separator funnel for some hours.

The homemade EC cell was made in Teflon and was placed above the sample, which was the working electrode (WE) of our system. In order to avoid solvent leakages, a Viton O-ring was interposed between the cell and the sample.

In addition to the WE, two Pt wires were inserted inside the EC cell: one wire, which turns around the overall cell, played the role of the counter electrode (CE) while the head of the second wire was used as a reference electrode (RE). More precisely, the latter was a quasi-reference because it did not exploit a redox couple. Nonetheless, the platinum quasi-reference (Pt-QRef) ensures good stability (within a few mV) when immersed in acid electrolytes, and a stable EC potential shift (+740 mV) with respect to the standard hydrogen electrode [50].

AFM images were collected by a commercial Keysight 5500 model. According to the sample's surface roughness and/or solid electrolyte interface evolution, the selected acquisition mode was contact or non-contact. In the former case, a constant laser deflection was used during the tip approach while, for the latter, a resonance frequency of about 130 kHz was found.

Raman spectroscopy was conducted ex situ before and after EC analysis. The samples were placed under a Nikon Eclipse Ni microscope of an NT-MDT Confotec NR500 confocal Raman spectrometer. A 632.8 nm laser (of approximately 23 mW) was exploited as an excitation source. The light was focused by a 100× objective directly on the sample. Here, the measured laser power was 5 mW because of multiple reflections of the laser beam on mirrors. Moreover, we carefully checked that no heating or surface damages to the samples were induced by the laser. The spectra were recorded with multiple scans, integrating the signal for an overall time that changed for each sample in order to optimize the spectrum.

4. Conclusions

Laser-induced graphene film on Kapton substrate represents an innovative, economic, and technologically important procedure for obtaining conductive circuits or electrodes on flexible materials (such as Kapton foils). In the Introduction of this study, we summarized the wide literature produced in recent years where these innovative devices have been successfully employed. Kapton foils have also found applications as electrodes (LIGE), and their EC characterization has been reported in the literature. Despite this fact, a comparative analysis of the LIGE performances with respect to other carbon-based electrodes is still missing. In this study, we reported an EC, microscopic (namely AFM), and spectroscopic (Raman technique) investigation of four electrodes (HOPG, graphite foil, glassy carbon, and LIGE) when immersed and used in a sulfuric electrolyte. HOPG is considered a model system because the intercalation processes observed on the electrode surface, when the oxygen evolution reaction is reached, are well reported in the literature and by the authors. Glassy carbon is a widely used electrode by comparison, due to its mechanical and chemical stability in corrosive environments. On the other hand, graphite foil has been exploited as a technological electrode in modern Li-batteries since its production is quite economic but, more importantly, it is a flexible electrode. LIGE was then compared to the above-mentioned electrodes to test its characteristics in analogous conditions.

The result of our study, summarized in Table 1, proves the stability of LIGE in acid electrolytes, a similarity in CV analysis (in particular with the graphite foil), and Raman features that recall what was observed on the glassy carbon electrode. In summary, LIGE collects the important and significant behaviors of the other carbonaceous electrodes and thus represents a concrete alternative in many innovative applications.

Table 1. Comparison table between HOPG, GF, GC and LIGE features.

Electrode	Cyclic-Voltammetry	AFM	Raman
HOPG	intercalation and de-intercalation features	blister evolution after anion intercalation	evolution of D and G_i peaks after the EC treatment
GF	oxidation and reduction peaks	surface swelling and pores	only D peak appearance after the CV
GC	no specific features	no significant changes related to the EC treatment	stable D and G peaks before and after the EC treatment
LIGE	oxidation and reduction peaks	too rough surface	stable D and G peaks before and after the EC treatment

Author Contributions: Conceptualization, C.F. and G.B.; methodology, B.S., C.F. and M.M.; validation, L.M. and E.M.; formal analysis, C.F.; investigation, B.S., C.F. and M.M.; resources, E.M. and C.D.N.; data curation, B.S. and C.F.; writing—original draft preparation, C.F., G.B., C.F., A.L.B. and L.D.; writing—review and editing, A.L.B.; supervision, G.B. All authors have read and agreed to the published version of the manuscript.

Funding: This work has been supported by Fondazione Cariplo, grant n° 2020-0977.

Acknowledgments: This work was carried out at Soli-Nano Σ lab (Politecnico di Milano). The authors are grateful to A. Lucotti, E. Gibertini, and M. Leone (Politecnico di Milano) for their useful discussions.

Conflicts of Interest: The authors declare no conflict of interest.

References

1. Simionescu, O.; Pachiu, C.; Ionescu, O.; Dumbrăvescu, N.; Buiu, O.; Popa, R.C.; Avram, A.; Dinescu, G. Nanocrystalline graphite thin layers for low-strain, high-sensitivity piezoresistive sensing. *Rev. Adv. Mater. Sci.* **2020**, *59*, 306–313. [CrossRef]
2. Tehrani, F.; Beltrán-Gastélum, M.; Sheth, K.; Karajic, A.; Yin, L.; Kumar, R.; Soto, F.; Kim, J.; Wang, J.; Barton, S.; et al. Laser-Induced Graphene Composites for Printed, Stretchable, and Wearable Electronics. *Adv. Mater. Technol.* **2019**, *4*, 1900162. [CrossRef]
3. Cardoso, A.R.; Marquesa, A.C.; Santos, L.; Carvalho, A.F.; Costad, F.M.; Martins, R.; Sales, M.G.F.; Fortunato, E. Molecularly-imprinted chloramphenicol sensor with laser-induced graphene electrodes. *Biosens. Bioelectron.* **2019**, *124–125*, 167–175. [CrossRef]
4. Zhu, J.; Liu, S.; Hu, Z.; Zhang, X.; Yi, N.; Tang, K.; Dexheimer, M.G.; Lian, X.; Wang, Q.; Yang, J.; et al. Laser-induced graphene non-enzymatic glucose sensors for on-body measurements. *Biosens. Bioelectron.* **2021**, *193*, 113606. [CrossRef]
5. Bauer, M.; Wunderlich, L.; Weinzierl, F.; Lei, Y.; Duerkop, A.; Alshareef, H.N.; Baeumner, A.J. Electrochemical multi-analyte point-of-care perspiration sensors using on-chip three-dimensional graphene electrodes. *Anal. Bioanal. Chem.* **2021**, *413*, 763–777. [CrossRef] [PubMed]
6. Santos, N.F.; Pereira, S.O.; Moreira, A.; Girão, A.V.; Carvalho, A.F.; Fernandes, A.J.S.; Costa, F.M. IR and UV Laser-Induced Graphene: Application as Dopamine Electrochemical Sensors. *Adv. Mater. Technol.* **2021**, *6*, 2100007. [CrossRef]
7. Hossain, M.F.; McCracken, S.; Slaughter, G. Electrochemical laser induced graphene-based oxygen sensor. *J. Electroanal. Chem.* **2021**, *899*, 115690. [CrossRef]
8. Barber, R.; Cameron, S.; Devine, A.; McCombe, A.; Pourshahidi, L.K.; Cundell, J.; Roy, S.; Mathur, A.; Casimero, C.; Papakonstantinou, P.; et al. Laser induced graphene sensors for assessing pH: Application to wound management. *Electrochem. Commun.* **2021**, *123*, 106914. [CrossRef]
9. Wan, Z.; Umer, M.; Lobino, M.; Thiel, D.; Nguyen, N.; Trinchi, A.; Shiddiky, M.J.A.; Gao, Y.; Li, Q. Laser induced self-N-doped porous graphene as an electrochemical biosensor for femtomolar miRNA detection. *Carbon* **2020**, *163*, 385–394. [CrossRef]
10. Chang, Z.; Zhu, B.; Liu, J.; Zhu, X.; Xu, M.; Travas-Sejdic, J. Electrochemical aptasensor for 17β-estradiol using disposable laser scribed graphene electrodes. *Biosens. Bioelectron.* **2021**, *185*, 113247. [CrossRef]
11. Jayapiriya, U.S.; Rewatkar, P.; Goel, S. Miniaturized polymeric enzymatic biofuel cell with integrated microfluidic device and enhanced laser ablated bioelectrodes. *Int. J. Hydrogen Energy* **2021**, *46*, 3183–3192.
12. Rewatkar, P.; Kothuru, A.; Goel, S. PDMS-Based microfluidic glucose biofuel cell integrated with optimized laser-induced flexible graphene bioelectrodes. *IEEE Trans. Electron Devices* **2020**, *67*, 1832–1838. [CrossRef]
13. Cameron, S.; Barber, R.; Scott, C.; Casimero, C.; Hegarty, C.; Loughlin, L.O.; Pourshahidi, K.; Papakonstantinou, P.; Roy, S.; Davis, J.; et al. Laser Scribed Polyimide as a Platform for Monitoring pH within Smart Bandages. In Proceedings of the 7th International Conference on Signal Processing and Integrated Networks (SPIN), Noida, India, 27–28 February 2020.

14. Kulyk, B.; Carvalho, A.F.; Santos, N.; Fernandes, A.J.; Costa, F.M. A short review on carbon-based nanomaterials and their hybrids. *Bol. Grupo Esp. Carbón* **2019**, *54*, 44–54.
15. Xu, G.; Jarjes, Z.A.; Desprez, V.; Kilmartin, P.A.; Travas-Sejdic, J. Sensitive, selective, disposable electrochemical dopamine sensor based on PEDOT-modified laser scribed graphene. *Biosens. Bioelectron.* **2018**, *107*, 184–191. [CrossRef] [PubMed]
16. Brahem, A.; Bouhamed, A.; Al-Hamry, A.; Ali, M.B.; Kanoun, O. Investigation of Hybrid Epoxy Composite Electrodes for Electrochemical Applications. In Proceedings of the 18th International Multi-Conference on Systems, Signals and Devices, Monastir, Tunisia, 22–25 March 2021.
17. Zaccagnini, P.; di Giovanni, D.; Gomez, M.G.; Passerini, S.; Varzi, A.; Lamberti, A. Flexible and high temperature supercapacitor based on laser-induced graphene electrodes and ionic liquid electrolyte, a de-rated voltage analysis. *Electrochim. Acta* **2020**, *357*, 136838. [CrossRef]
18. Song, B.; Moon, K.; Wong, C. Recent Developments in Design and Fabrication of Graphene-Based Interdigital Micro-Supercapacitors for Miniaturized Energy Storage Devices. *IEEE Trans. Compon. Packag. Manuf. Technol.* **2016**, *6*, 1752–1765. [CrossRef]
19. Santos, N.F.; Rodrigues, J.; Pereira, S.O.; Fernandes, A.J.S.; Monteiro, T.; Costa, F.M. Electrochemical and Photoluminescence Response of Laser-induced Graphene/Electrodeposited ZnO Composites. *Res. Sq.* **2021**. [CrossRef] [PubMed]
20. Duan, Y.; You, G.; Sun, K.; Zhu, Z.; Liao, X.; Lv, L.; Tang, H.; Xu, B.; He, L. The Advances in Wearable Textile-Based Micro Energy Storage Devices: Structuring, Application and Perspective. *Nanoscale Adv.* **2021**, *3*, 6271–6293. [CrossRef]
21. Lu, Z.; Wu, L.; Dai, X.; Wang, Y.; Sun, M.; Zhou, C.; Du, H.; Rao, H. Novel flexible bifunctional amperometric biosensor based on laser engraved porous graphene array electrodes: Highly sensitive electrochemical determination of hydrogen peroxide and glucose. *J. Hazard. Mater.* **2021**, *402*, 123774. [CrossRef] [PubMed]
22. Xu, R.; Liu, P.; Ji, G.; Gao, L.; Zhao, J. Versatile Strategy to Design Flexible Planar-Integrated Microsupercapacitors Based on Co_3O_4-Decorated Laser-Induced Graphene. *ACS Appl. Energy Mater.* **2020**, *3*, 10676–10684. [CrossRef]
23. Ren, M.; Zhang, J.; Tour, J.M. Laser-induced graphene synthesis of Co_3O_4 in graphene for oxygen electrocatalysis and metal-air batteries. *Carbon* **2018**, *139*, 880–887. [CrossRef]
24. Ren, M.; Zhang, J.; Tour, J.M. Laser-Induced Graphene Hybrid Catalysts for Rechargeable Zn-Air Batteries. *ACS Appl. Energy Mater.* **2019**, *2*, 1460–1468. [CrossRef]
25. Zhang, J.; Zhang, C.; Sha, J.; Fei, H.; Li, Y.; Tour, J.M. Efficient Water-Splitting Electrodes Based on Laser-Induced Graphene. *ACS Appl. Mater. Interfaces* **2017**, *9*, 26840–26847. [CrossRef]
26. Vanegas, D.C.; Patiño, L.; Mendez, C.; de Oliveira, D.A.; Torres, A.M.; Gomes, C.L.; McLamore, E.S. Laser Scribed Graphene Biosensor for Detection of Biogenic Amines in Food Samples Using Locally Sourced Materials. *Biosensors* **2018**, *8*, 42. [CrossRef]
27. Alhajji, E.; Zhang, F.; Alshareef, H.N. Status and Prospects of Laser-Induced Graphene for Battery Applications. *Energy Technol.* **2021**, *9*, 2100454. [CrossRef]
28. Ren, M.; Zhang, J.; Fan, M.; Ajayan, P.M.; Tour, J.M. Li-Breathing Air Batteries Catalyzed by MnNiFe/Laser-Induced Graphene Catalysts. *Adv. Mater. Interfaces* **2019**, *6*, 1901035. [CrossRef]
29. Hawes, G.F.; Rehman, S.; Pope, M.A. Rapid prototyping of electrochemical energy storage devices based on two dimensional materials. *Curr. Opin. Electrochem.* **2020**, *20*, 36–45. [CrossRef]
30. Pereira, S.O.; Santos, N.F.; Carvalho, A.F.; Fernandes, A.J.S.; Costa, F.M. Electrochemical Response of Glucose Oxidase Adsorbed on Laser-Induced Graphene. *Nanomaterials* **2021**, *11*, 1893. [CrossRef] [PubMed]
31. Sun, X.; Liu, X.; Li, F. Sulfur-doped laser-induced graphene derived from polyethersulfone and lignin hybrid for all-solid-state supercapacitor. *Appl. Surf. Sci.* **2021**, *551*, 149438. [CrossRef]
32. Aslam, S.; Sagar, R.U.R.; Liu, Y.; Anwar, T.; Zhang, L.; Zhang, M.; Mahmood, N.; Qiu, Y. Graphene decorated polymeric flexible materials for lightweight high areal energy lithium-ion batteries. *Appl. Mater. Today* **2019**, *17*, 123–129. [CrossRef]
33. Gao, J.; He, S.; Nag, A. Electrochemical Detection of Glucose Molecules Using Laser-Induced Graphene Sensors: A Review. *Sensors* **2021**, *21*, 2818. [CrossRef]
34. Lu, B.; Jin, X.; Han, Q.; Qu, L. Planar Graphene-Based Microsupercapacitors. *Small* **2021**, *17*, 2006827. [CrossRef]
35. Xu, G.; Aydemir, N.; Kilmartin, P.A.; Travas-Sejdic, J. Direct laser scribed graphene/PVDF-HFP composite electrodes with improved mechanical water wear and their electrochemistry. *Appl. Mater. Today* **2017**, *8*, 35–43. [CrossRef]
36. Han, T.; Nag, A.; Simorangkir, R.B.V.B.; Afsarimanesh, N.; Liu, H.; Mukhopadhyay, S.C.; Xu, Y.; Zhadobov, M.; Sauleau, R. Multifunctional Flexible Sensor Based on Laser-Induced Graphene. *Sensors* **2019**, *19*, 3477. [CrossRef] [PubMed]
37. Tiliakos, A.; Ceaus, C.; Iordache, S.M.; Vasile, E.; Stamatin, I. Morphic transitions of nanocarbons via laser pyrolysis of polyimide films. *J. Anal. Appl. Pyrolysis* **2016**, *121*, 275–286. [CrossRef]
38. Hossain, M.F.; Slaughter, G. Flexible electrochemical uric acid and glucose biosensor. *Bioelectrochemistry* **2021**, *141*, 107870. [CrossRef] [PubMed]
39. Jayapiriya, U.S.; Rewatkar, P.; Goel, S. Direct Electron Transfer based Microfluidic Glucose Biofuel cell with CO_2 Laser ablated Bioelectrodes and Microchannel. *IEEE Trans. NanoBiosci.* **2021**. [CrossRef] [PubMed]
40. Lin, J.; Peng, Z.; Liu, Y.; Ruiz-Zepeda, F.; Ye, R.; Samuel, E.L.G.; Yacaman, M.J.; Yakobson, B.I.; Tour, J.M. Laser-induced porous graphene films from commercial polymers. *Nat. Commun.* **2014**, *5*, 5714. [CrossRef]
41. Behrent, A.; Griesche, C.; Sippel, P.; Baeumner, A.J. Process-property correlations in laser-induced graphene electrodes for electrochemical sensing. *Microchim. Acta* **2021**, *188*, 159. [CrossRef]

42. Rewatkar, P.; Kothuru, A.; Goel, S. Laser-induced Flexible Graphene Bioelectrodes for Enzymatic Biofuel Cell. In Proceedings of the 13th IEEE International Conference of Nano/Molecular Medicine and Engineering, Gwangju, Korea, 21–24 November 2019.
43. Zanoni, J.; Moura, J.P.; Santos, N.F.; Carvalho, A.F.; Fernandes, A.J.S.; Monteiro, T.; Costa, F.M.; Pereira, S.O.; Rodrigues, J. Dual Transduction of H_2O_2 Detection UsingZnO/Laser-Induced Graphene Composites. *Chemosensors* **2021**, *9*, 102. [CrossRef]
44. Vashisth, A.; Kowalik, M.; Gerringer, J.C.; Ashraf, C.; van Duin, A.C.T.; Green, M.J. ReaxFF Simulations of Laser-Induced Graphene (LIG) Formation for Multifunctional Polymer Nanocomposites. *ACS Appl. Nano Mater.* **2020**, *3*, 1881–1890. [CrossRef]
45. Nayak, P.; Kurra, N.; Xia, C.; Alshareef, H.N. Highly Efficient Laser Scribed Graphene Electrodes for On-Chip Electrochemical Sensing Applications. *Adv. Electron. Mater.* **2016**, *2*, 1600185. [CrossRef]
46. Nasraoui, S.; Al-Hamry, A.; Anurag, A.; Teixeira, P.R.; Ameur, S.; Paterno, L.G.; Ali, M.B.; Kanoun, O. Investigation of Laser Induced Graphene Electrodes Modified by MWNT/AuNPs for Detection of Nitrite. In Proceedings of the 16th International Multi-Conference on Systems, Signals & Devices, Istanbul, Turkey, 21–24 March 2019.
47. Tai, M.J.Y.; Vasudevan, M.; Perumal, V.; Liu, W.W.; Mohamed, N.M. Synthesis of Laser Scribed Graphene Electrode with Optimized Power for Biosensing. In Proceedings of the IEEE Regional Symposium on Micro and Nanoelectronics (RSM), Pahang, Malaysia, 21–23 August 2019.
48. Yivlialin, R.; Bussetti, G.; Magagnin, L.; Ciccacci, F.; Duò, L. Temporal analysis of blister evolution during anion intercalation in graphite. *Phys. Chem. Chem. Phys.* **2017**, *19*, 13855–13859. [CrossRef]
49. Yivlialin, R.; Brambilla, L.; Accogli, A.; Gibertini, E.; Tommasini, M.; Goletti, C.; Leone, M.; Duò, L.; Magagnin, L.; Castiglioni, C.; et al. Evidence of graphite blister evolution during the anion de-intercalation process in the cathodic regime. *Appl. Surf. Sci.* **2020**, *504*, 144440. [CrossRef]
50. Bussetti, G.; Yivlialin, R.; Alliata, D.; Bassi, A.L.; Castiglioni, C.; Tommasini, M.; Casari, C.S.; Passoni, M.; Biagioni, P.; Ciccacci, F.; et al. Disclosing the Early Stages of Electrochemical Anion Intercalation in Graphite by a Combined Atomic Force Microscopy/Scanning Tunneling Microscopy Approach. *J. Phys. Chem. C* **2016**, *120*, 6088–6093. [CrossRef]
51. Goss, C.A.; Brumfield, J.C.; Irene, E.A.; Murray, R.W. Imaging the Incipient Electrochemical Oxidation of Highly Oriented Pyrolitic Graphite. *Anal. Chem.* **1993**, *65*, 1378–1389. [CrossRef]
52. Bussetti, G.; Yivlialin, R.; Ciccacci, F.; Duò, L.; Gibertini, E.; Accogli, A.; Denti, I.; Magagnin, L.; Micciulla, F.; Cataldo, A.; et al. Electrochemical scanning probe analysis used as a benchmark for carbon forms quality test. *J. Phys. Condens. Matter* **2021**, *33*, 115002. [CrossRef]
53. Li, H.Y.; Yu, Y.; Liu, L.; Liu, L.; Wu, Y. One-step electrochemically expanded graphite foil for flexible all-solid supercapacitor with high rate performance. *Electrochim. Acta* **2017**, *228*, 553–561. [CrossRef]
54. Pérez, S.; Rebollar, E.; Oujja, M.; Martín, M.; Castillejo, M. Laser-induced periodic surface structuring of biopolymers. *Appl. Phys. A* **2013**, *110*, 683–690. [CrossRef]
55. Ferrari, A.C. Raman spectroscopy of graphene and graphite: Disorder, electron–phononcoupling, doping and nonadiabatic effects. *Solid State Commun.* **2007**, *143*, 47–57. [CrossRef]
56. Ghanam, A.; Lahcen, A.A.; Beduk, T.; Alshareef, H.N.; Amine, A.; Salama, K.N. Laser scribed graphene: A novel platform for highly sensitive detection of electroactive biomolecules. *Biosens. Bioelectron.* **2020**, *168*, 112509. [CrossRef] [PubMed]

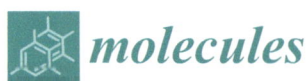

Article

Effect of Graphene Characteristics on Morphology and Performance of Composite Noble Metal-Reduced Graphene Oxide SERS Substrate

Tajana Kostadinova [1,2], Nikolaos Politakos [1], Ana Trajcheva [1,2], Jadranka Blazevska-Gilev [2,*] and Radmila Tomovska [1,3,*]

[1] POLYMAT, Facultad de Ciencias Químicas, University of the Basque Country UPV/EHU, Joxe Mari Korta Zentroa, Tolosa Etorbidea 72, 20018 Donostia-San Sebastián, Spain; tajana@tmf.ukim.edu.mk (T.K.); mikolaos.politakos@ehu.eus (N.P.); ana.trajcheva@polymat.eu (A.T.)
[2] Faculty of Technology and Metallurgy, Ss. Cyril and Methodius University in Skopje, Rudjer Boskovic 16, 1000 Skopje, North Macedonia
[3] Ikerbasque, Basque Foundation for Science, Maria Diaz de Haro 3, 48013 Bilbao, Spain
* Correspondence: jadranka@tmf.ukim.edu.mk (J.B.-G.); radmila.tomovska@ehu.eus (R.T.)

Citation: Kostadinova, T.; Politakos, N.; Trajcheva, A.; Blazevska-Gilev, J.; Tomovska, R. Effect of Graphene Characteristics on Morphology and Performance of Composite Noble Metal-Reduced Graphene Oxide SERS Substrate. *Molecules* **2021**, *26*, 4775. https://doi.org/10.3390/molecules26164775

Academic Editors: Gianlorenzo Bussetti and Luca Tortora

Received: 13 July 2021
Accepted: 2 August 2021
Published: 6 August 2021

Publisher's Note: MDPI stays neutral with regard to jurisdictional claims in published maps and institutional affiliations.

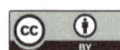

Copyright: © 2021 by the authors. Licensee MDPI, Basel, Switzerland. This article is an open access article distributed under the terms and conditions of the Creative Commons Attribution (CC BY) license (https://creativecommons.org/licenses/by/4.0/).

Abstract: Graphene/noble metal substrates for surface enhanced RAMAN scattering (SERS) possess synergistically improved performance, due to the strong chemical enhancement mechanism accounted to graphene and the electromagnetic mechanism raised from the metal nanoparticles. However, only the effect of noble metal nanoparticles characteristics on the SERS performance was studied so far. In attempts to bring a light to the effect of quality of graphene, in this work, two different graphene oxides were selected, slightly oxidized GOS (20%) with low aspect ratio (1000) and highly oxidized (50%) GOG with high aspect ratio (14,000). GO and precursors for noble metal nanoparticles (NP) simultaneous were reduced, resulting in rGO decorated with AgNPs and AuNPs. The graphene characteristics affected the size, shape, and packing of nanoparticles. The oxygen functionalities actuated as nucleation sites for AgNPs, thus GOG was decorated with higher number and smaller size AgNPs than GOS. Oppositely, AuNPs preferred bare graphene surface, thus GOS was covered with smaller size, densely packed nanoparticles, resulting in the best SERS performance. Fluorescein in concentration of 10^{-7} M was detected with enhancement factor of 82×10^4. This work demonstrates that selection of graphene is additional tool toward powerful SERS substrates.

Keywords: graphene aspect ratio; reduced graphene oxide; silver nanoparticles; gold nanoparticles; SERS

1. Introduction

Because of the graphene unique features, such as high electron mobility and high surface area, followed by exceptional mechanical, thermal, and electrical properties, it attracts a huge interest in various research fields, including materials science and engineering. One of the important applications of graphene is its utilization as a substrate for surface-enhanced Raman scattering (SERS) [1] that allows detection of a very low concentration of chemical or biological molecules. Raman signals are inherently weak, especially when the visible light excitation is used and therefore, a small number of scattered photons are used for the detection of the investigated molecules. However, by insertion of the investigated molecules onto the surface of the SERS substrate, a largely increased Raman scattering is induced because of two simultaneous effects. On the one hand, chemical enhancement mechanism, which occurs due to the established molecule-substrate interaction, building a charge transfer complex and facilitating the charge transfer [2–8]. On the other hand, in case of metal substrate, such as nano-cast gold (Au) or silver (Ag) surface, resonantly enhanced field allows an electromagnetic enhancement effect that much strongly enhances the Raman signal [9–14]. Additionally, graphene efficiently quenches the fluorescence resulting in improved quality of the probe molecule spectra [15,16]. As the chemical enhancement in SERS is deemed to arose from the creation of interaction due to vibrational coupling and creation of light-induced charge transfer among the molecule and the substrate, stronger the interaction higher is the chemical enhancement [17,18]. Graphene oxide (GO) and reduced graphene oxide (rGO) are progressing as adequate materials since their ubiquity has also been linked with greater SERS effects. It has been stated that single-layer graphene shows higher SERS signal enhancement in contrast to few-layer graphene [19].

Lately, several experimental attempts were reported concerning the enhancement of the SERS performance by connecting the plasmonic nanoparticles formed of silver and gold with graphene structures [20–27]. Song et al. [28] obtained detection of maximum 200–300 times average value enhanced SERS intensities from Ag nanoparticles on graphene sheet (GS) hybrid substrate compared to pure graphene. Nevertheless, Fan et al. [29] reported 2–3 times enhanced SERS excitations from hybrid nanostructure created of AgNP and GO with respect to neat AgNP. However, the performance of the metal nanoparticles is highly reliant on their dimension, structure, crystallinity, configuration, and formation geometry [30]. The effect of various variables on an achieved enhancement was studied. One of the most investigated was the size of the AgNP and Au nanoparticles (AuNP) and their aggregates [31–33], reporting that the average value of SERS enhancement factor is 1.6 times increased when the size distribution is reduced to half [28]. He et al. [34] studied the size of AgNP on the SERS enhancement. They reported that the SERS enhancement factor monotonically increases with augmentation of the particle size and the decrease of the distance between the particles in a dimer. As well, the shape of the AgNP and AuNPs was studied. In case when quasi-cubic AgNP were deposited onto graphene, the SERS enhancement factors were 6.53 times in average greater than that of spherical nanoparticles [28]. Zhang et al. [35] have designed GO-wrapped flower-like silver particles, and reported 3.5 times increased SERS signal based on the structure of the hybrid. An interesting study was conducted for dogbone-shaped gold nanoparticles used as colloidal SERS substrates, and it has been shown that the larger dogbone-shaped gold nanoparticles result in weaker limits of detection [36]. Dilong et al. [37] examined the SERS properties of Au nanoparticles with different sizes and shapes and reported that the Au nanospheres arrangements showed great SERS enhancement linked to their composition due to the presence of numerous SERS hot-spots among neighboring AuNPs generated by the electromagnetic coupling.

The control of substrate surface coverage with noble metal nanoparticles is an important parameter when fabricating active material as a SERS substrate. The proportional relation among the surface coverage and the increment of the intensity of SERS signal was presented [38]. When the coverage is doubled, the enhancement factor is as well nearly doubled [28]. Usually, the ultimate particle coverage decreases as the nanoparticle diameter increases. It has been demonstrated that the final particle coverage is decreased with increasing the particle size resulting in reduced hot-spots in the SERS excitation state and consequently decreasing the signal [25]. The responsibility for the highest SERS signal enhancement is related to the nanoscale gaps within nanoparticle dimers and the probe molecule adsorbed in these so-called "hot-spots" [28]. Ding et al. [39] demonstrated that the high coverage of AgNP onto GO led to enhanced SERS signal. This implies that the enhancement effect occurs due to the great electromagnetic coupling between two neighboring AgNPs with a very small gap, resulting in improved SERS signal.

It is clear that when hybrid SERS substrates were prepared, made of graphene-based materials and noble metal nanoparticles, the focus was placed on the quality, quantity, and structural characteristics of the nanoparticles, as well as their dispersion over graphene material. However, there are quite different graphene-based materials in size and thickness, level of oxidation, presence of heteroatoms, etc. The quality of graphene nanosheets by means of aspect ratio and presence of sp^3 C defects within the structure influences importantly the properties, especially the electrical conductivity, the capability of interactions, and mechanical resistance [40]. Therefore, one may expect that the interaction of different aspect ratio with different levels of functionalization of the surface will affect the interaction with metal nanoparticles, interactions with probe molecule, and subsequently, the activity as SERS substrate. This is especially true when simultaneous in situ production of noble metal nanoparticles and GO reduction is performed, which is the subject of the present work. For that aim, the different aspect ratio graphenes with importantly different oxidation level were decorated with Ag and Au nanoparticles and they were investigated as SERS substrate using fluorescein (Fl) as probe molecule. To the best of authors' knowledge, this is the first study where the effect of the different quality of graphene-based materials over the morphology of the SERS substrates was studied and provides useful information for selection of graphene material for designing a SERS substrate and optimization of their performance. Even though the graphene provides chemical enhancement to the hybrid substrate, which is much lower than the electromagnetic field enhancement from the NPs, the present work demonstrated that by variation of the graphene characteristics, the NPs structuring on the surface is influenced and thus, the SERS performance.

2. Materials and Methods

Two types of GO in aqueous dispersion were used (Table 1). The first one, supplied by Graphene Supermarket, (Ronkonkoma, NY, USA), (GOS), has the following characteristics: 60% single layer with concentration of 5 mg/mL, low aspect ratio of 1000 and lower content of oxygen functional groups, and other heteroatom (~20%). The second one was supplied by Graphenea, (San Sebastian, Spain), (GOG) with the following characteristics: about 14,000 aspect ratio, 95% one-layer platelets, with concentration of 4 mg/mL, high amount of oxygen functional groups, and heteroatoms ~50%.

Table 1. Properties and elemental analysis of GOG and GOS.

Properties	GOG	GOS
Concentration	4 mg/mL	5 mg/mL
Elemental Composition	Carbon: 49–56% Oxygen: 41–50% Hydrogen: 0–1% Nitrogen: 0–1% Sulfur: 2–4% (Up to 5% heteroatoms)	Carbon 79% Oxygen 20% (Up to 1% heteroatoms)
Lateral dimension	<10 µm	0.3–0.7 µm
Thickness	Monolayer content (measured in 0.05 wt%): >95%	1 atomic layer-at least 80%
Color	Yellow-brown	Brown
Aspect ratio (lateral dimension/diameter)	~14.000	~1000

Fluorescein (Fl, $C_{20}H_{12}O_5$) purchased from Fluka, (Fluka, Madrid, Spain), polyvinylpyrrolidone $(C_6H_9NO)n$ with average molar mass of 10,000 (PVP), silver nitrate ($AgNO_3$) ACS reagent, (Westborough, MA, USA), $\geq$99.0% and Gold(III) chloride hydrate 99.995% trace metals basis from Sigma Aldrich, (Madrid, Spain), L (+)-ascorbic acid, 99%, (AsA) from ACROS, (Madrid, Spain), were used as received. Milli-Q water was used in all experiments.

For synthesis of the hybrid SERS substrates, first aqueous dispersions were prepared by mixing GO and silver nitrate precursors for Ag nanoparticles (NP) and gold (III) chloride hydrate precursor for AuNP, according to the following procedure. About 50 mL GO aqueous dispersion was sonicated (Hielscher Sonicator-UIS250v, (Hielscher Ultrasonics GmbH, Teltow, Germany) with an amplitude of 70% and energy pulsed at 0.5 Hz at room temperature for 10 min in a 100 mL beaker under continuous agitation of 200 rpm, followed by addition of polyvinylpyrrolidone (PVP) solution (5 mg of PVP in 5 mL water). PVP with molar mass of 10,000 Da was added to assure colloidal stability in the aqueous dispersions during the reduction process. In this dispersion, 60 mL of the respective precursor in aqueous solution was added (60 mg precursor in 2 mL of water). After mixing, the reduction process was performed by ascorbic acid (AsA) reducing agent in concentration of 560 mg in 3 mL water, at room temperature for 72 h. AsA reduced simultaneously the GO and the respective precursor facilitating the growth of the nanoparticles in the dispersions that strongly adsorbed onto the rGO platelets. As a result, hybrid rGO nanoplatelets decorated with AgNP and AuNP were obtained, denoted as: rGOS-AgNP, rGOS-AuNP, rGOG-AgNP, and rGOG-AuNPs according to type of graphene and type of nanoparticles. Total of 4 µL of each of these dispersions was drop casted over glass rectangular substrates and left for drying at standard atmospheric conditions (20 °C and 55% relative humidity, Scheme 1).

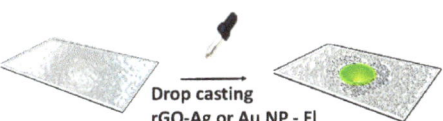

Scheme 1. Glass rectangular substrate and sample deposition by drop casting scheme.

The morphology of the composites was investigated by scanning electron microscopy (SEM, (Hitachi TM3030 tabletop model (Krefeld, Germany) at an accelerating voltage of 15 kV. The SEM instrument is equipped with EDX that was used to determine the elemental analysis and mapping of the hybrid substrates. The structure of the GO and distribution of silver and gold nanoparticles decorated onto GO surfaces were investigated with Philips TECNAI G2 20 TWIN transmission electron microscope (FEI, TEM, Barcelona, Spain). For the thermal degradation analysis (TGA) of the materials, a TGA500 apparatus (TA Instruments, Cerdanyola del Valles, Spain) was used. About 2 mg of each material was heated under oxygen ambient from 25 to 700 °C, at a heating rate of 10 °C/min. The SERS activity of the rGO-AgNP and rGO-AuNP hybrid structures was studied by Renishaw Raman Spectrometer (Renishaw, Barcelona, Spain) with an excitation wavelength of 532 nm, 1% of laser power (0.2 mW), 1 s acquisition time, and illumination range from 150 to 3500 cm^{-1}. The samples were captured using a 100× long-working distance objective lens and a CCD512 camera.

For SERS performance determination, Fl probe molecules were deposited over each of the hybrid films by drop casting 2 µL of Fl aqueous solution of different concentrations and were left overnight to dry (Scheme 1). Fl spectra onto the rGO/noble metal hybrids were determined up to 10^{-7} M. The blank sample was prepared by drop casting 4 µL Fl aqueous solution with concentration 10^{-1} M onto the neat glass substrate. At least three different spectra were collected for each Fl concentrations. The presented Raman spectra in the manuscript were normalized, using the characteristic peak of the glass substrate onto which the hybrids film were prepared and the Fl was deposited.

3. Results and Discussions

The reduction of neat GO in aqueous dispersion was performed with AsA reducing agent in presence of PVP (Mw of 10.000 Da) that sterically stabilized the rGO platelets in dispersions. The simultaneous reduction of GO and respective precursor for formation of Ag and Au nanoparticles resulted in the formation of rGO platelets decorated with AgNP or AuNP. The hybrid nanoplatelets were as well stabilized with PVP.

Elemental composition of all rGO-based materials was determined by EDX and the chemical composition by FTIR spectroscopy. The elemental composition of all materials is presented in Table S1, Supplementary Materials. These results showed that the reduction level is similar in all the samples independently of the presence of Ag or Au precursors, as the relative oxygen content is around 20% in all samples. Carbon content is lower for the composite samples than the neat ones, due to the presence of noble metal nanoparticles on their surface, the content of which is in the range of 7–12%. The exception is rGOG-AuNP material, which presented much lower reduction level and subsequently higher oxygen content and lower AuNP fraction in the composite. It is worth mentioning that the rGOS has similar oxygen content as the GOS (Table 1), which is probably the result of the presence of PVP used for colloidal stabilization of the reduced platelets.

FTIR spectra of the substrates are shown in Figure S1, Supplementary Materials. Both neat rGO materials present typical characteristic peaks of rGO, assigned as follows: ~1710 cm^{-1} (C=O stretching vibration), ~1620 cm^{-1} (C=C graphene domains), ~1400 cm^{-1} (OH deformation vibrations), and ~1030 cm^{-1} (C-O in epoxy). The same peaks appeared in composite substrates made of rGO and Ag or Au nanoparticles, however, certain shifts of each of these vibrations might be noticed with respect to the neat rGO materials, indicating changing of the chemical environment, likely due to the presence of nanoparticles. No important differences in chemical composition can be observed between the different types of rGO and nanoparticles.

In Figure 1 the characteristics of the rGOS hybrid nanoplatelets are shown. rGOS, with aspect ratio of 1000, is characterized with about 20% of oxygen content and about 3% of other heteroatoms, such as sulfur or nitrogen. Figure 1a presents SEM image of the neat rGOS material, in the inset of which, the EDX map is shown, presenting the elemental distribution on the surface of the film. The film is wrinkled and irregular and apparently, the rGOS platelets are covered with PVP, as the map in the inset shows high presence of nitrogen. The morphology of the hybrid rGOS films decorated with AgNP and AuNP are presented in Figure 1b,c, respectively.

Morphology of the hybrid films (Figure 1b,c) differs from that of neat rGOS, as the presence of nanoparticles influenced the drying process and the film quality. AgNP may be observed in Figure 1b (as white structures) in two different morphologies, along with spherical nanoparticles dendrimer-like crystals were observed. The size of the spherical nanoparticles is likely submicron, whereas the dendrimers are large structures of around 10 μm in average. The EDX map presented in the inset of Figure 1b shows that the surface of this hybrid is not covered completely with AgNP, as the graphene structure is still visible (carbon is denoted in red color in the EDX map). The dendrimer silver nanostructures have been observed previously [41], and their formation was explained by a diffusion-limited aggregate model. Namely, in case when growth rate of the nanoparticles is limited by the rate of diffusion of solute atoms to the interface, asymmetric growth of the nanoparticles occurred. Interestingly, such large crystal structures were not observed in case of rGOS-AuNP. As it is shown in Figure 1c, only tiny spherical nanoparticles distributed all over the rGO were obtained. According to the SEM image that represents very good coverage of surface of rGO with AuNP, the EDX-map in the inset of Figure 1c confirms the same, as almost no carbon atoms are visible on the surface of rGO. Even though, Table S1 in Supplementary Materials presents similar Ag and Au NP fractions (9% vs 10%, respectively), these fractions are mass fractions, which means much more moles of Au were presented onto the rGOS. Therefore, the higher quantity of Au nanoparticles along with their much smaller size is the main responsible factors for the higher coverage.

TGA curves of the nanostructures obtained in presence of oxygen are presented in Figure 1d. Except on thermal stability of the composite structures, TGA curves provide information on the chemical composition and interaction between the components. In Figure 1d three weight loss regions are observed. Until 100 °C, the weight loss is assigned to adsorbed water, whereas the weight loss observed between 100 °C and 225 °C corresponds to the oxygen functionalities presented onto the nanostructures. This loss is the largest for the neat rGO, indicating that the hybrid nanoplatelets contain importantly less oxygen functional groups. This means that, either in presence of nanoparticles' precursors the reduction of GO was more efficient, or the oxygen functionalities were spent in establishing interaction in rGO–nanoparticles, having the second explanation more probable. The degradation of PVP, adsorbed onto nanoplatelets to provide colloidal stability, occurred between 450 and 500 °C. The main loss, corresponding to the graphenic structure, occurred at temperatures higher than 500 °C. The presence of AgNP and AuNP onto the rGOS increased prominently the thermal stability of the hybrid platelets, and the main loss was postponed for about 150 °C, and in the case of AuNP the thermal reinforcement is even more prominent. This indicates that there is higher number of AuNP attached to the rGOS surface, as already shown by EDX (Table S1, Supplementary Materials).

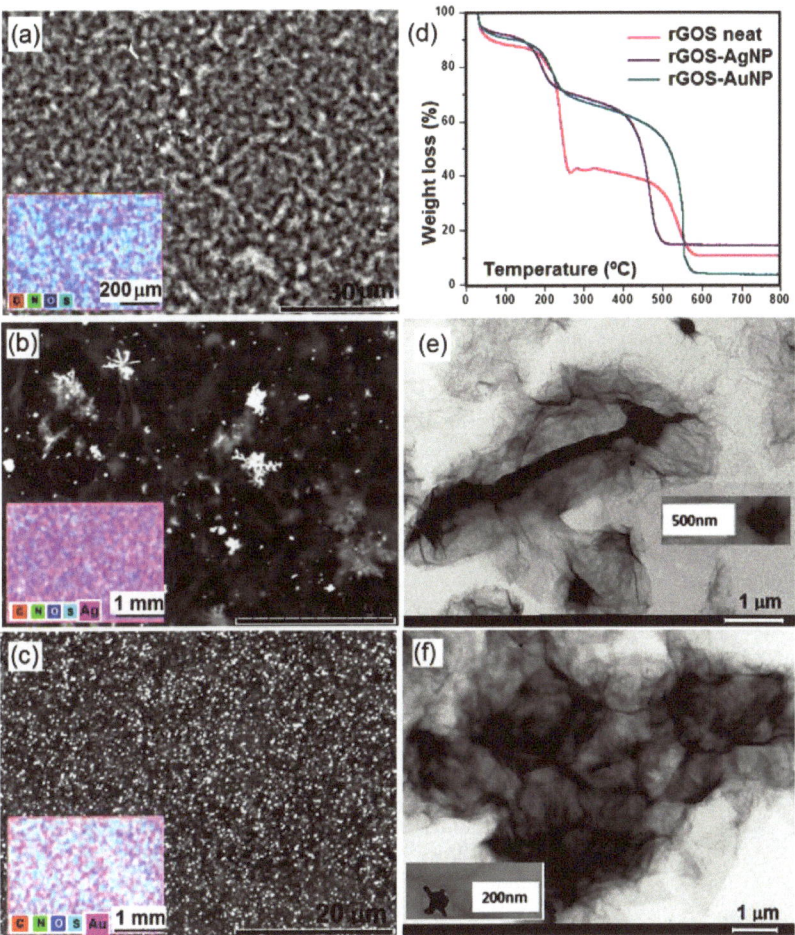

Figure 1. Characteristics of rGOS-AgNP and rGOS-AuNP hybrid films: (**a**) SEM image of neat rGOS, inset: EDX map of the same film; (**b**) SEM image of rGOS-AgNP film, inset: EDX map of the same film; (**c**) SEM image of rGOS-AuNP film, inset: EDX map of the same film; (**d**) TGA curves of hybrid films; (**e**) TEM image of rGOS-AgNP film; (**f**) TEM image of rGOS-AuNP film. In the insets of (**e**,**f**) single Ag and Au nanoparticle is shown, respectively.

The structure of the hybrids and the size and distribution of the nanoparticles onto the platelets are presented in TEM images (Figure 1e,f). In Figure 1e AgNP aggregates with diameter in a range of 200–500 nm distributed onto the rGO platelets may be observed, as shown in the enlarged image of individual particle in the inset of this figure. According to SEM image of the rGO-AuNP nanostructure (Figure 1f), AuNP are much smaller, therefore better distributed even on the nanoscale level. AuNP formed star-like aggregate with sizes in the range of 20–200 nm, as it is shown in the inset of Figure 1f. The rGO platelets are completely wrinkled and some re-aggregates may be observed (which may be result of the sample preparation).

To determine the SERS activity of the prepared films, the Fl probe molecules from aqueous solutions with different concentrations in a range of 10^{-1} to 10^{-13} M were deposited onto the investigated films formed on the glass substrate, followed by characterization by RAMAN spectroscopy. The obtained spectra were compared with these of Fl deposited onto a neat glass substrate and onto the rGOS neat film. The results are presented in Figure 2. It might be observed that the investigated Fl concentration in Figure 2 are up to 10^{-7} M, because bellow this concentration, the Fl was not detected and only characteristic peaks of rGO could be observed, as shown in Figure 2e.

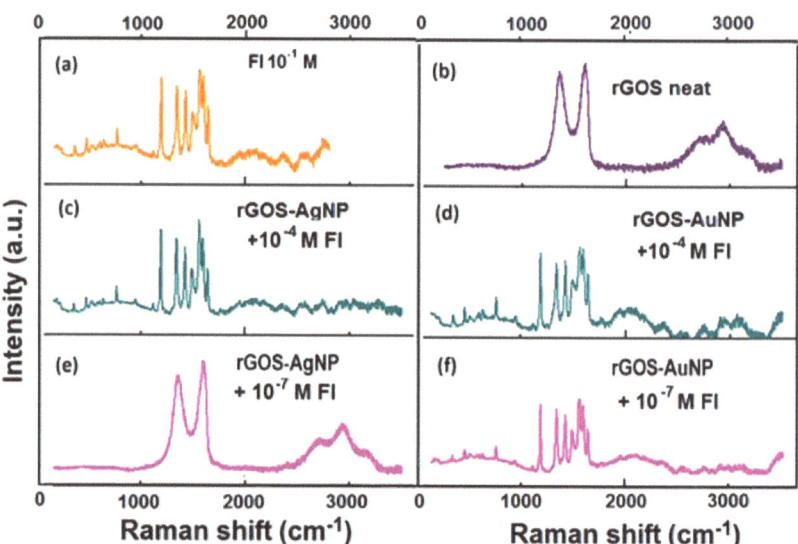

Figure 2. RAMAN spectra of Fl deposited in different concentration over the respective film: (**a**) Fl deposited from 10^{-1} M solution over a glass substrate; (**b**) neat rGOS film; (**c**) Fl deposited from 10^{-4} M solution over a rGOS-AgNP film; (**d**) Fl deposited from 10^{-4} M solution over a rGOS-AuNP film; (**e**) Fl deposited from 10^{-7} M solution over a rGOS-AgNP film; (**f**) Fl deposited from 10^{-7} M solution over a rGOS-AuNP film.

Fl deposited onto the glass substrate (Figure 2a, Scheme 1) presents the typical Fl Raman spectrum with skeletal vibration modes of the xanthene moiety that appears in the frequency range from 1000 to 1800 cm^{-1} [42] Raman spectrum of rGOS is presented in Figure 2b, where the characteristic D band at around 1348 cm^{-1} (originated from the defects in graphenic network) and the G band at around 1600 cm^{-1} (corresponding to the ordered sp^2 in plane vibration of carbon atoms) [43,44] is observed. The deposited Fl molecules onto the nanostructures containing AgNP onto the surface of rGO presented very nice spectra of Fl, up to Fl concentration of 10^{-4} M (Figure 2c). Further decrease of the Fl concentration deposited onto the nanostructured hybrid films of rGOS-AgNP remains undetectable in the RAMAN spectra, as only the rGO characteristic peaks appeared (Figure 2e). Enhancement factor (EF) was calculated using Equation (1) and the results are presented in Table 2.

$$EF = \frac{I_{SERS}}{I_{RAMAN}} \cdot \frac{[Fl]_{bulk}}{[Fl]_{SERS}} \qquad (1)$$

where I_{SERS} is the intensity of Fl characteristic peak at 1181.8 cm^{-1} in RAMAN spectra measured on the rGOS-AgNP, I_{RAMAN} is the intensity of the same peak in the RAMAN spectra of neat Fl; $[Fl]_{bulk}$ is the concentration of Fl deposited on the neat glass substrate and $[Fl]_{SERS}$ is the concentration of Fl deposited onto the SERS substrate, in this case rGOS-AgNP.

Table 2. EF values of the hybrid films made of rGOS combination with AgNPs and AuNPs.

Sample	rGOS-Ag	rGOS-Au	rGOS-Au	rGOG-Ag	rGOG-Au
[Fl]	10^{-4} M	10^{-4} M	10^{-7} M	10^{-4} M	10^{-4} M
EF	1373	1044	82×10^{-4}	908	1892

Table 2 shows that the EF for 10^{-4} M Fl onto rGOS-AgNP is 1373. The determined EF is rather modest and probably is due to the poor coverage of the rGOS with AgNP, large structures and large distance between them (poor coverage), limiting the electromagnetic enhancement effect.

On the other hand, the SERS activity of the hybrid substrate made of AuNPs deposited onto the rGOS nanoplatelets is presented in Figure 2d,f, for Fl concentration of 10^{-4} M and 10^{-7} M, respectively. For both concentrations strong SERS enhancement was obtained, giving rise to EF of 1044 for 10^{-4} M and EF of 82×10^4 for 10^{-7} M concentration of the Fl probe molecule. In this case, the substrate rGOS-AuNP has shown much higher detection capacity than the rGOS-AgNP, probably due to the important difference in the suface morphology and the molar quantity of AuNP. We think that two effects contribute toward this strong enhancement. Namely, as shown in Figure 1c and in the inset, the surface of the rGOS-AuNP film is almost completely covered by the nanosize AuNP. Such covarage ensure smaller distance between the nanoparticles, so called nanoscaled gaps [29] on the rGOS-AuNP than on rGOS-AgNP. Because of that, the former provides enhanced electomagnetic coupling effect between the neighbouring AuNPs [44] and consequently, the electromagnetic enhancement is better than for Ag-containing substrate. Nevertheless, as the TGA results suggested, likely strong interaction rGOS–AuNP were established, based on the important drop of the oxygen functional groups amount. The strong interaction decreased the distance substrate–probe molecule due to the vibrational coupling that creates a light-induced charge transfer complex [17,18], contributing to increase the chemical enhancement. Additional support was obtained by the star-like structure of the AuNP aggregates, as observed in TEM image (Figure 1f), as previously it was demonstrated that non-spherical AgNP positively affected the SERS effect [29].

In Figure 3a, the morphology of the neat rGOG sample is shown. According to the EDX map presented in the inset of Figure 2a, the rGOG surface is completely covered by PVP. The morphology of the composite samples rGOG-AgNP and rGOG-AuNP, displayed in Figure 3b,c, respectively, reveals non-regular spherical nanoparticles dispersed onto the surface of rGOG. The maps in the insets of both figures show uniform distribution of the nanoparticles throughout the whole rGOG sheets, however, much better for AgNP. If compared with the respective rGOS SEM images (Figure 1b,c), much more AgNPs with smaller size are distributed onto GOG-reduced platelets. This effect is probably a result of the increased oxidation of the initial GOG (50%) that established more interactions with the Ag+ ions during the in situ formation of the nanocomposite sample than GOS (20%). However, this effect is opposite in case of AuNPs. This can be because Au^{3+} ions are less prone to chemical interactions than Ag^+ ions, therefore the presence of the multiple functional oxygen groups on the GOG surface has rather negative effect on the AuNP–rGOG interactions. Consequently, the mechanism of coupling the rGOS and nanoparticles is distinct for Ag and Au. In case of Ag, the silver ions adsorbed on the GO surface and the nucleation of the nanoparticles occurred at the surface, whereas in case of Ag, the nanoparticles nucleated in the dispersion and are afterwards adsorbed on the rGOS surface. These results indicate that in case of AuNPs, more naked or less functionalized graphene surface is favorable for the synthesis of composite with well-distributed AuNP.

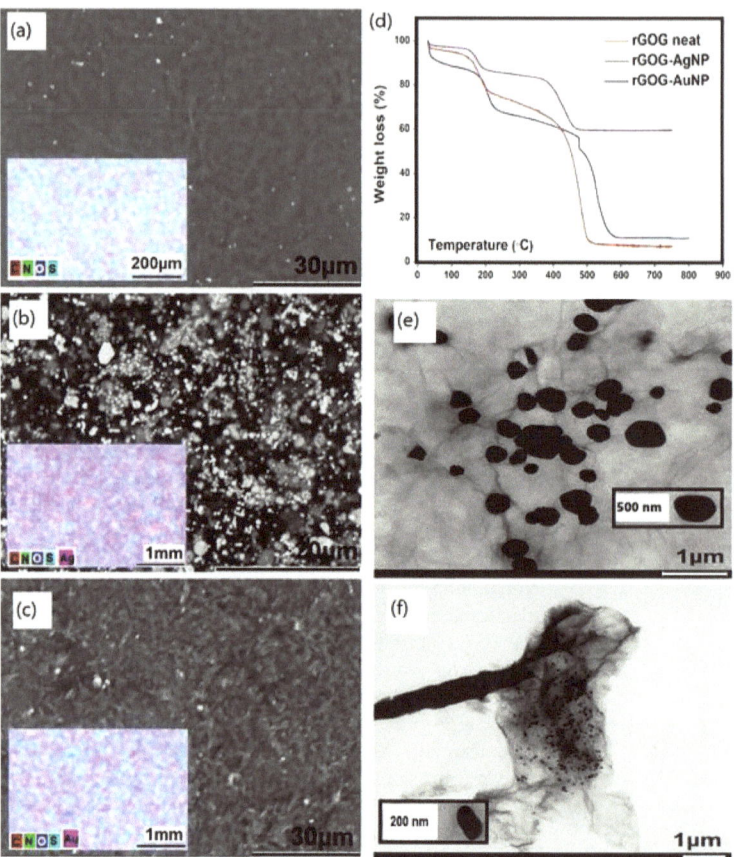

Figure 3. Characteristics of rGOG-AgNP and rGOG-AuNP hybrid films: (**a**) SEM image of neat rGOG, inset: EDX map of the same film; (**b**) SEM image of rGOG-AgNP film, inset: EDX map of the same film; (**c**) SEM image of rGOG-AuNP film, inset: EDX map of the same film; (**d**) TGA curves of hybrid films; (**e**) TEM image of rGOG-AgNP film; (**f**) TEM image of rGOG-AuNP film.

It is worth noting that the quality of graphene affects not only the distribution and aggregation of the nanoparticles formed on its surface, but also their morphology, probably due to the simultaneous reduction process of both graphene and the precursors. TEM images in Figure 3e present that AgNP forms large aggregates (200–800 nm) with a large distance between them, which means that the possibility for electromagnetic coupling between neighboring nanoparticles is rather low. Figure 1f reveals decreased particle size of AuNPs, which are packed closely onto some of the areas of the rGOG nanoplatelets. Finally, according to TGA results shown in Figure 3d, both nanocomposites presented important difference in the weight loss curves, which demonstrates presence of structural and compositional difference. The thermal degradation behavior is similar to the rGOS-based composites, thus three clear weight loss regions are observed. However, rGOG-AuNP shows similar behavior as the neat rGOG, indicating that the interaction between the AuNPs with the rGOG is not strong. There is very low amount of residuals after the TGA analysis, indicating low amount of AuNPs (according to Table S1, it is 7.3%), not strongly attached to rGOG. In case of rGOG-AgNP nanocomposite, significantly less oxygen functionalities were lost, accounting for better interaction of AgNP with rGOG with respect to AuNP and with respect to rGOS composites. The fact that rGOG is characterized by higher aspect ratios and lower thickness than rGOS means that at the same quantity, rGOG offers larger surface area, thus, lower coverage with nanoparticles is likely achieved than in case of rGOS. However, a very high amount of residual (~60%) indicates that AgNP were very strongly attached to the rGOG.

Figure 4 depicts the Raman spectra of the rGOG-based nanocomposite samples, compared with Fl deposited onto glass substrate and neat rGOG.

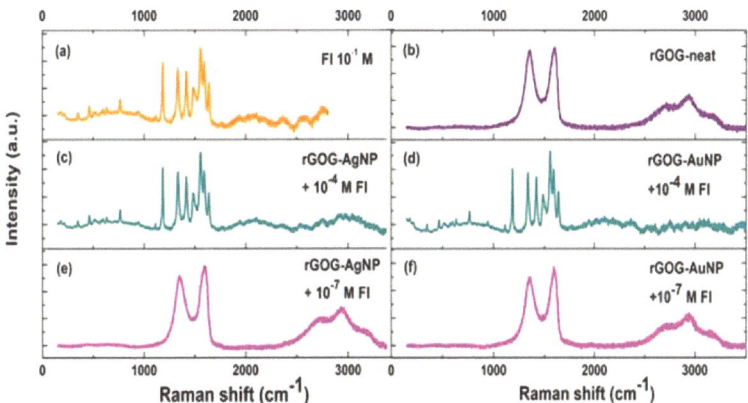

Figure 4. Raman spectra of Fl deposited in different concentration over the respective film: (**a**) Fl deposited from 10^{-1} M solution over a glass substrate; (**b**) neat rGOG film; (**c**) Fl deposited from 10^{-4} M solution over a rGOG-AgNP film; (**d**) Fl deposited from 10^{-4} M solution over a rGOG-AuNP film; (**e**) Fl deposited from 10^{-7} M solution over a rGOG-AgNP film; (**f**) Fl deposited from 10^{-7} M solution over a rGOG-AuNP film.

Comparing all the RAMAN spectra presented in Figure 4, it is clear that both nanocomposites rGOG-AgNP and rGOG-AuNP were able to detect Fl in as low molar concentration as 10^{-4}. The Fl spectra determined onto these nanocomposites substrates are clear, having all the characteristic peaks with higher intensity than the same in the Fl deposited onto glass substrate in a concentration of 0.1 M. The resulting EFs are 908 for rGOG-AgNP and 1892 for rGOG_AuNP (Table 2). Despite this strong enhancement, both nanocomposite substrates were not able to determine the 10^{-7} M concentration. The EF of rGOG-AgNP is similar to that of rGOS-AgNP; the result can be justified with the morphology and the composition of both samples. Namely, the AgNP formed onto rGOS surface are dendrimer-like structures with tens of microns dimensions, whereas on rGOG surface irregular spherical particles were formed with size in a range of 200–800 nm. Even though the last morphology is likely more prosperous for SERS activity, the large distance between the nanosized structures limits the detection to 10^{-4} M concentration, due to less possibility to establish the electromagnetic coupling. The rGOG-AuNP as well presented limited enhancement until 10^{-4} M Fl concentration. Moreover, its performance as SERS substrate is worse than rGOS-AuNP. Likely, it is due to the less established interaction between both rGOG and AuNP, and, because of the worst coverage of the surface of rGOG. The first effect accounts for the drop in chemical mechanism of enhancement, whereas the second one for the drop in electromagnetic mechanism.

4. Conclusions

The simultaneous reduction of GO in the presence of silver nitrate and gold (III) chloride hydrate resulted in successful modification on the surface of rGO with nanoparticles of silver and gold. Two types of colloidal GO were studied, one characterized with small aspect ratio (1000) and lower oxidation level (GOS, 20%) and the second one with much larger aspect ratio (14,000) and densely oxidized (GOG, 50%). The effect of these characteristics over the properties of the nanocomposites, was studied and related to their performance as SERS substrates. It was found that the characteristics of the GO affect importantly the properties and performance of the nanocomposites.

In case of AgNP onto lower aspect ratio GOS, the nanoparticles developed on the surface of its reduced form are with dendrimer-like morphology, few microns in size, and are less densely packed. Obviously, the nanoparticle nucleation points were the oxygen functionality. Because of that, in case of high aspect ratio and heavily functionalized GOG, the AgNP were smaller but more densely packed. Both of them presented very similar enhancement factor of about 1000 for detection of Fl molecules in concentration of 10^{-4} M. The similar behavior was attributed to the compensated effect of size and shape of AgNP, the distance between them, and the strong interactions. The aspect ratio obviously affected the coverage.

In case of AuNP, the effect of the quality and characteristics of GO were exactly opposite. Besides the light oxidation of GOS, the star-like aggregates of AuNP, developed onto rGOS, were more densely packed, than in case of GOG. As a consequence, the SERS performance of the smaller aspect ratio substrates based on GOS and AuNP presented the best performance for Fl detection, up to 10^{-7} M concentration with very high EF of 82×10^4. The limited enhancement effect of GOG-based substrate up to 10^{-4} M Fl concentration was attributed to lower coverage with AuNP and higher distance between them.

These results, for the first time to the best of the authors' knowledge, provide fundamental knowledge about the effect of the quality of graphene on the characteristics of in situ created hybrids with Ag and Au nanoparticles and their performance as SERS substrates.

Supplementary Materials: The following are available online. Table S1: Elemental analysis of all SERS substrate obtained by EDX. Figure S1: FTIR spectra of the neat rGO materials and their composites with Ag and Au nanoparticles.

Author Contributions: T.K. performed the experimental work, most of the characterization, and wrote the first draft; N.P. supervised the experimental work, participated in characterization of the materials, and in correction of manuscript; A.T. participated in characterization of the composites; J.B.-G. supervised the work and corrected the manuscript; R.T. conceptualized, planned, supervised the work and corrected the manuscript. All authors have read and agreed to the published version of the manuscript.

Funding: The authors gratefully acknowledged the financial support provided by NATO (SfP project G5244) and Basque Government (GV IT999-16).

Institutional Review Board Statement: Not applicable.

Informed Consent Statement: Not applicable.

Data Availability Statement: All data are already included in the main manuscript and in the Supporting information file.

Acknowledgments: The authors gratefully acknowledged the financial support provided by NATO (SfP project G5244) and Basque Government (GV IT999-16).

Conflicts of Interest: The authors declare no conflict of interest.

References

1. Kang, L.; Chu, J.; Zhao, H.; Xu, P.; Sun, M. Recent Progress in the Applications of Graphene in Surface-Enhanced Raman Scattering and Plasmon-Induced Catalytic Reactions. *J. Mater. Chem. C* **2015**, *3*, 9024–9037. [CrossRef]
2. Kim, J.; Jang, Y.; Kim, N.J.; Kim, H.; Yi, G.C.; Shin, Y.; Kim, M.H.; Yoon, S. Study of Chemical Enhancement Mechanism in Non-Plasmonic Surface Enhanced Raman Spectroscopy (SERS). *Front. Chem.* **2019**, *7*, 582. [CrossRef]
3. Liang, X.; Liang, B.; Pan, Z.; Lang, X.; Zhang, Y.; Wang, G.; Yin, P.; Guo, L. Tuning Plasmonic and Chemical Enhancement for SERS Detection on Graphene-Based Au Hybrids. *Nanoscale* **2015**, *7*, 20188–20196. [CrossRef]
4. Wu, D.; Liu, X.; Duan, S.; Xu, X.; Ren, B.; Lin, S. Chemical Enhancement Effects in SERS Spectra: A Quantum Chemical Study of Pyridine Interacting with Copper, Silver, Gold and Platinum Metals. *J. Phys. Chem.* **2008**, *112*, 4195–4204. [CrossRef]
5. Moore, J.E.; Morton, S.M.; Jensen, L. Importance of Correctly Describing Charge-Transfer Excitations for Understanding the Chemical Effect in SERS. *J. Phys. Chem. Lett.* **2012**, *3*, 2470–2475. [CrossRef] [PubMed]

6. Yu, X.; Cai, H.; Zhang, W.; Li, X.; Pan, N.; Luo, Y.; Wang, X.; Hou, J.G. Tuning Chemical Enhancement of SERS by Controlling the Chemical Reduction of Graphene Oxide Nanosheets. *ACS Nano* **2011**, *5*, 952–958. [CrossRef]
7. Morton, S.M.; Jensen, L. Understanding the Molecule-Surface Chemical Coupling in SERS. *J. Am. Chem. Soc.* **2009**, *131*, 4090–4098. [CrossRef]
8. Park, W.H.; Kim, Z.H. Charge Transfer Enhancement in the SERS of a Single Molecule. *Nano Lett.* **2010**, *10*, 4040–4048. [CrossRef] [PubMed]
9. Mock, J.J.; Norton, S.M.; Chen, S.Y.; Lazarides, A.A.; Smith, D.R. Electromagnetic Enhancement Effect Caused by Aggregation on SERS-Active Gold Nanoparticles. *Plasmonics* **2011**, *6*, 113–124. [CrossRef]
10. Lu, W.; Singh, A.K.; Khan, S.A.; Senapati, D.; Yu, H.; Ray, P.C. Gold Nano-Popcorn-Based Targeted Diagnosis, Nanotherapy Treatment, and in Situ Monitoring of Photothermal Therapy Response of Prostate Cancer Cells Using Surface-Enhanced Raman Spectroscopy. *J. Am. Chem. Soc.* **2010**, *132*, 18103–18114. [CrossRef]
11. Sun, Y.; Liu, K.; Miao, J.; Wang, Z.; Tian, B.; Zhang, L.; Li, Q.; Fan, S.; Jiang, K. Highly Sensitive Surface-Enhanced Raman Scattering Substrate Made from Superaligned Carbon Nanotubes. *Nano Lett.* **2010**, *10*, 1747–1753. [CrossRef]
12. Álvarez-Puebla, R.A.; Liz-Marzán, L.M. Environmental Applications of Plasmon Assisted Raman Scattering. *Energy Environ. Sci.* **2010**, *3*, 1011–1017. [CrossRef]
13. Senapati, T.; Senapati, D.; Singh, A.K.; Fan, Z.; Kanchanapally, R.; Ray, P.C. Highly Selective SERS Probe for Hg(II) Detection Using Tryptophan-Protected Popcorn Shaped Gold Nanoparticles. *Chem. Commun.* **2011**, *47*, 10326–10328. [CrossRef] [PubMed]
14. Yamamoto, Y.S.; Ozaki, Y.; Itoh, T. Recent Progress and Frontiers in the Electromagnetic Mechanism of Surface-Enhanced Raman Scattering. *J. Photochem. Photobiol. C Photochem. Rev.* **2014**, *21*, 81–104. [CrossRef]
15. Petreska, G.S.; Blazevska-Gilev, J.; Fajgar, R.; Tomovska, R. Surface-Enhanced Raman Scattering Activity of Ag/Graphene/Polymer Nanocomposite Films Synthesized by Laser Ablation. *Thin Solid Films* **2014**, *564*, 115–120. [CrossRef]
16. Xie, L.; Ling, X.; Fang, Y.; Zhang, J.; Liu, Z. Graphene as a Substrate to Suppress Fluorescence in Resonance Raman Spectroscopy. *J. Am. Chem. Soc.* **2009**, *131*, 9890–9891. [CrossRef]
17. Park, J.; Choi, Y.; Han, J.W.; Kim, J. Synthesis of Graphene Oxide-Silver Nanoparticle an Efficient Novel Antibacterial Agent Nanocomposites: An Efficient Novel Antibacterial Agent. *Curr. Nanosci.* **2016**, *12*, 762–773. [CrossRef]
18. Huang, J.; Zhang, L.; Chen, B.; Ji, N.; Chen, F.; Zhang, Y.; Zhang, Z. Nanocomposites of Size-Controlled Gold Nanoparticles and Graphene Oxide: Formation and Applications in SERS and Catalysis. *Nanoscale* **2010**, *2*, 2733–2738. [CrossRef] [PubMed]
19. Lee, J.; Shim, S.; Kim, B.; Shin, H.S. Surface-Enhanced Raman Scattering of Single-and Few-Layer Graphene by the Deposition of Gold Nanoparticles. *Chem. Eur. J.* **2011**, *17*, 2381–2387. [CrossRef]
20. Mehl, H.; Oliveira, M.M.; Zarbin, A.J.G. Thin and Transparent Films of Graphene/Silver Nanoparticles Obtained at Liquid-Liquid Interfaces: Preparation, Characterization and Application as SERS Substrates. *J. Colloid Interface Sci.* **2015**, *438*, 29–38. [CrossRef]
21. Lu, G.; Li, H.; Liusman, C.; Yin, Z.; Wu, S.; Zhang, H. Surface Enhanced Raman Scattering of Ag or Au Nanoparticle-Decorated Reduced Graphene Oxide for Detection of Aromatic Molecules. *Chem. Sci.* **2011**, *2*, 1817–1821. [CrossRef]
22. Lu, R.; Konzelmann, A.; Xu, F.; Gong, Y.; Liu, J.; Liu, Q.; Xin, M.; Hui, R.; Wu, J.Z. High Sensitivity Surface Enhanced Raman Spectroscopy of R6G on in Situ Fabricated Au Nanoparticle/Graphene Plasmonic Substrates. *Carbon N. Y.* **2015**, *86*, 78–85. [CrossRef]
23. Xu, W.; Mao, N.; Zhang, J. Graphene: A Platform for Surface-Enhanced Raman Spectroscopy. *Small* **2013**, *9*, 1206–1224. [CrossRef] [PubMed]
24. Sharma, S.; Prakash, V.; Mehta, S.K. Graphene/Silver Nanocomposites-Potential Electron Mediators for Proliferation in Electrochemical Sensing and SERS Activity. *TrAC Trends Anal. Chem.* **2017**, *86*, 155–171. [CrossRef]
25. Fan, Z.; Kanchanapally, R.; Ray, P.C. Hybrid Graphene Oxide Based Ultrasensitive SERS Probe for Label-Free Biosensing. *J. Phys. Chem. Lett.* **2013**, *4*, 3813–3818. [CrossRef]
26. Du, Y.; Zhao, Y.; Qu, Y.; Chen, C.H.; Chen, C.M.; Chuang, C.H.; Zhu, Y. Enhanced Light-Matter Interaction of Graphene-Gold Nanoparticle Hybrid Films for High-Performance SERS Detection. *J. Mater. Chem. C* **2014**, *2*, 4683–4691. [CrossRef]
27. Zhang, L.; Jiang, C.; Zhang, Z. Graphene Oxide Embedded Sandwich Nanostructures for Enhanced Raman Readout and Their Applications in Pesticide Monitoring. *Nanoscale* **2013**, *5*, 3773–3779. [CrossRef]
28. Song, H.; Li, X.; Yoo, S.; Wu, Y.; Liu, W.; Wang, X.; Liu, H. Highly Sensitive Surface Enhanced Raman Spectroscopy from Ag Nanoparticles Decorated Graphene Sheet. *J. Nanomater.* **2014**, *2014*, 538024. [CrossRef]
29. Fan, W.; Lee, Y.H.; Pedireddy, S.; Zhang, Q.; Liu, T.; Ling, X.Y. Graphene Oxide and Shape-Controlled Silver Nanoparticle Hybrids for Ultrasensitive Single-Particle Surface-Enhanced Raman Scattering (SERS) Sensing. *Nanoscale* **2014**, *6*, 4843–4851. [CrossRef]
30. Gentile, A.; Ruffino, F.; Grimaldi, M.G. Complex-Morphology Metal-Based Nanostructures: Fabrication, Characterization, and Applications. *Nanomaterials* **2016**, *6*, 110. [CrossRef]
31. Tzounis, L.; Contreras-Caceres, R.; Schellkopf, L.; Jehnichen, D.; Fischer, D.; Cai, C.; Uhlmann, P.; Stamm, M. Controlled Growth of Ag Nanoparticles Decorated onto the Surface of SiO2 Spheres: A Nanohybrid System with Combined SERS and Catalytic Properties. *RSC Adv.* **2014**, *4*, 17846–17855. [CrossRef]
32. Hong, S.; Li, X. Optimal Size of Gold Nanoparticles for Surface-Enhanced Raman Spectroscopy under Different Conditions. *J. Nanomater.* **2013**, *2013*, 790323. [CrossRef]
33. Yang, Y. SERS Enhancement Dependence on the Diameter of Au Nanoparticles. *J. Phys. Conf. Ser.* **2017**, *844*, 012030. [CrossRef]

34. He, R.X.; Liang, R.; Peng, P.; Norman Zhou, Y. Effect of the Size of Silver Nanoparticles on SERS Signal Enhancement. *J. Nanoparticle Res.* **2017**, *19*, 267. [CrossRef]
35. Zhang, C.Y.; Hao, R.; Zhao, B.; Fu, Y.; Zhang, H.; Moeendarbari, S.; Pickering, C.S.; Hao, Y.W.; Liu, Y.Q. Graphene Oxide-Wrapped Flower-like Sliver Particles for Surface-Enhanced Raman Spectroscopy and Their Applications in Polychlorinated Biphenyls Detection. *Appl. Surf. Sci.* **2017**, *400*, 49–56. [CrossRef]
36. Saute, B.; Narayanan, R. Solution-Based Direct Readout Surface Enhanced Raman Spectroscopic (SERS) Detection of Ultra-Low Levels of Thiram with Dogbone Shaped Gold Nanoparticles. *Analyst* **2011**, *136*, 527–532. [CrossRef] [PubMed]
37. Liu, D.; Li, C.; Zhou, F.; Zhang, T.; Zhang, H.; Li, X.; Duan, G.; Cai, W.; Li, Y. Rapid Synthesis of Monodisperse Au Nanospheres through a Laser Irradiation-Induced Shape Conversion, Self-Assembly and Their Electromagnetic Coupling SERS Enhancement. *Sci. Rep.* **2015**, *5*, 1–9. [CrossRef]
38. Wang, L.; Sun, Y.; Li, Z. Dependence of Raman Intensity on the Surface Coverage of Silver Nanocubes in SERS Active Monolayers. *Appl. Surf. Sci.* **2015**, *325*, 242–250. [CrossRef]
39. Ding, G.; Xie, S.; Liu, Y.; Wang, L.; Xu, F. Graphene Oxide-Silver Nanocomposite as SERS Substrate for Dye Detection: Effects of Silver Loading Amount and Composite Dosage. *Appl. Surf. Sci.* **2015**, *345*, 310–318. [CrossRef]
40. Choi, W.; Lahiri, I.; Seelaboyina, R.; Kang, Y.S. Synthesis of Graphene and Its Applications: A Review. *Crit. Rev. Solid State Mater. Sci.* **2010**, *35*, 52–71. [CrossRef]
41. Wang, L.; Roitberg, A.; Meuse, C.; Gaigalas, A.K. Raman and FTIR Spectroscopies of Fluorescein in Solutions. *Spectrochim. Acta-Part. A Mol. Biomol. Spectrosc.* **2001**, *57*, 1781–1791. [CrossRef]
42. Zainy, M.; Huang, N.M.; Vijay Kumar, S.; Lim, H.N.; Chia, C.H.; Harrison, I. Simple and Scalable Preparation of Reduced Graphene Oxide-Silver Nanocomposites via Rapid Thermal Treatment. *Mater. Lett.* **2012**, *89*, 180–183. [CrossRef]
43. Vijay Kumar, S.; Huang, N.M.; Lim, H.N.; Marlinda, A.R.; Harrison, I.; Chia, C.H. One-Step Size-Controlled Synthesis of Functional Graphene Oxide/Silver Nanocomposites at Room Temperature. *Chem. Eng. J.* **2013**, *219*, 217–224. [CrossRef]
44. Carbone, K.; Paliotta, M.; Micheli, L.; Mazzuca, C.; Cacciotti, I.; Nocente, F.; Ciampa, A.; Dell'Abate, M.T. A Completely Green Approach to the Synthesis of Dendritic Silver Nanostructures Starting from White Grape Pomace as a Potential Nanofactory. *Arab. J. Chem.* **2019**, *12*, 597–609. [CrossRef]

MDPI AG
Grosspeteranlage 5
4052 Basel
Switzerland
Tel.: +41 61 683 77 34

Molecules Editorial Office
E-mail: molecules@mdpi.com
www.mdpi.com/journal/molecules

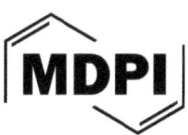

Disclaimer/Publisher's Note: The title and front matter of this reprint are at the discretion of the Guest Editors. The publisher is not responsible for their content or any associated concerns. The statements, opinions and data contained in all individual articles are solely those of the individual Editors and contributors and not of MDPI. MDPI disclaims responsibility for any injury to people or property resulting from any ideas, methods, instructions or products referred to in the content.

www.ingramcontent.com/pod-product-compliance
Lightning Source LLC
LaVergne TN
LVHW072356090526
838202LV00019B/2563